PHYSICALFITNESS
&WELLNESS

Second Canadian Edition

Jerrold S. Greenberg   University of Maryland

George B. Dintiman   Virginia Commonwealth University

Barbee Myers Oakes   Wake Forest University

Jennifer D. Irwin   University of Western Ontario

Don Morrow   University of Western Ontario

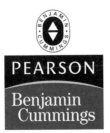

PEARSON

Benjamin
Cummings

Toronto

National Library of Canada Cataloguing in Publication

Physical fitness & wellness / Jerrold S. Greenberg ... [et al.]. — 2nd
Canadian ed.
Includes index.

ISBN 0-205-36587-6

1. Physical fitness. 2. Health. 3. Exercise. I. Greenberg, Jerrold S. II. Title: Physical fitness and health.
RA781.P525 2004   613.7   C2003-902626-4

ISBN 0-205-36587-6

Vice President, Editorial Director: Michael J. Young
Senior Acquisitions Editor: Kelly Torrance
Marketing Manager: Marlene Olsavsky
Associate Editor: Eleanor MacKay
Production Editor: Judith Scott
Copy Editor: Laurel Sparrow
Production Coordinator: Andrea Falkenberg
Photo Research: Susan Wallace-Cox
Page Layout: Joan M. Wilson
Art Director: Mary Opper
Interior and Cover Design: Alex Li
Cover Image: David Stoecklein/CORBIS/MAGMA

Statistics Canada information is used with the permission of the Minister of Industry, as Minister responsible for
Statistics Canada. Information on the availability of the wide range of data from Statistics Canada can be obtained
from Statistics Canada's Regional Offices, its World Wide Web site at http://www.statcan.ca, and its toll-free access
number 1-800-263-1136.

2 3 4 5   08 07 06 05 04

Printed and bound in the USA.

PEARSON
Benjamin
Cummings

Contents

4 PRINCIPLES OF EXERCISE 65

5 EXPLORING CARDIORESPIRATORY FITNESS 89

6 IMPROVING MUSCULAR STRENGTH AND ENDURANCE 117

7 FLEXIBILITY 143

15 DESIGNING A PROGRAM UNIQUE FOR YOU: PHYSICALLY ACTIVE LIFSTYLE FOR A LIFETIME 363

Preface

THERE ARE A WIDE VARIETY of books on the topic of physical fitness, but only a limited number that include concepts of physical fitness under the larger "umbrella" of wellness.

Moreover, we were unable to find a book on physical fitness and wellness that was grounded in solid Canadian content. Given these limitations and interests, we made certain to incorporate into this text all the usual fitness content in a way that was sensitive to and appreciative of the diversity of readers in Canadian society.

We certainly discuss concepts that one might expect to find in a book concerned with physical fitness. There are, for example, sections on the principles of exercise, on cardiorespiratory fitness, on muscular strength and endurance, on flexibility, and so forth. However, we have tried to discuss physical fitness in the full context of wellness in a concerted effort to expand traditional perspectives of fitness beyond merely training the body. Our perspective relates physical fitness to health and well-being in a more complete wellness lifestyle approach. Thus, we also discuss topics such as nutrition, weight control, stress and stress management, chemicals and drugs, heart disease and disease prevention, and exercise injury prevention/treatment. To be fit in body without being healthy and well is not to have enjoyed the journey toward a full and complete life.

As Canadians, we share some similarities with our US neighbours, but we are not Americans and some contextual aspects of wellness and health promotion are different in Canada. Diversity, we would suggest, is more characteristic of Canadians. For example, while Canada has two official languages, English and French, many Canadians have other native tongues including Italian, Greek, Cantonese, Mandarin, Korean, Arabic, Spanish, Urdu, Portuguese, Polish, and Ukranian along with a host of other languages. As the second largest country in the world in terms of land mass, our extensive plains, vast mountain ranges, and numerous lakes and rivers provide unique and diverse opportunities for participating in a variety of year-round and seasonal activities. Canadians have enjoyed a system of universal health care which ensures that all of us, regardless of our economic situation, are entitled to receive the medical attention we require.

With a two-tier health care system looming on the horizon, however, promoting our personal health and wellness will become increasingly important. It remains to be seen how efficacious and equitable this new system will be.

Much of our uniqueness is missed in the American textbooks we so often use to teach our Canadian students. We have sought to bring a very Canadian perspective to the content and spirit of this book. We honour Canadian **Wellness Heroes**; we highlight the important and excellent research conducted in Canada on Canadians; and we offer suggestions and insights for incorporating what we know about the health and wellness needs of Canadians into our uniquely Canadian lifestyles. At the same time, by virtue of our proximity to the United States, we do share a lot of commonalties with that country and there are aspects of physical fitness and wellness that have no political or geographic boundaries. For example, American-based research such as their *Surgeon General's Report on Physical Activity and Health* is outstanding in its comprehensiveness and implications for North Americans in general. Thus, we have been careful to include all relevant and important information for Canadians seeking to maintain and improve their lifestyles.

In addition to the more traditional approaches to the topic of physical fitness, we have updated information unique to this book. In recognition that researchers continue to find knowledge of physical fitness insufficient in itself to motivate people to become fit and to maintain adequate lifelong levels of physical fitness and wellness, we have updated the chapter on **Behavioural Change and Motivational Techniques**. These well-researched strategies are further described throughout the text in examples of how they might be used to overcome barriers to fitness and wellness. Most of the chapters have a **Behavioural Change and Motivational Strategies** box that describes obstacles specific to that chapter's content, obstacles that can interfere with achieving fitness and higher level wellness, and strategies for behavioural change that can be employed in overcoming such barriers.

We also know that changing behaviour can be easier if role models exist to reflect and symbolize the potential for change and lifestyle growth. For this reason, we have updated our "Wellness Heroes." These sidebars describe people who have achieved diverse and/or higher levels of wellness. Such descriptions or stories are designed to inspire and expand readers' perceptions of the full potential of human capabilities whether from the life perspective of a corporate executive, high level athlete or secondary school student.

We were also exasperated by the mis- and myth-conceptions about fitness and wellness that we have encountered. Too much inaccurate information exists and is passed on as valid. For this reason, we updated our **Myth and Fact Sheet** box in each chapter. These boxes present general misconceptions related to the content of the chapter together with correct factual information about these misconceptions. The Myth and Fact sheets might serve to stimulate discussions about other misconceptions, debunking such information at the same time as they provide strategies and methods that can be used to find and evaluate the validity of fitness and wellness information. Similarly, an important and unique feature of this book remains the **Diversity Issues** feature. These boxes present issues specific to the content of the chapter and also incorporate issues relating to ethnic, racial, cultural, sexual and socio-economic diversity and physical capability. This feature directs attention throughout the book to the existence of and the value in our differences and similarities. We refrain from grouping everyone into the majority cultural norm, and we recognize our diversities, including our Canadian uniqueness, as strengths rather than interferences in working toward healthier lifestyles.

Along with "Canadianizing" *Physical Fitness and Wellness*, further we maintained our focus on the spirit of the whole area of wellness in the book. In each chapter, we emphasize the importance of engaging in physical activity as a lifestyle process and of developing and using the tools to do so. The provision of methods and suggestions for utilizing the information within each chapter to hone fitness and wellness decision-making has been an important goal of this edition.

Finally, we want to point out that the chapter on **Nutrition** remains one of the most substantially altered chapters from the American edition of Physical Fitness and Wellness. We provided guidance for good decision-making with particular emphasis placed on Canadian information about eating habits, nutritional intake, and proper use of Canada's Guide to Healthy Eating. We also offer insights for incorporating good nutrition into everyday living. Similarly, the **Weight and Fat Management** chapter is considerably revised from the American edition. To offer the best guidance about maintaining a healthy physical body and to help combat what we refer to as the "Thinderella syndrome," we focus on body composition management more than on weight control. In this chapter, for example, we incorporate Canadian information and findings/direction from the National Population Health Survey as well as from the "Vitality Movement."

NEW TO THIS EDITION

The second Canadian edition of *Physical Fitness and Wellness* incorporates many valuable suggestions from instructors and students. We have strengthened and refined each chapter by including more Canadian data, revising and updating content based on the most current available research, and by providing up to date references and web-based resources. In response to reviewer feedback, we have added a completely new feature: **Study Questions**. These questions appear at the end of each chapter and are designed to stimulate discussion and assist students in testing their knowledge of key chapter concepts.

In summary, we have made the following additions and revisions to this edition:

- **Study Questions** at the end of each chapter
- Updated tables, figures, and box features
- More use of Canadian data
- Updated chapter end references
- New and updated weblinks
- More detailed coverage of the following areas:
  - Behaviour change and motivational techniques and theories (Chapter 3)
  - Maintaining your fitness program (Chapter 3)
  - Fitness concepts (Chapter 4)
  - Nutritional health habits (Chapter 8)
  - Anorexia (Chapter 9)
  - Chemical use in physical fitness (Chapter 11)
  - Tobacco and Smoking (Chapter 11)
  - Cancer screening (Chapter 13)

SUPPLEMENTS

Instructor's Manual and Test Item File with Transparency Masters and Video Guide

This comprehensive supplement provides everything a health and wellness instructor will need to teach from this exciting text. Included in the Instructor's Manual section are chapter outlines, objectives and summaries, key terms and concepts, suggested answers to study questions, lecture and lab activity outlines, discussion questions, suggested student activities, supplementary readings, and supplementary videos and other media materials. The Test Item File provides 50 questions for each chapter with multiple choice, true-false, fill-in, and essay type questions to choose between. In order to further assist instructors with lecture material, all the figures from the text have been reproduced as PowerPoint slides on the Instructor's Resource CD-ROM.

Instructor's Resource CD-ROM

The Instructor's Resource CD-ROM is a comprehensive supplement containing PowerPoint slides of all the figures from the text as well as electronic files of the Instructor's Manual and Test Item File.

Acknowledgements

WE EXTEND OUR gratitude to the staff at Pearson Education Canada for their work in producing this revised edition of *Physical Fitness and Wellness, Second Canadian Edition.* We would like to dedicate this book to the students, past and present, who comprise the Kinesiology/Health Sciences first-year "superclass" in Wellness-Lifestyle Analysis at the University of Western Ontario. Some 1100 students enrol in this superclass each year and every group has been an inspiration to our faculty. By continually providing us with the ideas, insights, and resources, we have been able to develop and enhance the way we teach our classes, conduct our research and provide the best possible learning environment.

This second edition is again testament to the importance of critical analysis of lifestyle wellness. We are delighted that this book represents a part of our efforts, personal and professional, to promote health and wellness and to contribute to this important area of study. From our perspective, it is important that people in all societies have an opportunity as well as the resources to live their lives creatively and wholly. We believe having an understanding of wellness and physical fitness is an integral part of establishing that kind of life, and we hope this new edition will be helpful in that endeavour.

We would also like to thank the following reviewers for their thoughtful comments on the first Canadian edition and drafts for the second edition:

- Kristal Anderson (University of Saskatchewan)
- Bonnie Gordon (University of British Columbia)
- Mark Lund (Grant McEwan College)
- Dru Marshall (University of Alberta)
- Barbara Pimento (George Brown College)
- Duane Schadd (Conestoga College)
- Angie Thompson and (University of Saskatchewan)
- Gordon Wilcox (Algonquin College)
- Ilse Wong (University of Lethbridge)

Jennifer Irwin and Don Morrow

1

Physical Fitness, Health, and Wellness

CHAPTER OBJECTIVES

By the end of this chapter, you should be able to:

1. Define and differentiate among physical fitness, health, and wellness.
2. Discuss the contributions of the Ottawa Charter for Health Promotion.
3. Describe the benefits of being physically active.
4. Discuss the relationship between physical fitness and self-esteem.

INEZ WAS A university athlete. Her basketball team always had a winning record, and she was a major reason they were so good. Still, that was long ago. Today, Inez is in her 50s, and an automobile accident has left her without the use of her legs. She still participates in sports, though. She plays wheelchair basketball in her leisure time and coaches a community centre soccer team on the weekends. She may not be able to run a mile, but she certainly can shoot foul shots. She may not be able to demonstrate a soccer kick, but she sure can motivate the girls she coaches.

Several years had passed—five to be exact—since Rodney and I had last seen each other. I was looking forward to catching up on old times. When I asked the standard "How have you been?" Rodney replied that he had never felt better. He had taken up jogging and was now running 80 kilometres a week. He had given up cigarette smoking, become a vegetarian, and had more confidence than ever.

In spite of his reply, I needed further assurance. He looked like death warmed over. His face was gaunt, his body emaciated. His clothes were baggy, creating a sloppy appearance. He had an aura of tiredness about him.

"How's Cynthia?" I asked.

"Fine," Rodney replied. "But we are no longer together. She just couldn't accept the time I devoted to running, and her disregard for her own health was getting on my nerves. She is still somewhat overweight, you know, and I started viewing her differently when I became healthier myself."

You may know an Inez, a Rodney, or someone like them. Are they healthy? This is a complicated question, one that this chapter explores, first by defining physical fitness, health, and wellness and then by differentiating among them.

Physical fitness is defined differently by different people. In this text, we define it as the ability to meet life's physical demands and still have enough energy to respond to unplanned events; fitness is a product of physical activity. There are five basic components of physical fitness: cardiorespiratory endurance, muscular strength, muscular endurance, flexibility, and body composition. Participation in sports activities that can improve these fitness components often requires certain motor skills. Consequently, motor skills (such as agility, balance, coordination, power, speed, and reaction time) are often included in physical fitness programs. However, it is possible to develop the five basic components of physical fitness without proficiency in these and other motor skills. That is why someone who is not a natural athlete can still be extremely fit.

COMPONENTS OF PHYSICAL FITNESS

Elsewhere in this book, we will discuss developing the five basic components of physical fitness. First, however, we must define these components.

Cardiorespiratory Endurance

To engage in physical activity, even breathing, requires oxygen. Without oxygen, it would be impossible to burn the food you need for energy. To supply oxygen to the various parts of the body requires a transport system. The body's transport system consists of lungs, heart, and blood vessels. When you breathe, you inhale air that contains oxygen into the lungs. The lungs absorb oxygen into their blood vessels and transport it to the heart, where it is pumped out through other blood vessels to all parts of the body. The more efficiently and effectively you transport oxygen, the greater your cardiorespiratory endurance (*cardio* for heart and *respiratory* for lungs and breathing)—the ability to supply and use oxygen, over a period of time and in sufficient amounts, to perform normal and unusual activities.

Muscular Strength and Endurance

The maximal pulling force of a muscle or a muscle group to perform an action once is called **muscular strength**.

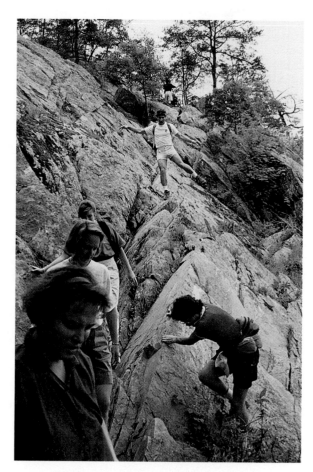

Exercising outdoors is an invigorating way to enhance spiritual health while at the same time improving physical health.

The ability of a muscle to contract repeatedly or to sustain a contraction is called **muscular endurance**. Lifting a load or moving an object depends on muscular strength. Doing that repeatedly over time requires muscular endurance. In spite of tremendous cardiovascular endurance, without sufficient muscular strength or endurance you may not be able to do the things you wish to do.

Flexibility

The range of motion around a joint, or more simply the degree to which you can move your limbs with smoothness and efficiency, is **flexibility**. Flexibility is important in performing exercise efficiently, safely, and enjoyably. Without adequate flexibility, you might not be able to stretch far, might overstress a muscle or ligament, and might even feel uncomfortable moving. Flexibility is probably the component of physical fitness that is most overlooked; yet the consequences of ignoring flexibility can be pain and discomfort, injury, and poor health.

◼ Body Composition

Your body contains some parts that are made up of fats and others that are not. The fat component is usually referred to as **fat weight**, and fat in relation to the body as a whole is referred to as **percent body fat**. The nonfatty component is called **lean body mass. Body composition** is the relationship between these two components. In the past, people relied on height–weight charts to evaluate body composition. We now realize that someone can weigh much more than a chart based on height says is appropriate but still have good body composition. This can happen because the person is muscular and has a good deal of lean body mass. Conversely, someone at just the right weight according to a height chart could in actuality be overweight because of too much fatty tissue and not enough lean body mass.

*H*EALTH AND WELLNESS

What do you imagine when you think of health? If someone told you Aaron was really healthy, what picture of Aaron would you have in your mind? If you were asked to elaborate on your health, what would you say? We will help you answer that question, but first try listing five ways in which you could improve your health.

We are willing to bet you listed ways to improve your *physical* health. You probably listed ways to prevent your contracting heart disease such as eating less fatty foods or exercising more, or ways to prevent cancer by not smoking cigarettes and getting regular checkups. Yet physical health is not the total picture; other components of health are just as important. These include:

1. **Social health** This is the ability to interact well with people and the environment, to have satisfying interpersonal relationships.

2. **Mental health** This is the ability to learn and grow intellectually. Life's experiences as well as more formal structures (for example, schools) enhance mental health.

3. **Emotional health** This is the ability to control emotions so that you feel comfortable expressing them and you can express them appropriately. Conversely, it is the ability not to express emotions when it is inappropriate to do so.

4. **Spiritual health** This is a belief in some unifying force, which will vary from person to person but will have the concept of faith at its core. Faith is a feeling of connection to other humans, of a purpose to life, and of a quest for meaning in life.

So health is not simply caring for your body. It concerns your social interactions, mind, feelings, and spirit. Often, we decide to give up health in one area to gain greater health in another. For example, when you decide you're just not up to exercising today, you may choose to improve your emotional health (to seek relaxation) at some expense to your physical health. When you decide to study instead of spending time with your friends, you may be choosing mental over social health. We make decisions like these about our health all the time even though we do not express them in these terms.

Now you can appreciate that physical fitness is just one component of health. In fact, it is just one component of physical health, which, in turn, is a component of overall health. **Health**, then, is an individual's total physical, social, emotional, mental, and spiritual status, and health is separate and distinct from illness, as shown in the continuum in Figure 1.1.

Note that the continuum is a dotted, rather than a solid, line. Each dot is made up of the five health components shown in Figure 1.2, and therefore everyone has some degree of health no matter where he or she is located on the continuum.

Imagine that each health dot, as depicted in Figure 1.2, is a tire on the vehicle in which you travel through life. If the tire is properly inflated, you will have a smooth ride; if it is not, the ride will be bumpy. The same is true for your *health tire*. If you do not pay

---

Physical fitness The ability to meet life's physical demands and still have enough energy to respond to unplanned events; a product of regular physical activity.

Muscular strength The maximal amount of force a muscle can exert for one repetition.

Muscular endurance A muscle's ability to continue submaximal contractions against resistance.

Flexibility The range of motion around a joint or the ability to move limbs smoothly and efficiently.

Fat weight The weight of your body fat.

Percent body fat The percentage of your body weight made up of fat.

Lean body mass The nonfatty component of your body.

Body composition The relationship between your fat weight and your lean body mass.

Health The total of your physical, social, emotional, mental, and spiritual status.

DIVERSITY ISSUES

Canadian Special Olympics

The Canadian Special Olympics (CSO) 2002 Summer Games in Prince Albert, Saskatchewan, hosted 980 athletes and 320 coaches, as well as volunteers and staff, from all provinces and each territory. The year 2002 marked the 34th anniversary of the Special Olympics movement pioneered by Canadian research scientist Dr. Frank Hayden through his work with the Kennedy Foundation.

The Special Olympics is a worldwide program supporting sports training and competition for people with a mental disability. As a community-based program, local sports clubs are key organizations that facilitate the continuation of the program through their training facilities' organizational support. Club competitions and local meets occur on a regular basis, and athletes advance through a cycle of provincial games to compete in both national and world games and championships. To provide Canadians with the opportunity to compete in either a national or an international event each year, both the national winter and summer games and the world winter and summer competitions take place every four years.

Today, over 20 000 Canadian athletes participate in training and competition organized by 11 provincial and territorial CSO chapters, coordinated by a national office and sustained by the efforts of over 6000 registered volunteers and about 60 staff members across the country. Those involved help to provide an opportunity for mentally disabled athletes to appreciate their abilities, and to learn to build on the confidence developed through their acquisition of sports skills and the application of those skills in competition.

The official Special Olympics winter sports include cross-country and alpine skiing, figure skating, speed skating, snowshoeing, and floor hockey. Official Special Olympics summer sports consist of athletics, aquatics, bowling, gymnastics, and soccer. Other sports are curling, broomball, power lifting, and softball.

The Mission of the Canadian Special Olympics

The mission of the Canadian Special Olympics is to ensure that a full continuum of sport opportunities are available to people with mental disabilities. The following are the mission's supporting principles:

- Special Olympics provides sport opportunities directly for athletes with mental disabilities and links them with other organizations, providing integrated sport opportunities.
- Special Olympics is a sports program. It involves both physical training and the matching of strength, endurance, and physical skills in formalized settings with structured rules.
- The practice of grouping athletes for competition on the basis of their abilities is fundamental and critical to the Special Olympics program. This practice ensures that all athletes experience equitable competition.
- Training and preparation are essential to meaningful participation in sport and are indispensable elements of any Special Olympics program.
- Special Olympics uses sport to assist people with a mental disability to become all that they can be—physically, mentally, socially, emotionally—and to become accepted, respected, and productive members of society.
- Special Olympics may contain elements of play, recreation, or physical education and should assist athletes in participating meaningfully and successfully in all dimensions of a physically active lifestyle.
- Special Olympics rewards dedication, preparation, effort, and spirit ("doing your best" both in training and in competition). Success is measured by the effect of the experience on the athlete. ✦

Source: Adapted from information at *Canadian Special Olympics,* CSO Web site **http://cso.on.ca**

Figure 1.1 ✦ The Health–Illness Continuum

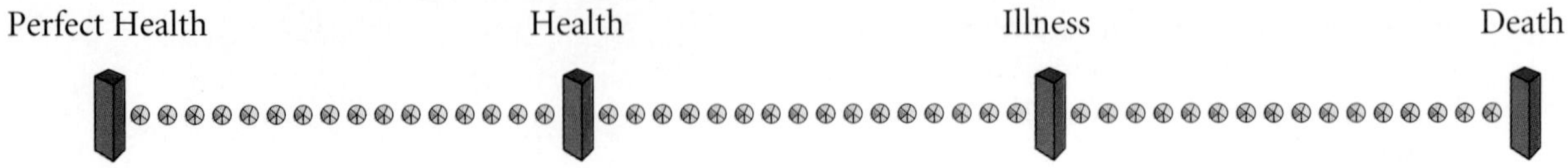

Perfect Health   Health   Illness   Death

Figure 1.2 ✦ A Single Health–Illness Continuum Dot

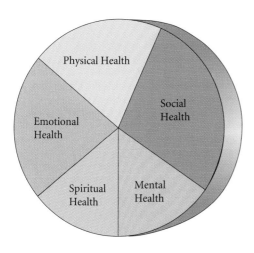

Figure 1.3 ✦ An Asymmetrical Dot on the Health–Illness Continuum

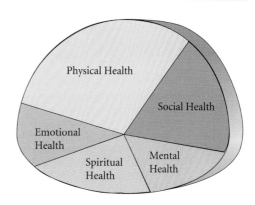

enough attention to your health and all its components, improving (inflating) them when you can, you will experience conditions that make life more difficult and dissatisfying. For example, if you do not exercise frequently enough or properly, you may become fatigued easily or be susceptible to various illnesses.

If you overdo any one component of health at the expense of the others, you may wind up with a tire like the one in Figure 1.3. That tire is *out of round* and will not provide a smooth ride. That health tire has expanded physical health to the detriment of the other aspects of health. Here is where Rodney, introduced at the beginning of this chapter, comes to mind. He expanded his physical health but was no longer married and looked emaciated. He had no time for interacting with friends (social health), reading (mental health), or enjoying nature or participating in religious traditions (spiritual health). Even though he was more physically fit, he was not arguably healthier. Further, he did not possess a very high level of wellness. We refer to **wellness** as having your health tire *in round*, that is, having the components of health adequately inflated and balanced, paying attention to and improving all aspects of health without exaggerating any one. Inez, the other person we introduced at the beginning of this chapter, did not have the use of her legs, but she did participate in physical activity at the level at which she was capable. She even learned about soccer so she could coach a local team. Inez probably possessed a higher level of wellness than the physically advantaged Rodney. That is why you need to focus on your social, mental, emotional, and spiritual health as you read about physical fitness in this book. We will help you do that by regularly presenting the health and wellness implications of the content discussed.

◼ Health Objectives for the Nation

The major causes of death at the beginning of the twentieth century were diseases passed from one person to another or resulting from unsanitary practices (tuberculosis, pneumonia, influenza). The incidence of these diseases has, for the most part, been drastically reduced through the development of proper waste disposal and sewage systems, quarantines, and other community and legislative actions.

The killers of today (Figure 1.4) do not lend themselves to such remedies. These conditions (heart disease, cancer, stroke) are more the result of lifestyle than of a microorganism. In a democratic society, we cannot legislate lifestyle. For significant decreases to occur in these diseases, people must voluntarily change unhealthy behaviours (cigarette smoking, lack of regular physical activity, lack of proper amounts of sleep, abuse of alcohol and other drugs, consumption of foods high in saturated fats, and so forth). Medical researchers estimate that 20 percent of the risk for heart disease, cancer, and stroke can be attributed to heredity, another 20 percent to environmental factors, 10 percent to inadequate health care, and an alarming 50 percent to unhealthy lifestyles.

Health Canada, in cooperation with the Canadian Society for Exercise Physiology, has recognized the need to encourage and promote healthier lifestyles for all Canadians. To that end, the federal government has published a very user-friendly manual entitled *Canada's*

Wellness Having the components of health balanced and at sufficient levels.

Figure 1.4 ✦ Current Primary Causes of Death in Canada

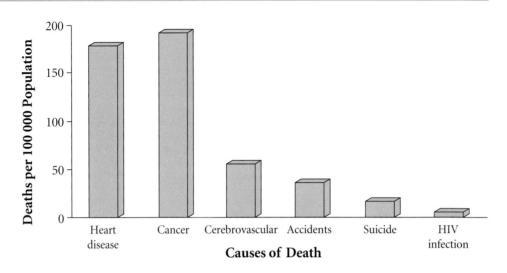

Source: Adapted from the Statistics Canada publication *Births and Deaths*, Catalogue No. 84-210, 1997.

Physical Activity Guide to Healthy Active Living. The *Guide* recommends participating in moderate physical activity for at least 30 minutes, four or more days each week. To gain the health benefits of physical activity, these 30 minutes can take place all at once or can be accumulated in three or more 10-minute periods. The *Guide* contains a variety of practical and physical activity-specific suggestions directly related to the wider federal goals for health promotion first established in the Ottawa Charter for Health Promotion (see Table 1.1).

WHAT PHYSICAL FITNESS CAN DO FOR YOU

As we have discussed, physical fitness can make you healthier and help you to achieve high-level wellness. And, as you will soon see, it can even help you feel better about yourself and be more self-assured.

◼ The Benefits of Physical Activity

A friend of ours likes to kid that he gets his exercise serving as a pallbearer at the funerals of his jogger friends. Aside from simply being contentious, he is expressing an important point: Exercise itself will not guarantee a long life. Heredity sets limits on how long you will live, but within these limits is a range. Regular physical activity of sufficient duration and intensity can help you reach your upper limits. This is demonstrated in the studies of Harvard alumni by Paffenbarger and colleagues (1986). Paffenbarger found that mortality rates were lower for

physically active alumni. By age 80, the amount of additional life attributed to adequate exercise, compared to sedentariness, was between one and two plus years. The multiple-risk-factor intervention trial (MRFIT) study involved over 12 000 men and also found that the most physically active men lived longer than the least physically active (Leon and Connett, 1991). Further, the MRFIT study indicated that *any* activity (not just vigorous activity) for 30 minutes, five times a week, decreased the risk of coronary heart disease, although more strenuous physical activity was more protective. Blair and associates (1989) found that the death rate increased as fitness level decreased. Two of the major reasons for lower death rates of exercisers can be explained by our knowledge that exercise can help prevent "certain kinds of cancer" (Freidenreich, 1999; Powell et al., 1989; Rockhill et al., 1999; Wyrwich and Wolinsky, 2000; Krucoff, 1992) and coronary heart disease (Donahue et al., 1988), the leading causes of death in Canada. Researchers have found an increase in natural killer (NK) cell activity among people who exercise as seldom as once per week (Kusaka, Kondou, and Morimoto, 1992). NK cells help prevent cancer.

Physical activity can both prevent illness and disease and help rehabilitation. In this way, it enhances physical health. Because we will discuss the relationship between physical activity and health in more detail elsewhere in this book, suffice it to say here that among the illnesses and diseases that physical activity can help prevent are the nation's leading killers: heart disease, cancer, and stroke. And this sort of activity can help prevent, and serve as a treatment for, hypertension (high blood pressure), itself a major cause of heart disease and stroke.

Table 1.1 ✦ The Ottawa Charter for Health Promotion: First International Conference on Health Promotion, Ottawa, Canada, 1986

The Ottawa Charter was perhaps the most significant form of public policy recognizing the significance of *health promotion* as a process rather than as a set of risk factors or outcomes, or as the "softer" side of medicine.

"Health promotion is the process of enabling people to increase control over, and to improve, their health."

The Charter identified the following resources and strategies:

- Health is a resource for everyday life, not the goal of living.
- The fundamental conditions/resources of health are:
  - Peace
  - Shelter
  - Education
  - Food
  - Income
  - A stable economic system
  - Sustainable resources
  - Social justice
  - Equity

- Strategies for change in the attitude toward health promotion:
  - Build healthy public policy
  - Create supportive environments
  - Strengthen community action
  - Develop personal skills
  - Reorient health skills

The end result of the Charter conference was the creation of a Framework for Health Promotion (1986) with a challenge to government, society, and individuals to pursue a "health for all" goal by the year 2000.

Provincial responses to the Charter and Framework policy documents included:

- A vibrant "healthy community" project in British Columbia
- The establishment of three Centres for Health and Well-Being in Alberta
- A partners-for-all community health promotion project in Manitoba

Ontario and Quebec have been slower to respond to the concept and implementation of health promotion programs, and Atlantic Canada has been slow to move toward such a policy due to economic inequities. Saskatchewan has a decades-old community coalition health promotion system.

The 1986 Charter and Framework documents were reinvigorated with a new federal policy, the 1996 Action Statement for Health Promotion, which:

- Recommits to the Charter and Framework.
- Stresses health as a process once again.
- Attempts to empower individuals, communities, and organizations via education about decision-making for health promotion.

In the early 2000s, Canadian politicians and policymakers continue to work on enhancing Canadians' health and well-being through seeking strategies that will both foster health promotion initiatives and maintain Canada's universal health care system.

Sources: The Ottawa Charter for Health Promotion, as found on the World Health Organization website: **www.who.int/hpr/archive/docs/ottawa.html**.

One reason physical activity is so helpful in preventing and treating various conditions is that it helps people control their weight. Overweight, obesity, and malnutrition are implicated in numerous states of ill health. These conditions are also related to the amount of cholesterol in the blood (serum cholesterol), which can clog arteries leading to the heart or brain, thereby resulting in a heart attack or stroke. Some cholesterol, however, is actually helpful because it picks up blood fats and deposits them outside of the body. This *good* cholesterol is called high-density lipoprotein (HDL). Exercise increases the amount of HDL in the blood (Shepard, 1989). It also decreases the amount of bad cholesterol (low-density lipoprotein [LDL]) that accumulates on the blood vessel walls, which can eventually block the flow of blood to the heart and other body parts.

In addition, regular exercise can be an extremely effective means of managing stress and mood disturbances (ACSM, 2000; Barabasz, 1991; Brevard and Ricketts, 1996; DiLorenzo et al., 1999; McGuigan, 1999; Moore et al., 1999; Sothern et al., 1999). In this way, it improves emotional health. As we will discuss in

WELLNESS HEROES

Ed Buffett

Ed Buffett is chair and CEO of Buffett Taylor and Associates Ltd., a leading Canadian employee benefits and wellness consulting firm. He has served as the chair of the board of governors of the Whitby General Hospital and the chair of the board of the Durham Foundation. Ed is a member of McMaster University's board of governors and of the board of directors of the Wellness Councils of America (WELLCOA). In 1997, he hosted the Toronto Health Summit, which gave rise to the creation of the Wellness Council of Canada for which he now acts as chair. Ed's story as a "wellness hero" is fascinating.

At the age of 14, he started to smoke cigarettes and ultimately became a three-pack-a-day smoker. An accomplished athlete, Ed was a member of the Ontario Juvenile Hockey Championship team in the early 1960s and attended university on a football scholarship in the United States. An avowed workaholic in the workforce, Ed put in 12-to-15-hour days seven days a week. Throughout his 40s, Ed often ate only one meal per day, typically late in the evening. In October 1994, at the age of 51, Ed suffered a major heart attack that "flatlined" on his electrocardiogram twice during that day. This event completely altered the course of Ed's daily life.

After the attack and during his rehabilitation, he became determined to take an unfortunate incident and a poor choice of lifestyle and turn them into an opportunity both in relation to his business pursuits and as a means of making a meaningful contribution to society. He began to read voraciously on preventive health measures. In the course of that research, he came into contact with Bill Kaiser Sr., the founder of WELLCOA, and WELLCOA's president, Dr. David Hunnicutt. Ed became convinced that there was a definite need for a similar organization here in Canada, and confirmed this by conducting the first comprehensive Canadian Wellness Survey in 1996 (now published every three years). Armed with a mass of data from this survey, he hosted a Toronto summit that drew some 42 major Canadian employers as well as six of the top representatives of WELLCOA. Drawing on 15 years of experience from the latter organization, Ed worked very hard to promote WELCAN, as he called the new organization, and deliver the wellness message

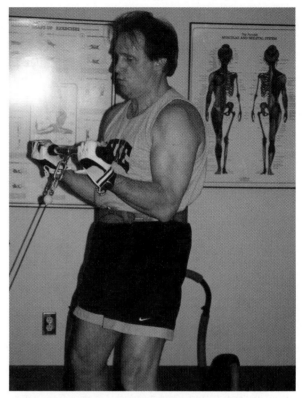

Ed Buffett, president and CEO of Buffett Taylor and Associates Ltd. and founder of the Wellness Council of Canada. Ed exercises an hour and a half every morning, has a healthy diet, listens to his body, and works to manage his time.

at every opportunity throughout North America. Moreover, he individually bore many of the costs associated with the formulation and establishment of WELCAN, because he was convinced of the value it could provide to employers and employees throughout Canada.

Today, WELCAN comprises more than 200 member organizations, including founding members such as Shoppers Drug Mart, Telus, Clarica Life, and several school boards. The organization provides its members with a monthly newsletter, *The Well Workplace*, as well as a number of regular publications of interest to wellness coordinators and preventive health care practitioners. It also sponsors "well workplace" awards to reinforce initiatives, and sponsors a biannual conference on worksite wellness and health promotion. WELCAN also serves as a forum for the exchange of wellness and health promotion ideas and initiatives.

Clearly, Ed Buffett has been a most significant individual in promoting Canadian wellness and certainly deserves the title "Wellness Hero." ✦

Chapter 10, stress changes the body so that it is prepared to respond to a threat. It is geared up for some physical reaction. Exercise uses the built-up stress by-products and the body's preparedness to do something physical. The result is a sense of stress relief. Exercise also enhances the production of brain neurotransmitters (endorphins) that make you feel better and less stressed.

The rehabilitative benefits of exercise are almost notorious. It wasn't too long ago that people needing surgery or women having given birth were restricted to a hospital bed for days and sometimes weeks. That is no longer the case. The benefits of physical activity in recuperating from many conditions are now well recognized. Take the case of a man we know who had a triple bypass operation in which three of the blood vessels supplying his heart were found to be obstructed. The obstructed sections were bypassed with blood vessels grafted from his legs. Shortly after the operation, he was expected to get out of bed and walk around. Although he was nervous at first, he soon learned that physical movement helped him get back to his regular routine. His muscular strength returned sooner than he expected, his blood circulation was enhanced by muscular contractions forcing pressure on the blood vessel walls, and his mood improved dramatically.

Physical activity can even help elderly people live longer (Rakowski and Mor, 1992) and postpone the effects of aging. As people get older, they become susceptible to conditions that can restrict their activities, even to the extent that they become dependent on others to tie their shoes, transport them, and shop for them. A life of regular physical activity can postpone this dependency by providing elders with the necessary muscular strength and endurance, cardiorespiratory endurance, and flexibility to manage their own affairs. Several health studies have identified how physical activity can combat the physical and cognitive effects of aging, and thus help Canadians age youthfully. The benefits of physical activity specific to aging are as follows (information from the Canadian Fitness and Lifestyle Research Institute's Web page "Physical Activity a Fountain of Youth"):

- Cardiovascular fitness declines by 1 percent per year after the age of 25, but moderate to intense aerobic exercise improves cardiovascular fitness and alleviates the percentage decline.

- Physically active adults have increased memory and reaction times, which are common concerns for aging people.

- Training programs lead to significant strength increases in older adults (up to 200 percent), which can reverse functional impairments and improve the outlook for independent living.

- Balance and confidence can be enhanced through physical activity. Falls are of great concern to the elderly, and strengthening the muscles in the ankles and legs can decrease the risk of falling.

- Physical activity has a moderating effect on high blood pressure.

- Physical activity helps decrease the risk of heart disease, the nation's major killer.

- Stretching exercises increase joint mobility and improve flexibility, an especially important benefit for older adults. Gains in flexibility can facilitate everyday tasks such as tying shoes, climbing stairs, reaching into cupboards, etc.

Physical activity has additional benefits that are often overlooked. For example, several researchers have found that workers who are physically fit are absent from the job less frequently (Steinhardt, Greenhow, and Stewart, 1991; Tucker, Aldana, and Friedman, 1990). In addition, people who are physically fit are less apt to experience depression and are more likely to feel in control of their lives (Brandon and Lofton, 1991).

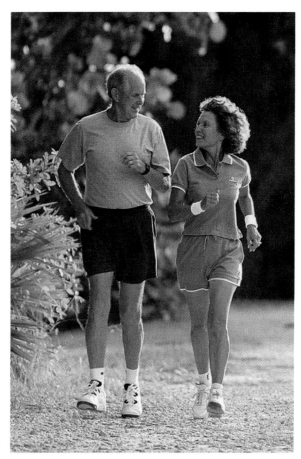

The MRFIT study demonstrated that people who exercise regularly can add years to their life, and life to their years.

Myth and Fact Sheet

Myth	Fact
1. The most important component of your overall health is your physical health.	1. Health consists of more than just physical health. It includes social, emotional, mental, and spiritual health as well. Different people will value different components of health during different stages of their lives. This is not wrong, but simply a matter of shifting values. Who is to say which component of health is more important than another for any individual?
2. Wellness and health are one and the same.	2. Health refers to the degree to which you have the five components of health. Wellness means having the five components of health in balance. No one component is exaggerated at the expense of any other. Consequently, health and wellness are not synonymous.
3. Someone who is good at basketball is physically fit.	3. Though someone may be skilled at a particular sport, this does not mean that the person is physically fit. Someone who can shoot baskets or hit a tennis ball may not be able to run a long distance or may not possess upper-body muscular strength or muscular endurance. Further, that individual may not be flexible or agile. To be physically fit, you need to work on all of these fitness components.
4. Because the leading causes of death result from unhealthy lifestyles, there is little the Canadian government can do to make people healthier.	4. Through Health Canada, the Canadian government has developed a wide variety of guides and materials to encourage Canadians to adopt healthier lifestyles and thereby live better-quality lives. See, for example, Health Canada's home page **www.hc-sc.gc.ca** for a complete list of these materials together with instructions for downloading copies for yourself.
5. Being physically fit makes you healthier, but you probably won't feel any different about yourself.	5. If you become physically fit, you will feel better about yourself and your self-esteem will improve. You will develop more confidence, feel less depressed, and experience a sense of more control in your life. The benefits of physical fitness go well beyond the healthy changes that occur within your body. They include improvements in your mind and your spirit as well.

Physical activity can also improve spiritual health. For example, when you are exercising outdoors, you have the opportunity to experience nature and all its wonders—to feel the rush of air on your face and the heat of the sun on your skin, to hear the sound of the birds and of the wind rustling through the leaves, and to sense the exhilaration of your body performing physical movement. In this way, you can feel connected—body, mind, and spirit—to a unifying force. And if you engage in physical activity with other people, you improve your social health in addition to all the other components of health.

Health Benefits of Moderate Physical Activity

The evidence supporting the benefits of physical activity has been accumulating for many years, and in years to come this list is likely to become longer still. Among the benefits of physical activity touted by a variety of researchers are the following:

- Improves potential for reaching life expectancy.
- Promotes heart health and reduces risk of heart disease.

- Improves probability of remaining diabetes-free for life.
- Reduces the risk of coronary heart disease, stroke, and hypertension (Salonen, Puska, and Tuomelehto, 1982).
- Helps reduce blood pressure in people who already have high blood pressure.
- Improves posture and balance, and enhances body composition (Health Canada and the Canadian Society for Exercise Physiology, Cat. No. H39-429/1998).
- Promotes better self-esteem, a sense of relaxation, and an overall feeling of well-being (Health Canada and the Canadian Society for Exercise Physiology, Cat. No. H39-429/1998).
- Reduces the risk of developing osteoporosis (Damilakis et al., 1999), back injuries and gallstones (Sothern et al., 1999), and certain types of cancer (Wyrwich and Wolinsky, 2000).
- Helps build and maintain healthy bones, muscles, and joints.
- Helps older adults become stronger and better able to move about without falling.
- Enhances independent living later on in life (Health Canada and the Canadian Society for Exercise Physiology, Cat. No. H39-429/1998).

Canada's Physical Activity Guide to Healthy Active Living outlines the exercise time and effort level needed to stay healthy, along with examples of activities for each level (Table 1.2). People who are now inactive and decide to engage in moderate physical activity can gain the above benefits, and have more

Table 1.2 ✦ Physical Activity for Health Benefits

EFFORT, TIME NEEDED	EXAMPLES OF ACTIVITIES
Light, 60 minutes	Light walking Volleyball Easy gardening Stretching
Moderate, 30–60 minutes	Brisk walking Biking Raking leaves Swimming Dancing Water aerobics
Vigorous, 20–30 minutes	Aerobics Jogging Hockey Basketball Fast swimming Fast dancing

physical energy and alertness, better self-esteem, and the ability to perform daily tasks more easily. Even greater benefits can be derived from activities requiring greater intensity, duration, or frequency.

An excerpt from *Canada's Physical Activity Guide to Healthy Active Living* suggests different ways Canadians can build physical activity into their daily lives (see Appendix C).

◼ Self-Esteem and Physical Activity

Physical activity also has the potential of giving you more confidence and making you feel better about yourself. We call this **self-esteem**. These benefits occur for several reasons. First, regular exercise helps maintain body weight and develop a positive body image. Feeling good about how your body looks and feels will translate into feeling good about yourself.

Second, physical activity often provides challenges that are faced and overcome. That is one of the advantages of competitive sports activities. Being successful at these challenges will give you confidence to face other

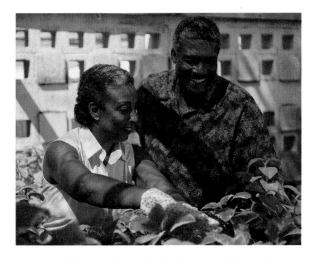

Even gardening can be an effective fitness activity, and can contribute especially to social and spiritual health.

Self-esteem The amount of regard you hold for yourself; the amount of value you place on yourself.

challenges in your life. And yet not all challenges are mastered. Physical activity also allows you to fail to meet the challenge but recognize that life goes on. You have probably heard someone say that you cannot hit a home run if you do not step up to the plate. When you bat, however, you can also strike out. So what? Striking out, or trying and failing, can be a more effective learning and growth experience than succeeding. After all, if you succeed, by definition you were able to do whatever it was anyhow. Only when you fail can you learn what you need to adjust to become better.

Lastly, physical activity improves endurance and strength. This allows you to perform activities more effectively and for longer periods of time. Being able to perform in this way can make you more confident and less likely to avoid events that are physically challenging. The result will be greater self-esteem and, as a result, better emotional health.

Your Personal Physical Fitness Profile

The first step in achieving the benefits of physical fitness is to assess where you begin. What level of physical fitness are you at now? Which components of physical fitness do you want to maintain and which do you want to improve? We help you perform such an assessment in the next chapter. In addition, throughout this book, we include questionnaires, scales, physical tests to evaluate components of fitness, and even measures of psychosocial factors (such as self-esteem) related to decisions to exercise. We also provide lab activities in each chapter that are designed to help you learn more about yourself and about physical fitness. By the time you finish reading this book, you will have enough information about yourself to plan an effective fitness program, one that is based on your personal fitness profile and will meet your personal fitness goals.

Summary

■ Components of Physical Fitness

Physical fitness encompasses cardiorespiratory endurance, muscular strength, muscular endurance, flexibility, and body composition. It also includes the motor skills of agility, balance, coordination, power, speed, and reaction time.

■ Health and Wellness

Health consists of five components: physical, social, mental, emotional, and spiritual. Physical fitness is but one component of physical health, albeit an important one.

Wellness is maintaining the components of health in sufficient amounts and in balance with one another. An ideal state of wellness is one in which no one component of health is emphasized at the expense of any other component.

In the past, the conditions causing the deaths of the most people in Canada were passed from one person to another or were the result of unsanitary practices. Tuberculosis and pneumonia are examples. Today, most deaths are the result of lifestyle practices such as cigarette smoking, lack of exercise, inadequate sleep, and poor nutrition. Changes in these practices are up to individuals; governments cannot legislate these changes.

The federal government challenged Canadians to achieve "health for all" by the year 2000, and Health Canada developed a variety of guides and resources to assist Canadians in achieving this goal. In the early 2000s we have not reached this goal but continue to work toward it—in part, by using the previously developed guides. Several of these guides are specific to physical fitness and physical activity, and others are tangentially related.

■ What Physical Fitness Can Do for You

Physical activity can improve physical health by decreasing LDLs (bad cholesterol) and increasing HDLs (good cholesterol), by preventing or reducing high blood pressure, by helping to maintain desirable weight and lean body mass, and by preventing some cancers.

Physical activity can also improve emotional health by helping to manage stress, spiritual health by focusing on nature and bodily sensations, and social health by exercising with other people. In addition, physical activity can help diminish and postpone the effects of aging and aid in recuperation from illnesses and medical procedures. Further, physical activity can make you feel more confident and thereby improve your self-esteem. It can also improve self-esteem by helping to maintain recommended body weight and a desirable body image and by providing challenges that develop confidence and the realization that, even if the challenges are not successfully overcome, significant learning occurs. Self-esteem is also enhanced when endurance and strength are developed so you can perform daily activities effectively and for longer periods of time.

STUDY QUESTIONS

1. Briefly define physical fitness and its five basic components.

2. List five benefits of physical activity.

3. Define health and provide a brief description of each of its five components. How does health relate to wellness?

4. Referring to the definition of physical fitness, identify three aspects of your life in which you benefit from physical fitness (e.g., I can get myself from one class to another in a short time by walking across campus quickly).

5. To what extent do we take our physical fitness for granted? Provide examples. How might this change as we age?

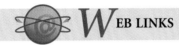

WEB LINKS

Health Canada Home Page
www.hc-sc.gc.ca

The Ottawa Charter for Health Promotion
www.hc-sc.gc.ca/hppb/phdd/docs/charter/index.html

Canadian Institute for Health Information
www.cihi.ca

Health Canada's Health Promotion Online
www.hc-sc.gc.ca/hppb/hpo/

Active Ontario
www.activeontario.org

Plan of Action for Healthy Living
www.activeliving.ca/activeliving/alc/toward_summary.html

Canadian Health Network
www.canadian-health-network.ca/

Alberta Centre for Active Living
www.centre4activeliving.ca

REFERENCES

American College of Sports Medicine. *ACSM's Guidelines for Exercise Testing and Prescription*, 6th Edition. Philadelphia: Lippincott, Williams & Wilkins, 2000.

Barabasz, M. "Effects of Aerobic Exercise on Transient Mood State." *Perceptual and Motor Skills* 73 (1991): 657–658.

Blair, Steven N., Harold W. Kohl, Ralph S. Paffenbarger, Debra G. Clark, Kenneth J. Cooper, and Larry W. Gibbons. "Physical Fitness and All-Cause Mortality: A Prospective Study of Healthy Men and Women." *Journal of the American Medical Association* 262 (1989): 2395–2401.

Brandon, Jeffrey E., and J. Mark Lofton. "Relationship of Fitness to Depression, State and Trait Anxiety, Internal Health Locus of Control, and Self-Control." *Perceptual and Motor Skills* 73 (1991): 563–568.

Brevard, P.B., and C.D. Ricketts. "Residence of College Students Affects Dietary Intake, Physical Activity, and Serum Lipid Levels." *Journal of the American Dietetic Association* 96 (1996): 35–38.

Damilakis, J., K. Perisinakis, G. Kontakis, E. Vagios, and N. Gourtsoyiannis. "Effect of Lifetime Occupational Physical Activity on Indices of Bone Mineral Status in Healthy Postmenopausal Women." *Calcified Tissue International*, 64, 2 (1999): 112–116.

DiLorenzo, T.M., E.P. Bargman, R. Stucky-Ropp, G.S. Brassington, P.A. Frensch, and T. LaFontaine. "Long-Term Effects of Aerobic Exercise on Psychological Outcomes." *Preventive Medicine*, 28, 1 (1999): 75–85.

Donahue, Richard P., Robert D. Abbott, Qwayne M. Reed, and Katsuhiko Yano. "Physical Activity and Coronary Heart Disease in Middle-Aged and Elderly Men: The Honolulu Heart Program." *American Journal of Public Health* 78 (1988): 683–685.

Health Canada and the Canadian Society for Exercise Physiology. *Canada's Physical Activity Guide to Healthy Active Living*. Minister of Supply and Services Canada (1998). Catalogue Number H39-429/1998-1E. ISBN 0-662-86627-7.

Krucoff, Carol. "Exercise and Cancer: Moderate Activity May Help Reduce Risk of Some Tumors." *Washington Post Health*, January 14, 1992, p. 16.

Kusaka, Yukinori, Hiroshi Kondou, and Kanehisa Morimoto. "Healthy Lifestyles Are Associated with Higher Natural Killer Cell Activity." *Preventive Medicine* 21 (1992): 602–615.

Leon, Arthur S., and John Connett. "Physical Activity and 10.5 Year Mortality in the Multiple Risk Factor Intervention Trial (MRFIT)." *The International Journal of Epidemiology* 20 (1991): 690–697.

McGuigan, F.J. *Encyclopedia of Stress.* London: Allyn & Bacon, 1999.

Moore, K.A., M.A. Babyak, C.E. Wood, M.A. Napolitano, P. Khatri, W.E. Craighead, S. Herman, R. Krishman, and J.A. Blumenthal. "The Association Between Physical Activity and Depression in Older Depressed Adults." *Journal of Aging and Physical Activity*, 7, 1 (1999): 55–61.

Paffenbarger, Ralph S., Robert T. Hyde, Alvin L. Wing, and Chung-Cheng Hsieh. "Physical Activity, All-Cause Mortality, and Longevity of College Alumni." *New England Journal of Medicine* 314 (1986): 605–613.

Powell, K.E., C.J. Caspersen, J.P. Koplan, and E.S. Ford. "Physical Activity and Chronic Disease." *American Journal of Clinical Nutrition* 49 (1989): 999–1006.

Rakowski, William, and Vincent Mor. "The Association of Physical Activity with Mortality Among Older Adults in the Longitudinal Study of Aging." *Journal of Gerontology* 47 (1992): M122–M129.

Rockhill, B., W.C. Willett, D.J. Hunter, J.E. Manson, S.E. Hankinson, and G.A. Colditz. "A Prospective Study of Recreational Physical Activity and Breast Cancer Risk." *Archives of Internal Medicine* 159 (1999): 2290–2296.

Salonen, J.T., P. Puska, and J. Tuomelehto. "Physical Activity and Risk of Myocardial Infarction, Cerebral Stroke and Death: A Longitudinal Study in Eastern Finland." *American Journal of Epidemiology* 115 (1982): 526–537.

Shepard, Roy J. "Nutritional Benefits of Exercise." *Journal of Sports Medicine* 29 (1989): 83–90.

Sothern, M.S., M. Loftin, R.M. Suskind, J.N. Udall, and U. Blecker. "The Health Benefits of Physical Activity in Children and Adolescents: Implications for Chronic Disease Prevention." *European Journal of Pediatrics*, 158, 4 (1999): 271–274.

Steinhardt, Mary, Linda Greenhow, and Joy Stewart. "The Relationship of Physical Activity and Cardiovascular Fitness to Absenteeism and Medical Care Claims Among Law Enforcement Officers." *American Journal of Health Promotion* 5 (1991): 455–460.

Tucker, Larry A., Steven G. Aldana, and Glenn M. Friedman. "Cardiovascular Fitness and Absenteeism in 8,301 Employed Adults." *American Journal of Health Promotion* 5 (1990): 140–145.

U.S. Public Health Service. *Physical Activity and Health: A Report of the Surgeon General.* Washington, DC: U.S. Department of Health and Human Services, 1996.

Wyrwich, K.W., and F.D. Wolinsky. "Physical Activity, Disability, and the Risk of Hospitalization for Breast Cancer Among Older Women." *Journal of Gerontology. Series A, Biological Sciences and Medical Sciences* 55, 7 (2000): M418–M421.

Lab Activity 1.1

Assessing Your Health Risk

INSTRUCTIONS: *The U.S. government developed this questionnaire to help people assess their health behaviour and risk of ill health. Notice that it has six sections. Complete one section at a time, by circling the number corresponding to the answer that describes your own behaviour. Then add up the circled numbers to determine your score for each section. Write your score in the lines provided at the ends of the sections. Interpret your score with the table found on on page 18.*

✦ Cigarette Smoking	Almost Always	Sometimes	Almost Never
1. I avoid smoking cigarettes.	(2)	1	0
2. I smoke only low-tar and low-nicotine cigarettes, or I smoke a pipe or cigars only.	(2)	1	0

Your Cigarette Smoking Score: ___4___

✦ Alcohol and Drugs	Almost Always	Sometimes	Almost Never
1. I avoid drinking alcoholic beverages, or I drink no more than one or two a day.	(4)	1	0
2. I avoid using alcohol or other drugs (especially illegal drugs) as a way of handling stressful situations or my problems.	(2)	1	0
3. I am careful not to drink alcohol when I am taking certain medicines (for example, medicine for sleeping, pain, colds, and allergies).	(2)	1	0
4. I read and follow the label directions when I use prescribed and over-the-counter drugs.	(2)	1	0

Your Alcohol and Drugs Score: ___10___

(continued)

Lab Activity 1.1 *(continued)*
Assessing Your Health Risk

✦ **Eating Habits**

	Almost Always	Sometimes	Almost Never
1. I eat a variety of foods each day, such as fruits and vegetables, whole grain breads and cereals, lean meats, dairy products, dry peas and beans, and nuts and seeds.	4	(1)	0
2. I limit the amount of fat, especially saturated fat, and cholesterol I eat (including fats in meats, eggs, butter, cream, shortenings, and organ meats such as liver).	(2)	1	0
3. I limit the amount of salt I eat by not adding salt at the table, avoiding salty snacks, and making certain my meals are cooked with only small amounts of salt.	2	(1)	0
4. I avoid eating too much sugar (especially frequent snacks of sticky candy or soft drinks).	2	(1)	0

Your Eating Habits Score: _____5_____

✦ **Exercise and Fitness**

	Almost Always	Sometimes	Almost Never
1. I maintain a desired weight, avoiding overweight and underweight.	3	(1)	0
2. I do vigorous exercise for 15–30 minutes at least three times a week (examples include running, swimming, and brisk walking).	(3)	1	0
3. I do exercises that enhance my muscle tone for 15–30 minutes at least three times a week (examples include yoga and calisthenics).	2	(1)	0
4. I use part of my leisure time participating in individual, family, or team activities that increase my level of fitness (such as gardening, bowling, golf, or baseball).	2	(1)	0

Your Exercise and Fitness Score: _____6_____

✦ **Stress Control**	Almost Always	Sometimes	Almost Never
1. I enjoy the school or other work I do.	2	(1)	0
2. I find it easy to relax and express my feelings freely.	2	(1)	0
3. I recognize early, and prepare for, events or situations likely to be stressful for me.	2	1	(0)
4. I have close friends, relatives, or others with whom I can talk about personal matters and call on for help when it is needed.	2	(1)	0
5. I participate in group activities (such as religious or community organizations) or hobbies that I enjoy.	(2)	1	0

Your Stress Control Score: ___5___

✦ **Safety**	Almost Always	Sometimes	Almost Never
1. I wear a seat belt while I am riding in a car.	(2)	1	0
2. I avoid driving while I am under the influence of alcohol and other drugs. I also avoid getting in a car with someone driving who is under the influence of alcohol or other drugs.	(2)	1	0
3. I obey the traffic rules and the speed limit when I am driving and ask others to do so when I am a passenger in a car with them.	(2)	1	0
4. I am careful when I am using potentially harmful products or substances (such as household cleaners, poisons, and electrical devices).	(2)	1	0
5. I avoid smoking in bed.	(2)	1	0

Your Safety Score: ___10___

(continued)

Your Health Score

INSTRUCTIONS: *After you have totaled your score for each of the six sections, circle the number in each column below that matches your score for that section of the test.*

CIGARETTE SMOKING	ALCOHOL AND DRUGS	EATING HABITS	EXERCISE AND FITNESS	STRESS CONTROL	SAFETY
(10)	(10)	10	10	10	(10)
9	9	9	9	9	9
8	8	8	8	8	8
7	7	7	7	7	7
6	6	6	(6)	6	6
5	5	(5)	5	(5)	5
4	4	4	4	4	4
3	3	3	3	3	3
2	2	2	2	2	2
1	1	1	1	1	1
0	0	0	0	0	0

✦ Interpreting Your Score

Scores of 9 or 10 are excellent! Your answers show that you are aware of the importance of this area to your health. More important, you are putting your knowledge to work by practicing good health habits. Even so, you may want to consider areas in which your health habits can be improved.

Scores of 6 to 8 indicate that your health practices in this area are good but that there is room for improvement. Look again at the items you answered with "sometimes" or "almost never." What changes can you make to improve your score?

Scores of 3 to 5 mean your health risks are showing. You should ask your instructor for more information about the health risks you are facing. Your instructor will probably be able to help you decrease these risks. *An exception is the cigarette smoking section, for which a score of 3 to 4 is excellent.* Review your responses to the cigarette smoking items to better interpret their meaning.

Scores of 0 to 2 for all sections *except the cigarette smoking section* mean you may be taking serious, unnecessary risks with your health. Maybe you are not aware of the risks and what to do about them. Consult with a health expert or your instructor to improve your health. For the cigarette smoking section, scores of 0 to 1 mean you may be taking unnecessary risks with your health. Review your responses to these items to better interpret their meaning.

2

Assessing Your Present Level of Fitness

CHAPTER OBJECTIVES

By the end of this chapter, you should be able to:

1. Indicate when it is appropriate to obtain a medical examination prior to beginning an exercise program or test.

2. List the components of a good medical evaluation.

3. List the major components of a fitness appraisal.

4. Measure and analyze your cardiorespiratory endurance, muscular strength and endurance, flexibility, nutrient intake, and body composition.

KIM'S EXCUSE FOR avoiding a regular exercise program is one that is voiced by many university students: "I get enough exercise in my part-time job at the department store and my daily routine. I'm already fit. Why should I use my valuable time exercising more?" Unfortunately, there are few, if any, active occupations, including that of a university student, that develop cardiorespiratory endurance, muscular strength, muscular endurance, and flexibility and that control body weight and fat. One way for Kim to find out if she possesses an adequate level of health-related fitness is to complete the test battery described in this chapter to see whether she scores in the average or above-average category on each item.

THE MEDICAL EVALUATION

There is an abundance of literature regarding the need for medical evaluation before beginning a program of regular exercise. There are also a number of areas of disagreement among experts concerning what the components of such a medical evaluation should be, who should receive one, and even whether an evaluation is necessary at all. These viewpoints will be presented as objectively as possible to help you make a decision about your need for such an examination.

The Need for a Medical Evaluation

Most physicians indicate that a physical examination is necessary for individuals over the age of 40, those with symptoms of heart disease or other medical ailments, and those who have previously been sedentary. Some physicians favour a comprehensive exam; others prefer only general screening.

The Canadian Society for Exercise Physiology recommends that individuals planning to begin an exercise program self-determine their need to see a physician first by filling out the Physical Activity Readiness

Figure 2.1 ✦ Physical Activity Readiness Questionnaire (PAR-Q)

Physical Activity Readiness Questionnaire - PAR-Q (revised 2002)

PAR-Q & YOU

(A Questionnaire for People Aged 15 to 69)

Regular physical activity is fun and healthy, and increasingly more people are starting to become more active every day. Being more active is very safe for most people. However, some people should check with their doctor before they start becoming much more physically active.

If you are planning to become much more physically active than you are now, start by answering the seven questions in the box below. If you are between the ages of 15 and 69, the PAR-Q will tell you if you should check with your doctor before you start. If you are over 69 years of age, and you are not used to being very active, check with your doctor.

Common sense is your best guide when you answer these questions. Please read the questions carefully and answer each one honestly: check YES or NO.

YES	NO		
☐	☐	1.	**Has your doctor ever said that you have a heart condition and that you should only do physical activity recommended by a doctor?**
☐	☐	2.	**Do you feel pain in your chest when you do physical activity?**
☐	☐	3.	**In the past month, have you had chest pain when you were not doing physical activity?**
☐	☐	4.	**Do you lose your balance because of dizziness or do you ever lose consciousness?**
☐	☐	5.	**Do you have a bone or joint problem (for example, back, knee or hip) that could be made worse by a change in your physical activity?**
☐	☐	6.	**Is your doctor currently prescribing drugs (for example, water pills) for your blood pressure or heart condition?**
☐	☐	7.	**Do you know of any other reason why you should not do physical activity?**

If you answered

YES to one or more questions

Talk with your doctor by phone or in person BEFORE you start becoming much more physically active or BEFORE you have a fitness appraisal. Tell your doctor about the PAR-Q and which questions you answered YES.

- You may be able to do any activity you want — as long as you start slowly and build up gradually. Or, you may need to restrict your activities to those which are safe for you. Talk with your doctor about the kinds of activities you wish to participate in and follow his/her advice.
- Find out which community programs are safe and helpful for you.

NO to all questions

If you answered NO honestly to all PAR-Q questions, you can be reasonably sure that you can:

- start becoming much more physically active – begin slowly and build up gradually. This is the safest and easiest way to go.
- take part in a fitness appraisal – this is an excellent way to determine your basic fitness so that you can plan the best way for you to live actively. It is also highly recommended that you have your blood pressure evaluated. If your reading is over 144/94, talk with your doctor before you start becoming much more physically active.

DELAY BECOMING MUCH MORE ACTIVE:

- if you are not feeling well because of a temporary illness such as a cold or a fever – wait until you feel better; or
- if you are or may be pregnant – talk to your doctor before you start becoming more active.

PLEASE NOTE: If your health changes so that you then answer YES to any of the above questions, tell your fitness or health professional. Ask whether you should change your physical activity plan.

Informed Use of the PAR-Q: The Canadian Society for Exercise Physiology, Health Canada, and their agents assume no liability for persons who undertake physical activity, and if in doubt after completing this questionnaire, consult your doctor prior to physical activity.

No changes permitted. You are encouraged to photocopy the PAR-Q but only if you use the entire form.

NOTE: If the PAR-Q is being given to a person before he or she participates in a physical activity program or a fitness appraisal, this section may be used for legal or administrative purposes.

"I have read, understood and completed this questionnaire. Any questions I had were answered to my full satisfaction."

NAME ____________________

SIGNATURE ____________________ DATE ____________________

SIGNATURE OF PARENT or GUARDIAN (for participants under the age of majority) ____________________ WITNESS ____________________

Note: This physical activity clearance is valid for a maximum of 12 months from the date it is completed and becomes invalid if your condition changes so that you would answer YES to any of the seven questions.

CSEP SCPE © Canadian Society for Exercise Physiology Supported by: Health Canada Santé Canada

continued on other side...

Source: Physical Activity Readiness Questionnaire (PAR-Q), © 2002. Reprinted with permission from the Canadian Society for Exercise Physiology, **www.csep.ca/forms.asp**

Questionnaire (PAR-Q) (Figure 2.1). If any of the health questions contained in PAR-Q receive a Yes response, persons aged 15–69 are advised to consult a physician prior to engaging in a new exercise program.

Health Canada advises that most people under 60 years of age do not need a medical examination prior to beginning a gradual and sensible exercise program, because sedentary living is a far more dangerous practice than exercising without a physician's approval, many people do not take the time to secure an examination, and a recommended medical exam can be nothing more than another excuse to avoid exercise.

Certainly, it is desirable for everyone to have a complete medical examination before a physical fitness evaluation and the start of a new exercise program to increase safety and aid in the exercise prescription. It is also generally accepted that certain categories of people face risk when engaging in fitness programs without a medical examination.

Components of the Ideal Medical Evaluation

Although the exact content of the ideal evaluation depends on the history and symptoms of each individual, common areas include a medical history that asks questions about your own and your family's history of diabetes and coronary heart disease and associated risk factors such as hypertension, stress, smoking, eating habits, current activity level, and physical disabilities. If symptoms indicate the need, the examination may also include measurement of blood pressure, listening to the sounds of the heart and lungs, determination of the resting pulse rate, a chest X-ray, **blood lipid analysis**, a resting **electrocardiogram (ECG)**, and a **graded exercise test (stress test)**.

The results of this medical evaluation should be discussed with the patient, and any restrictions on physical activity or fitness testing should be identified at that time. Remember that the fact that your physical activity may have limits does not mean you should avoid exercise. This book provides you with a number of sound exercise choices that will meet your fitness needs without endangering your health.

THE FITNESS APPRAISAL

In addition to the medical evaluation, it is also important to appraise your present level of **health-related fitness**, to monitor your body's response to exercise, to prepare your individualized program, and to monitor your progress.

Specific tests in this section are classified and described according to each component of health-related fitness: cardiorespiratory endurance, muscular strength, muscular endurance, flexibility, nutrition, and body

composition. Several tests are provided in each area to allow you to make appropriate choices depending on the facilities and equipment available, your specific likes and dislikes, and physical and emotional factors that may cause you to favour one test over another. For a more comprehensive analysis of your health-related fitness, we recommend taking a larger number of tests. The proper techniques to administer each test are also described in this section.

To help you interpret your scores, test norms and standards are provided in Lab Activity 2.1: Your Physical Fitness Profile, next to where your scores are recorded. In this Lab, we have also attempted to provide a "health interpretation" for your fitness scores based on the various test norm categories into which you fall. In addition to comparing your scores to those of other university students of a similar age, we analyze the health implications of your scores.

During your fitness appraisal, **stop any test** immediately if: you begin to feel chest pains, faintness, or dizziness; you develop an excruciating headache; or you cannot get enough air. If you notice any other disturbing sensations, do not complete the test. If any of these symptoms appear, consult a physician to determine their causes. It may be that your fitness level simply is so low that your body cannot handle strenuous activity, or a medical problem may exist. To avoid endangering your health and to eliminate worry, it is important to have the problem diagnosed.

Cardiorespiratory Assessment

All sound exercise programs place primary emphasis on cardiorespiratory endurance. The publicity surrounding the benefits of exercise in combating the nation's leading killer (heart disease), justified or not, is probably responsible for the emphasis on improving the functioning of the heart, circulatory system, and lungs.

Blood lipid analysis Examination and study of the fats present in the blood.

Electrocardiogram (ECG) A tracing of the electrical currents involved in the cycles of a heartbeat.

Graded exercise test (stress test) Test designed to monitor the electrical activity of the heart; it is performed by walking on a treadmill that is slowly being elevated to increase the workload.

Health-related fitness An adequate or above-average level of achievement, based on test scores, in components such as cardiorespiratory endurance, muscular strength and endurance, flexibility, and body composition that has been associated with the prevention of certain diseases and disorders, high energy, and a high level of wellness.

MYTH AND FACT SHEET

Myth	Fact
1. A physical examination isn't necessary for university students who are feeling all right.	1. It is quite common for young adults to feel good and still possess high blood pressure and/or high blood cholesterol. These "silent" killers afflict adults of all ages and are only detected through regular checkups. Although you may have no reason to suspect that you are afflicted with such ailments, an examination may uncover them in their early stages when treatment is most effective. Still, the majority of university students probably do not need a complete physical examination prior to beginning an exercise program. For those who are overweight or obese, have been inactive for several years, have a family history of health problems, experience any of the danger signs described in this chapter during activity, or have not seen a physician for several years, an examination may be indicated.
2. Cardiorespiratory fitness testing is too dangerous.	2. Each of the running tests (4.8-kilometre walk, and 12-minute run) are run–walk tests that allow you to go at your own safe pace. You can also stop at any time during the Harvard step test if you experience difficulty. The tests are not dangerous if performed properly. If you have been inactive for more than a year or have never engaged in aerobic exercise, you have several choices. First, you can skip these tests, assume that your cardiorespiratory fitness rating is poor, and choose a beginner's aerobic exercise program that allows you to progress slowly and safely to higher levels. Second, you can undertake a two-to-three-week preconditioning program of walking and jogging to prepare yourself for the 4.8-kilometre test. Finally, you can choose to stop and walk during any or all of the tests as long as you give your best effort.
3. Fitness testing will make you too sore to function the next day.	3. When sedentary people complete tests that require maximum effort, they do experience considerable soreness the next day. The areas of soreness show which muscles you have not been using. Many instructors eliminate the problem of soreness by using a two-to-three-week preconditioning program before performing any maximum-effort fitness testing.
4. You know enough about your fitness level already and do not need to be tested.	4. You may have a good feel for some aspects of your physical fitness. On the other hand, standardized tests may be just what you need to compare yourself to others of your age and to highlight the areas in which you need the most improvement. Test results often provide strong motivation for individuals to begin an exercise program.
5. You're fit enough—too much exercise will cause athlete's heart and jeopardize your health.	5. "Athlete's heart," or "sportherz," is a term used by a Swedish researcher who detected enlarged heart muscles among skiers in 1899. As the years passed, the term gained momentum and was used incorrectly to refer to an abnormally large heart brought on by exercise. Because of this myth, some people actually became concerned that exercise would damage their hearts and result in disability or death. Aerobic exercise does develop the heart muscle more fully and cause it to become heavier and larger. It also causes the heart to pump more blood per beat (stroke volume) and per minute (cardiac output) and to become a more efficient organ. Cardiac changes that occur from aerobic exercise are both natural and healthy, and it is highly unlikely that proper aerobic exercise will cause damage to a healthy heart.

Exercise that overloads the **oxygen-transport system** (aerobic activity) leads to an increase in cardiorespiratory endurance and the muscular strength and endurance of some large muscle groups.

Run–Walk Tests You can assess your cardiorespiratory endurance using a **run–walk test**—either the 4.8-kilometre walk or the 12-minute run.

The 12-minute run and 4.8-kilometre walk can be completed indoors or outdoors. Begin by measuring off a 1-to-5-kilometre course on a track or other flat area where you can run or walk. After an adequate warm-up consisting of 8–12 minutes of walking and jogging followed by 4–5 minutes of stretching, your objective is to complete the distance as quickly as possible by running, walking, or combining the two. You can easily time yourself in the *4.8-kilometre walk test* on the track or a grass or sidewalk area that has been accurately measured. Record your times and ratings in Lab Activity 2.1 at the end of this chapter.

The *12-minute test* is best performed on a 400-metre track or other measured area that allows the tester to determine the exact distance you cover in 12 minutes. Markers can be placed every 10 to 25 metres on the course with a spotter assigned to each runner to improve the accuracy of scoring. After proper warm-up and stretching, you stand on the starting line and await the signal to run and walk as many laps as possible around the course within the time period. When the allotted time expires, the tester blows a whistle, signalling the spotter, who has also been counting the laps, to mark the distance to the nearest 10 metres. In the meantime, you should continue to jog or walk for a 4-to-5-minute cool-down period.

Cycling and Swimming Tests If you prefer to swim or cycle, you can determine your level of cardiorespiratory endurance using a **cycling or swimming test**—either the 12-minute swimming test or the 12-minute cycling test. You should first complete an adequate warm-up consisting of swimming or slow pedaling followed by 4 to 5 minutes of stretching. Both tests are completed in the same manner in a swimming pool or on a premeasured road course with total metres recorded at the point time expires in the swimming test and total kilometres (to the nearest tenth) in the cycling test. Scores and rating categories are recorded in Lab Activity 2.1.

The Harvard Step Test An alternative assessment method that accurately identifies your cardiorespiratory fitness level is the **Harvard step test**. Since test results are based on accurate resting and exercise heart rates, it is important to improve your skill in this area by completing Lab Activity 2.2: Determining Your Resting and Exercise Heart Rate. To complete the test, get a

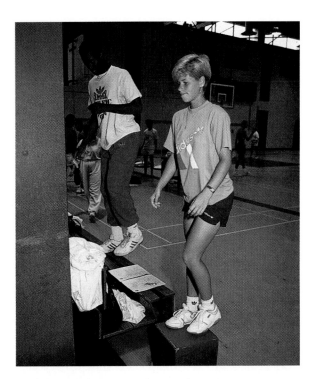

The Harvard step test is one way to determine your cardiorespiratory endurance. It involves stepping up and down repeatedly and then measuring the pulse rate to determine how fast the heart recovers.

sturdy 45-centimetre bench or stool and a wristwatch with a second hand and then follow these procedures:

1. Step on the bench first with one foot and then with the other until you are standing erect with the knees unbent. Then step down with one foot followed by the other to return to the starting position.

2. Step at a cadence that will result in 30 such repetitions each minute (one every 2 seconds) for 4 (females) or 5 (males) minutes.

3. At the end of the 4-or-5-minute period, sit down.

Oxygen-transport system The ability of the body to take in and use oxygen at the tissue level during physical activity.

Run–walk tests Field tests designed to measure cardiorespiratory endurance (aerobic fitness).

Cycling and swimming tests Field tests designed to measure cardiorespiratory endurance (aerobic fitness).

Harvard step test Test designed to measure cardiorespiratory endurance (aerobic fitness).

DIVERSITY ISSUES

Exercise for Everyone

In Canada, culture has a strong influence on whether we choose to exercise on a regular basis or to avoid such activity in our daily lives. Differences in exercise involvement exist between various age groups, between males and females, between education levels, and across household income and employment status levels. We know from data provided by Statistics Canada (2000) that physical activity is engaged in more frequently by men than by women. We also know that the most frequent exercise age groups, men and women combined, are first ages 35 to 44, then 25 to 34, then 45 to 54. In short, contrary to conventional thinking about highly physically active youth, the ages from 15 to 19 and 20 to 24 are not among the top three exercise frequency groups in our country. Furthermore, only about 60 percent of all Canadians report that they exercise (that is, do calisthenics, jogging, racquet sports, team sports, dance classes, or brisk walking) for at least 15 minutes, three times per week. Of greater concern is the fact that some 22 percent of all Canadians exercise less than once per week or never. This is particularly disconcerting given Health Canada's recommendation to engage in physical activity for 30 minutes each day, five days per week.

In our attempt to convert everyone to a physically active lifestyle, we sometimes overlook some deep-rooted factors that influence behaviour. Studies show that Canadians are generally more physically active the higher the level of education they have attained; conversely, Canadians are more likely to be sedentary the lower their level of formal education. The same data confirm that in our country, the more affluent (by household income level) we are, the more physically active we tend to be. Thus, socioeconomic levels, sex, age, and probably many other factors influence the decision to be sedentary or physically active. Perhaps we need a more all-encompassing or holistic approach in order to understand the wide variety of factors involved in promoting exercise for everyone.

Source: Data partly adapted from Statistics Canada Publication, National Population Health Survey Public Use Microdata files Household component, 1998–1999, Catalogue 82M0009, December, 2000

4. After waiting exactly 1 minute, take your pulse or have a partner take your pulse for 30 seconds, and record that number.

5. Wait an additional 30 seconds before taking your pulse once again for a 30-second period, and record that number.

6. Repeat Step 5 in 30 seconds. You will now have taken your pulse between 1 and 1½ minutes, 2 and 2½ minutes, and 3 and 3½ minutes after completing the step test.

7. Using the total of the three pulse counts, compute the formula:

$$\text{Index} = \frac{\text{Duration of exercise in seconds} \times 100}{2 \times \text{Sum of 3 pulse counts in recovery}}$$

Once again, record your scores in Lab Activity 2.1, and determine your cardiorespiratory fitness level from Table C in the Lab.

■ Muscular Strength Assessment

In the laboratory, muscular strength, the absolute maximum force that a muscle can generate, is measured using elaborate and expensive equipment. Dynamometers, cable tensiometers, and force transducers and recorders have all been used this way. One problem with such methods is the need to test numerous muscle groups to obtain an accurate measure in the legs, the abdomen, and the arms. These muscles cover such diverse body parts, however, that you can safely assume that their levels of muscular strength are representative of total body strength.

You can also measure the strength and endurance of practically any muscle group by using free weights or a variety of weight machines. In some cases, you can test yourself; in others, such as the 1-RM testing using barbells, you will need a *spotter* to assist you throughout the movement.

1-RM (Repetitions Maximum) Testing Free weights are commonly used to determine your **1-RM** (maximum amount of weight you can lift one time) for a particular muscle group.

The *bench press* and *shoulder press* accurately measure the strength of your triceps, pectoralis, and deltoid muscles; the *arm curl* measures bicep muscle strength; and the *leg press* determines the strength of the quadriceps muscle group. For each test, a weight is selected that can be lifted comfortably. Additional weight is then added in subsequent trials until the weight is found that can be lifted correctly only one time. If the weight can be lifted more than once, additional weight is added until a true 1-RM is determined. Approximately three trials with a 2-to-3-minute rest interval between trials are needed to determine the 1-RM for each muscle group. Because the resistance to be overcome in 1-RM testing is heavy, it is important to use one or two spotters to protect you from injury should you be unable to complete the lift. (Chapter 6 discusses the proper technique for these tests.) Record your scores in Lab Activity 2.1.

■ Muscular Endurance Assessment

There is a great difference between muscular endurance and muscular strength and therefore between the kinds of tests that apply to these components. Strength tests determine the maximum amount of weight that can be moved one time, whereas endurance tests measure continuous work by determining the total number of times a specific weight can be moved.

You can evaluate the muscular endurance of your abdominal area, arms, and shoulders by completing the curl test (men and women) and one of the following: the pull-up (men) or flexed-arm hang test (women) or the push-up (men) or modified push-up test (women).

Abdominal Endurance Although it is difficult to obtain a pure, isolated measurement of the abdominal region, the 1-minute *abdominal curl test* provides a fairly accurate score. To prepare for the test, place a strip of tape 7–8 centimetres wide across a mat (see Figure 2.2). Lie on your back with your knees flexed, both feet flat on the floor as close to the hips as possible, and your fingertips at the edge of the strip. On signal, curl forward until your fingertips move forward the width of the tape (from the front to the back of the tape), then curl back until both shoulder blades touch the mat. Your shoulder blades should lift from the mat with each repetition while your lower back and feet remain on the mat. Record the number of curls completed in one minute and your rating in Lab Activity 2.1.

Arm and Shoulder Muscular Endurance You can complete the *pull-up test* for men by grasping an adjustable horizontal bar with your palms facing away from the body. Now raise your body until your chin clears the top of the bar, then slowly lower yourself to a full hang without any pause as many times as you can (see Figure 2.3). Your body must return to a stretch position (elbows locked) each time. Deliberate swinging, resting, or leg kicking is not permitted. Table F in Lab Activity 2.1 will help you evaluate the strength and endurance of your arms and shoulders.

The *modified pull-up test* for women closely resembles the pull-up for men. You grasp an adjustable horizontal bar with your palms facing away from your body at a level that is just even with the base of the sternum (breastbone). Place your body under the bar until a 90-degree

Figure 2.2 ✦ Abdominal Curls

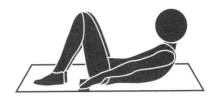

angle is formed at the point where your arms and chest join. Only your heels support the weight of your lower body (see Figure 2.3). You score one point each time you pull your chin over the bar and return your body to the support position with your arms fully extended.

The *push-up test* for men begins with your arms and back straight and your fingers forward. Lower your chest to the floor until your elbows form a right angle and your upper arms are parallel to the floor (the chest must almost touch the floor) before returning to the starting position (see Figure 2.4). The *modified push-up test* for women is performed in a similar manner but with the knees rather than the toes supporting the body (see Figure 2.4). Again, record your scores and ratings in Lab Activity 2.1.

■ Flexibility Assessment

Flexibility is an important component of fitness. It involves the ability to move the body throughout a range of motion and stretch the muscles and tissues around skeletal joints. *Canada's Physical Activity Guide to Healthy Active Living* recommends flexibility training 4 to 7 days a week to keep your muscles relaxed and joints mobile. Many people do not realize how inflexible they are.

The shoulder reach, trunk flexion, and trunk extension tests provide an excellent indication of body flexibility.

Shoulder Reach You can complete the *shoulder reach test* by standing against a pole or a projecting corner, raising your right arm, and reaching down behind your back as far as possible. At the same time, reach up from behind with your left hand and try to overlap the palm of your right hand (see Figure 2.5). Have a partner measure, in centimetres, how much the fingers on your right hand overlap the fingers of your left hand. If you overlap, place a plus sign in front of the amount of overlap in Lab Activity 2.1; if the fingers of your right and left hands do not touch, place a minus sign in front of the amount of

1-RM The maximum amount of weight that can be lifted one time.

Figure 2.3 ✦ Pull-ups and Modified Pull-ups

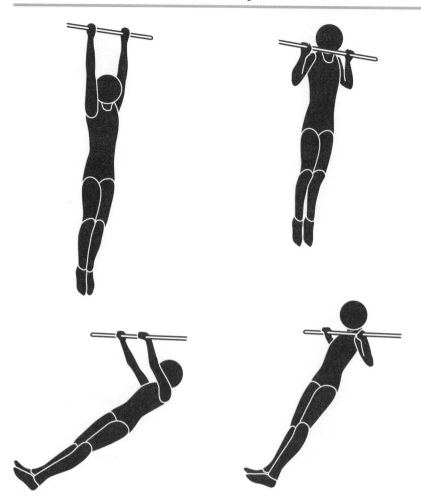

Figure 2.4 ✦ Push-ups and Modified Push-ups

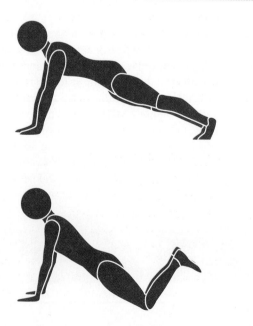

the gap. If the fingers of one hand just barely touch those of the other, give yourself a score of zero. Repeat this test with your arms reversed; that is, the arm that first reached down over the shoulder will now reach up from behind the back.

Trunk Flexion The *trunk flexion test* measures your ability to flex your trunk and stretch the back of your thigh muscles. To begin, remove your shoes and sit with your legs straight and your feet flat against a box positioned against a wall. Place a ruler on top of the box. Place one hand on top of the other so your middle fingers are together and the same length. While your partner keeps your knees from bending, lean forward and place your hands on top of the box. Slide your hands along the measuring scale as far as possible without bouncing and hold that position for at least 3 seconds (see Figure 2.5). Repeat the test two more times and record your highest score to the nearest centimetre in Lab Activity 2.1. Your score is the number of centimetres beyond the edge of the box you can stretch (use a plus

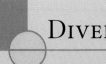

DIVERSITY ISSUES

The Canadian Physical Activity, Fitness and Lifestyle Appraisal (CPAFLA)

Fitness appraisal in Canada has a strong tradition and varied background. The existence of a wide variety of appraisal mechanisms and systems led to the publication of the *Canadian Standardized Test of Fitness* (CSTF) in 1979. This manual was revised several times throughout the 1980s, but in all its forms it has sought to provide a simple, safe, and standardized approach to assessing the main components of fitness in apparently healthy individuals.

The fourth and current edition of the CSTF rightfully is titled *Canadian Physical Activity, Fitness and Lifestyle Appraisal* (CPAFLA). The CPAFLA was developed in accordance with the most up-to-date research, which recognizes the health benefits of moderate physical activity and the relationship between lifestyle behaviours and health. This manual and its attendant course certification stem from a straightforward and systematic approach outlining the proper procedures for the appraisal and counselling of Canadians aged 15 to 69 while emphasizing health benefits of physical activity. In short, the Canadian appraisal system has broadened its perspective from a narrow physical fitness focus to a more all-encompassing lifestyle approach. Major differences between the CSTF and the CPAFLA are:

CSTF	CPAFLA
• Performance-related	• Health-related
• Emphasis on fitness	• Emphasis on physical
• Focus on prescribed	activity
exercise	• Considers broader,
• Tests and measures	lifestyle issues
• Assumed readiness for	• Information and advice
behaviour change	• Recognizes/helps
	"nonmovers"

CPAFLA certification involves an approximately 40-hour course (two weekends) that covers such topics as understanding behaviour change, healthy physical activity participation, healthy lifestyle, basic exercise physiology, and health-related fitness, and includes appraisal tools, case studies, and references.

For more information on how to take this course, contact: Canadian Society for Exercise Physiology, 202–185 Somerset Street West, Ottawa, Ontario K2P 0J2. ✦

Sources: Adapted from The Canadian Physical Activity, Fitness and Lifestyle Appraisal Manual, 2nd ed. (Ottawa: Health Canada, 1998). Additional information from Dr. Don Paterson representing the Canadian Society for Exercise Physiology.

Figure 2.5 ✦ Flexibility

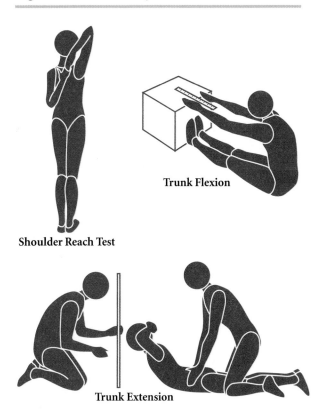

Shoulder Reach Test

Trunk Flexion

Trunk Extension

sign in front of that value) or the number of centimetres short of the edge of the box you can reach (use a minus sign in front of that value). If you can reach only to the edge of the box, give yourself a score of zero. Care should be taken to warm up before this test to avoid back strain.

Trunk Extension To determine the flexibility of your back, complete the *trunk extension test.* Lie on the floor face-down with a partner applying pressure on your upper legs and buttocks. Clasp your hands behind your neck, raise your head and chest off the ground as high as possible, and hold that position for 3 seconds (see Figure 2.5). Ask your partner to measure the distance to the nearest centimetre between your chin and the floor. Again, enter this value in Lab Activity 2.1.

■ Nutritional Assessment

Numerous IBM- and Macintosh-compatible software programs are available to analyze your dietary intake accurately. Regardless of the software you choose, you will need to record your dietary intake (food and drink) carefully over a 3-to-7-day period, noting portion sizes, brand names of products whenever they are available, fast-food products, and other information that you will code later according to the specifications of the software documentation.

Figure 2.6 ✦ Nomogram for BMI

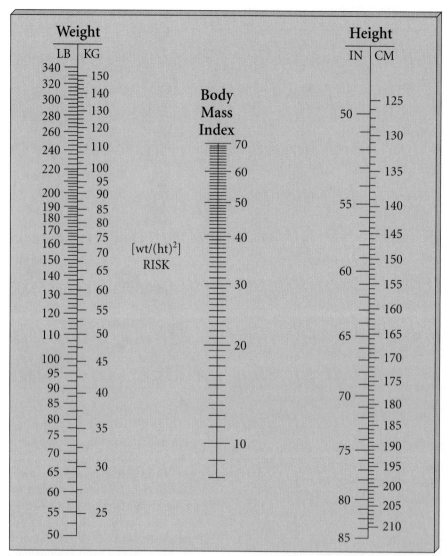

◼ Body Composition Assessment

Numerous tests are available to measure your body's composition. Height–weight charts, discussed in Chapter 9, are perhaps the least accurate method of providing an indication of associated health risks except for the very obese individual. Three practical tests—body mass index, waist-to-hip ratio, and skinfold measures—provide an adequately precise assessment of your body composition and the associated health risks.

1. **Body mass index (BMI)** A more sensitive indicator of body composition and health risks than body weight is provided by the **body mass index**.

BMI has previously been deemed a reliable and valid indicator of body composition for university students who are neither heavily muscled nor suffering from severe muscle atrophy (as would be the case for someone with anorexia nervosa, for example) (Otte, Hassler, Brogowski, Bowen, and Mayhew, 2000). You can determine your BMI using Figure 2.6 by placing a dot at your exact height in centimetres in the column to the right and another dot at your exact weight in kilograms in the column to the left, drawing a straight line to connect the two dots, and recording the number where the line intersects the vertical column in the middle. Keep in mind that weights and heights are

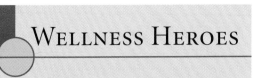

WELLNESS HEROES

Marnie McBean

Marnie McBean was not a stereotypical Olympic athlete in terms of lifestyle and life choices. McBean competed in the sport of rowing, which demands great cardiovascular and muscular endurance and overall body strength, and shares the distinction (with her rowing partner, Kathleen Heddle) of being the only Canadian to have won three Olympic gold medals in any sport. While competing, McBean was adamant that she made choices about her Olympian lifestyle, not absolute or drastic sacrifices: "Rowing is my priority; I do have to make choices about how much time to train like an Olympian and how much time to spend as a normal person."

For over 13 years, Marnie achieved phenomenal successes in international rowing. After winning a bronze medal at the 1986 World Junior Championships, she dominated North American, International, and World Cup regattas in pairs, double sculls, single sculls, straight fours, and quadruple sculls, and in the eight-oared events. At the Barcelona games in 1992, she won two gold medals in the pairs and eights; at the Atlanta games four years later, she won gold in the double sculls event and a bronze medal in the quadruple sculls.

Although she had to withdraw from the Sydney 2000 games due to a back injury, McBean still remains active, having climbed Mount Kilimanjaro in 2002. That same year, she received the Thomas Keller Medal for an "outstanding career in rowing." Currently, McBean works as a motivational and teamwork speaker, and still contributes to the sport of rowing through various fundraising activities.

The life of an Olympian is far from glamorous. McBean trained three to seven hours a day, six days a week; every four years, she got one "real" holiday. Her hands were always rough and callused from the countless kilometres rowed and kilograms lifted. Every morning she woke up with a goal for rowing that was anywhere from one day to four years away.

Yet while Marnie knows many elite-level athletes who sacrifice everything for their sport, her attitude was less spartan. For the most part, her diet was well balanced; but all food was a sometimes food, and she ate any kind of cheesecake (a personal favourite), hamburgers, and occasionally fried chicken, and she loves beer and dancing.

For all the work and dedication, rowing was always a thrill. In her words, "I feel I get to play when I'm on the water." ✦

Sources:
1. "Marnie McBean Receives 2002 Thomas Keller Medal," off *WorldRowing.com* Web site, September 21, 2002, accessed May 30, 2003 **www.worldrowing.com/news/fullstory. sps?iNewsID=22310&itype=iCategoryID=;**
2. "Canadian Olympian Marnie McBean to Climb Mount Kilimanjaro," off Yahoo Web site, July 5, 2002, accessed May 30, 2003 **http://ca.sports.yahoo.com/020705/6/nh5d.html**
3. Personal interview with the authors

determined without clothing. A BMI greater than 27.2 for men or 26.9 for women indicates a need for weight reduction. Traditional weight tables and the BMI provide only rough estimates of what people should weigh. For example, Sonia is 168 centimetres tall, weighs 83 kilograms, and has a BMI of about 31.0.

2. **Waist-to-hip ratio** This provides an indication of the way you store fat. Obese people who tend to store large amounts of fat in the abdominal area, rather than around the hips and thighs, are at higher risk for coronary heart disease, high blood pressure, congestive heart failure, strokes, and diabetes. To provide an accurate and practical indicator, the waist-to-hip ratio test was devised by a panel of scientists appointed by the National Academy of Sciences and the Dietary Guidelines Advisory Council for the U.S. Departments of Agriculture and Health and Human Services. For a waist-to-hip ratio of 1.0 or higher in men and 0.85 or higher in women, the panel recommends fat loss. For example, John has a 102-centimetre waist and a 97-centimetre hip. His ratio of 1.05 (102 ÷ 97) is indicative of increased risk for disease.

3. **Skinfold measures** At various sites on the body, these provide an accurate indicator of your percentage of body fat. The four-site skinfold test described in Chapter 9 is designed for both university men and women.

Body mass index (BMI) A method of determining overweight and obesity by dividing body weight (in kilograms) by height (in centimetres) squared; this method is considered superior to height–weight table ranges.

BEHAVIOURAL CHANGE AND MOTIVATIONAL STRATEGIES

There are many excuses for not starting an exercise program. Here are some common barriers (roadblocks) and strategies for overcoming them.

Roadblock	Behavioural Change Strategy
Like many other men and women, you do not like undergoing a medical examination. The setting makes you feel so uncomfortable and embarrassed that you will do almost anything to avoid it.	These feelings are quite natural. Fortunately, there are ways to make the experience less traumatic. Consider informing your physician that you want to begin an exercise program and would feel better knowing that there are no medical contraindications. Your physician may know enough about your medical history to give you the green light over the phone. If not, make an appointment with your physician to have the tests you want completed, and make it clear that these are the only tests you need at this time and that you are not interested in other examination procedures.
You detest running and would never choose that form of aerobic exercise. In fact, the mere thought of running 2.5 kilometres to complete the aerobic test may be a turnoff and destroy your motivation to begin a program.	Many people dislike running as a form of exercise. Fortunately, there are other valuable aerobic choices as beneficial as jogging or running. You can also assess your cardiorespiratory endurance without running. Review the Harvard step test described in this chapter. Find a bench and complete the test in your gym. Many step classes at fitness centres use this method as a complete workout. You can complete the test alone. If you dislike physical tests, avoid both the 2.5-kilometre and the Harvard step test, and select an aerobic exercise program that has a beginner's level and slowly progresses toward more advanced fitness.
You are self-conscious about the amount of fat on your body and do not want anyone to measure you with skinfold calipers.	This is a common concern, and you have the right to avoid such tests of body composition. The following options will still provide you with some type of assessment. 1. Borrow a skinfold caliper for an hour or two and ask a relative or a close friend to take the measurements. 2. Find equipment to perform hydrostatic (underwater) weighing. A school physical education or biology department might have this kind of equipment. Then you need only put on a bathing suit and submerge yourself in water. 3. Avoid any specific test of body composition, and apply your own *pinch-an-inch* method to various body parts. If you are pinching an inch (about 2.5 centimetres), you are now aware that you possess too much fat in that area. If this occurs in more than two areas, it is an indication that your total body fat is too high.
List other roadblocks you are experiencing that seem to be reducing the effectiveness of the fitness assessment phase of your program.	Now list the behavioural change strategies that can help you overcome these roadblocks. Read ahead in Chapter 3 for help with behavioural change and motivational techniques.

1. _____	1. _____
2. _____	2. _____
3. _____	3. _____

PUTTING IT ALL TOGETHER

Your fitness profile is complete. You can now evaluate your physical fitness in absolute terms (Are you satisfied with your levels of each component?) or in relative terms (Are you happy with how you compare with others?). Wellness requires information. Where are you now? Where do you want to be? How can you get there? Now that you have identified your current fitness level, you can decide on what goals you need to set for your-

self. For example, if you are not satisfied with your cardiorespiratory fitness, read the rest of this book with a view toward improving that component. You can do the same for muscular strength and endurance, flexibility, or body composition. This book contains the means for you to be successful at enhancing your level of physical fitness. All you need to do is apply them. Always keep in mind that improving one aspect of your health or fitness should not result in the decline of another component. It is important to strive for a balance in all components of physical fitness.

SUMMARY

The Medical Evaluation

Not all experts agree whether everyone starting an exercise program should obtain a medical evaluation. Even when there is agreement in this area, experts may disagree concerning exactly what the examination should entail. We recommend a medical examination after age 45 and at any age when identifiable risk or disease is present. The content of the evaluation depends on the age of the patient and the symptoms present and may include taking a medical history, measuring blood pressure, listening to the sound of the heart and lungs, determining resting pulse rate, having a chest X-ray, administering a resting ECG and a graded exercise test, and administering blood tests for blood fats and the ratio between high- and low-density lipoproteins. We also believe that you should decide whether you need a medical examination before you start exercise testing and an exercise program based on your knowledge of your personal health, present physical fitness level, and medical history.

The Fitness Appraisal

The ideal health-related fitness appraisal should include measures of cardiorespiratory endurance, muscular

strength and endurance, flexibility, nutrition, and body composition. This chapter allows you and your instructors to choose from a number of tests in each area depending on individual interest, equipment, and the amount of time available for assessment. *Cardiorespiratory endurance* can be measured with any one or more of the following tests: the 4.8-kilometre walk or the 12-minute run; the 12-minute swimming or cycling test; and the Harvard step test. The 1-RM (amount of weight that can be lifted one time) measures *muscular strength* through one or more of the following tests: bench press, military press, two-arm curl, and leg press. *Muscular endurance* is determined through such tests as the abdominal curl, pull-ups (men) or modified pull-ups (women), and push-ups (men) or modified push-ups (women). *Flexibility* is measured through the use of the shoulder reach, trunk flexion, and trunk extension tests. Tests designed to measure *body composition* include body mass index (BMI), waist-to-hip ratio, and skinfold measures (explained in detail in Chapter 9). Nutritional analysis is best completed through the use of numerous software programs that analyze dietary intake over a period of three days.

For an accurate evaluation of your health-related fitness, it is important to give your best effort on each test while staying alert to physical signs of overexertion.

STUDY QUESTIONS

1. Is it important to obtain a medical evaluation prior to beginning an exercise routine? Explain your answer.

2. Define the components of the ideal medical evaluation.

3. Identify the six assessment components in appraisal of a person's present level of health-related fitness. Provide examples for each assessment.

4. Briefly describe the three practical tests involved in measuring body composition.

5. Briefly describe the tests involved in measuring cardiorespiratory endurance.

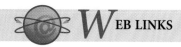

WEB LINKS

Canadian Society for Exercise Physiology
www.csep.ca/

Canadian Active Living
www.activeliving.ca

Canadian Fitness and Lifestyle Research Institute
www.cflri.ca/

Canada's Physical Activity Guide
www.paguide.com

Canadian Association for the Advancement of Women and Sport and Physical Activity
www.caaws.ca

Canadian Centre for Activity and Aging
www.uwo.ca/actage/

REFERENCES

British Columbia Fitness Appraisal Certification and Accreditation (BCFACA), 2000. **www.bcfaca.bc.ca/index. html**

Otte, A., J. Hassler, J. Brogowski, J.C. Bowen, and J.L. Mayhew. "Relationship of Body Mass Index and Predicted Percent Fat in College Men and Women." *Missouri Journal of Health, Physical Education, Recreation, and Dance* 10 (2000): 23–29.

Lab Activity 2.1

Your Physical Fitness Profile

INSTRUCTIONS: *This Lab allows you to choose from a number of different tests within each of the major areas of health-related fitness. After you complete a test, consult the norm tables or standards and record your rating in the space provided to the left. Summarize your health-related fitness profile by completing Section VII.*

✦ I. Cardiorespiratory Fitness

Health Interpretation: Scores on any of these tests that place you in the Poor or Very Poor category, near the 5th percentile or below, or below the standards provided for the 4.8-kilometre walk and 12-minute swimming or cycling tests are considered UNHEALTHY. You should strive to meet the minimum standards suggested or achieve scores that place you at the 50th percentile or above or that rate you at least Average or Fair in cardiorespiratory fitness. Scores that place you in the Superior or Excellent category or at the 95th percentile or above classify you as ATHLETICALLY FIT.

Test	Test Standards (Norms)
A. 12-Minute Run Test	**See Table A.**

Score _____

Rating _____

(continued)

Lab Activity 2.1 *(continued)*
Your Physical Fitness Profile

Test	Test Standards (Norms)
B. 4.8-Kilometre Walk Test, 12-Minute Swimming or Cycling Test	**See Table A.**

Score _____

Rating _____

Table A ✦ Standards for Classification of Good Fitness for 4.8-Kilometre Walk, 12-Minute Swimming, and 12-Minute Cycling Tests for Ages 13–60+

TEST	AGE					
	13–19	*20–29*	*30–39*	*40–49*	*50–59*	*60+*
Males						
4.8-kilometre walking (minutes & seconds)	33:00–37:30	34:00–38:30	35:00–40:00	36:30–42:00	39:00–45:00	41:00–48:00
12-minute swimming (metres)	640–731	549–639	503–593	457–548	411–502	366–456
12-minute cycling (kilometres)	12.35–14.95	11.7–14.27	11.05–13.62	10.4–12.97	9.1–11.67	7.8–10.37
Females						
4.8-kilometre walking (minutes & seconds)	35:00–39:30	36:00–40:30	37:30–42:00	39:00–44:00	42:00–47:00	45:00–51:00
12-minute swimming (metres)	549–639	457–548	411–502	366–456	320–411	274–365
12-minute cycling (kilometres)	9.75–12.32	9.1–11.67	8.45–11.02	7.8–10.37	6.5–9.07	5.2–7.77

Note: Lower times or greater distances place the individual in the Excellent fitness category and higher times or lesser distances place the individual in the Fair–Very Poor fitness categories.

Source: Adapted from *The Aerobics Program for Total Well-Being* by Kenneth H. Cooper, MD., MPH. © 1982 by Kenneth H. Cooper. Used by permission of Bantam Books, a division of Bantam Doubleday Dell Publishing Group, Inc.

Test	Test Standards (Norms)

C. 12-Minute Run

Score _____

Rating _____

See Table B.

Table B ✦ Norms for 12-Minute Run (Metres)
(Minutes and Seconds) for Ages 13–18

	MALES	FEMALES
PERCENTILE	*12-Minute Run*	*12-Minute Run*
95	3015	2239
75	2633	1920
50	2370	1702
25	2108	1483
5	1726	1165

Source: Adapted from *AAHPERD Youth Fitness Test Manual* (Reston, VA: AAHPERD, 1976).

D. Harvard Step Test

Score _____

Rating _____

See Table C.

Table C ✦ Ratings for Harvard Step Test

SCORE	RATING
Below 55	Poor
55–64	Low average
65–79	Average
80–89	Good
90 and above	Excellent

✦ II. Muscular Strength

Health Interpretation: Scores on the 1-RM strength tests are optimal values for your body weight. Your weight-training program should elevate you to these optimal levels within a period of 3–6 months. Reaching these levels provides a number of health- and performance-related benefits, such as increased muscle mass, increased basal metabolism (calorie expenditure at rest), more energy, reduced chance of soft-tissue injury (muscles, tendons, ligaments), and improved ease in performance of daily movements (getting out of a car or chair, lifting objects, going up steps). A program that helps you reach and then maintain these values will also help prevent the loss of lean muscle tissue as you age.

(continued)

Lab Activity 2.1 *(continued)*
Your Physical Fitness Profile

Test	Test Standards (Norms)
A. Bench Press	**See Table D.**

Score _____

Rating _____
     (above or below optimal scores)

B. Shoulder Press   **See Table D.**

Score _____

Rating _____
     (above or below optimal scores)

C. Biceps Curl   **See Table D.**

Score _____

Rating _____
     (above or below optimal scores)

D. Leg Press   **See Table D.**

Score _____

Rating _____
     (above or below optimal scores)

Table D ✦ Optimal Strength Values for Various Body Weights (based on 1-RM test)

BODY WEIGHT (kg)	BENCH PRESS		SHOULDER PRESS		BICEPS CURL		LEG PRESS	
	Male	*Female*	*Male*	*Female*	*Male*	*Female*	*Male*	*Female*
36	31.8	27.6	24.9	18.1	18.1	13.6	72.6	54.4
45	38.6	31.8	31.8	22.7	22.7	15.9	90.7	68.0
54	47.6	38.6	36.3	27.6	27.6	18.1	108.9	81.6
64	56.7	45.4	43.1	29.5	31.8	22.7	127.0	95.3
73	65.8	52.2	49.9	34.0	36.3	27.6	145.2	108.9
82	72.6	56.7	54.4	38.6	40.8	29.5	163.3	122.5
91	81.6	63.5	61.2	43.1	45.4	31.8	181.4	136.1
95	90.7	70.3	68.0	47.6	49.9	34.0	199.6	149.7
109	102.1	77.1	72.6	52.2	54.4	38.6	217.7	163.3

Note: Data in kilograms; obtained on Universal Gym apparatus; applicable ages 17 to 30.

Source: Adapted from *Health and Fitness Through Physical Activity* by Michael Pollock, Jack Wilmore, and Samuel Fox III (New York: Macmillan College Publishing Company, 1978). © 1978 by Allyn and Bacon. Reprinted/adapted by permission.

✦ III. Muscular Endurance

Health Interpretation: Scores on the muscular endurance tests have health implications similar to those of the fitness and strength tests discussed previously. Low scores in the abdominal curl tests may also increase the possibility of lower-back problems in the future. Ratings that place you in the Low or Very Low or Poor or Very Poor categories on any of these tests are considered UNHEALTHY. You should strive to achieve scores that place you in at least the Average or Moderate categories by engaging in regular muscular endurance training (see Chapter 6). Ratings of Excellent or Very High place you in the category of ATHLETICALLY FIT.

Test	Test Standards (Norms)
A. Abdominal (Curls)	**See Table E.**
Score _____	
Rating _____	**Table E** ✦ Norms for Abdominal Curls for Ages 18–30

Table E ✦ Norms for Abdominal Curls for Ages 18–30

	SCORE	
RATING	*Males*	*Females*
Excellent	96 and above	89 and above
Good	82–95	76–88
Average	68–81	63–75
Poor	54–67	49–62
Very poor	53 and below	48 and below

Source: G. Robbins, D. Powers, and S. Burgess, *A Wellness Way of Life* (Dubuque, IA: Brown, 1991). Reproduced with the permission of the McGraw-Hill Companies.

Test	Test Standards (Norms)
B. Arm and Shoulder	**See Table F.**
Pull-ups (men) Score _____	
Modified pull-ups (women) Score _____	

Table F ✦ Performance Standards for Pull-ups and Modified Pull-ups

RATING	PULL-UPS	MODIFIED PULL-UPS
Excellent	13 or above	30 or above
Good	10–12	25–29
Average	5–9	16–24
Poor	0–4	0–15

(continued)

Lab Activity 2.1 *(continued)*
Your Physical Fitness Profile

Test	Test Standards (Norms)
Push-ups (men) Score _____	**See Table G.**
Modified push-ups (women) Score _____	

Table G ✦ Ratings for Push-ups and Modified Push-ups

	RATING				
AGE	*Very High*	*High*	*Moderate*	*Low*	*Very Low*
Push-ups					
15–29	Above 54	45–54	35–44	20–34	Below 20
30–39	Above 44	35–44	25–34	15–24	Below 15
40–49	Above 39	30–39	20–29	12–19	Below 12
Over 50	Above 34	25–34	15–24	8–14	Below 8
Modified Push-ups					
15–29	Above 48	34–48	17–33	6–16	Below 6
30–39	Above 39	25–39	12–24	4–11	Below 4
40–49	Above 34	20–34	8–19	3–7	Below 3
Over 50	Above 29	15–29	6–14	2–5	Below 2

✦ IV. Flexibility

Health Implications: Scores on the flexibility tests have numerous health implications in terms of injury prevention, lower-back pain, and the ease with which people of all ages perform routine tasks such as dressing, tying shoes, bending, lifting, and even moving efficiently. Scores that place you in the category of Below Average are considered UNHEALTHY. You can easily improve your range of motion by following one of the flexibility-training programs discussed in Chapter 7. It is important to at least reach the Average category shown in Table H. Scores 10–20 percent higher than the Above Average rating place you in the category of ATHLETICALLY FIT.

Test	Test Standards (Norms)
A. Shoulder Reach	**See Table H.**

Score _____

Rating _____

Test	Test Standards (Norms)
B. Trunk Flexion	**See Table H.**
Score _____	
Rating _____	
C. Trunk Extension	**See Table H.**
Score _____	
Rating _____	

Table H ✦ Flexibility Interpretations

RATING	SHOULDER REACH (RUP/LUP)	TRUNK FLEXION	TRUNK EXTENSION
Men			
Above average	6+/3+	11+	15+
Average	4–5/0–2	7–10	8–14
Below average	Below 4/below 0	Below 7	Below 8
Women			
Above average	7+/6+	12+	23+
Average	5–6/0–5	7–11	15–22
Below average	Below 5/below 0	Below 7	Below 15

✦ V. Body Composition

Health Interpretation: Body composition scores have numerous health-related implications. Unacceptable BMI scores, waist-to-hip ratio scores, and skinfold measures (percentage of body fat) are associated with a higher risk of atherosclerosis, hypertension, diabetes, heart/lung difficulties, early heart attack and stroke, numerous other chronic and degenerative disorders, some types of cancer, and higher death rates at all ages. Scores on any of the following tests that place you in categories such as Severe Overweight or Morbid Obesity (BMI test), higher waist-to-hip ratios, and Very High Fat or Obese (skinfold measures) are considered UNHEALTHY. It is important to strive for so-called normal levels of body fat—Average or Ideal. The literature does not support the notion of increased health benefits by achieving the very low levels found in some endurance athletes. In fact, the essential fat in the human body is considered to be approximately 3–4 percent for men and 12–14 percent for women. It is quite unrealistic and potentially unhealthy to achieve lower fat levels than these.

(continued)

Lab Activity 2.1 *(continued)*
Your Physical Fitness Profile

Test	Test Standards (Norms)
A. Body Mass Index	**See Table I.**
Score _____	
Rating _____	

Table I ✦ BMI Values for Men and Women

	MEN	WOMEN
Underweight	< 20.7	< 19.1
Acceptable weight	20.7–27.8	19.1–27.3
Overweight	27.8	27.3
Severe overweight	31.1	32.3
Morbid obesity	45.4	44.8

Source: From the 1983 Metropolitan Life Insurance Company tables, designed by B. T. Burton and W. R. Foster, Health Implications of Obesity, an NIH Consensus Development Conference, *Journal of the American Dietetic Association* (1985) 85: 1117–1121. © 1983 Metropolitan Life Insurance Company. All rights reserved. Reproduced by permission.

Test	Test Standards (Norms)
B. Waist-to-Hip Ratio	**See Table J.**
Score _____	
Rating _____	

Table J ✦ Waist-to-Hip Ratio Scores

	RATIO	RECOMMENDATION
Men	1.0 or higher	Weight loss
Women	0.85 or higher	Weight loss

Test	Test Standards (Norms)
C. Skinfold Measures	**See page 219 in Chapter 9.**
Score _____	
Rating _____	

✦ VI. Nutrition

The best procedure for determining the status of your dietary intake is to keep careful records of all food and fluid intake for 3–4 days (2–3 weekdays and 1 weekend day) by carefully recording this information on the forms accompanying the nutritional analysis software available at your school's Department of Health and Physical Education. Chapter 8 also provides less accurate methods of identifying some obvious shortcomings in your diet. Careful recordkeeping and nutritional analysis software can often identify nutrient deficiencies that can be corrected before symptoms develop.

1. List the deficient areas identified:

   a. _____

   b. _____

   c. _____

   d. _____

   e. _____

   f. _____

   g. _____

2. List a plan of action and specific food and fluid items that will help correct deficiencies:

   a. _____

   b. _____

   c. _____

   d. _____

   e. _____

   f. _____

   g. _____

✦ VII. Summary

List those components of health-related fitness in which you rated:

1. Above Average or Superior

   a. _____

   b. _____

   c. _____

   d. _____

   e. _____

(continued)

Lab Activity 2.1 *(continued)*
Your Physical Fitness Profile

    2. Average

        a. _____

        b. _____

        c. _____

        d. _____

        e. _____

    3. Poor or Very Poor (unhealthy)

        a. _____

        b. _____

        c. _____

        d. _____

        e. _____

Lab Activity 2.2

Determining Your Resting and Exercise Heart Rate

INSTRUCTIONS: *Resting and exercise heart rate can often provide useful information about your fitness level and training method. It is therefore important to learn how to obtain these measures accurately by following these steps.*

1. Lie down for 15 minutes in a comfortable place. Be sure not to eat or drink for at least three hours before starting this activity. If you have not given up smoking, do not smoke for at least 30 minutes prior to starting this activity.

2. After the rest period and while you are still lying down, take your pulse at the carotid artery on either side of the neck or use the radial pulse at the thumb side of your wrist. Since your thumb has its own pulse and will cause inaccurate readings, use only the fingers to find and count the pulse. Count for an entire minute. The resulting number is your resting heart rate.

3. To determine your postexercise heart rate, stop at the end of your next aerobic workout and take your carotid or radial pulse for only 6 seconds. Add a 0 to determine the number of beats per minute. The 30- and 60-second pulse count should not be used at the end of a workout since the heart slows down rapidly during that lengthy period.

4. Record your resting and postexercise pulse below.

   Date _____   Date _____

   Resting heart rate _____   Resting heart rate _____

   Postexercise heart rate _____   Postexercise heart rate _____

   Date _____   Date _____

   Resting heart rate _____   Resting heart rate _____

   Postexercise heart rate _____   Postexercise heart rate _____

5. Repeat this activity every month to measure your progress. Your resting heart rate will continue to decline as you become more aerobically fit. This is a direct result of an increase in both stroke volume (more blood pumped per beat) and cardiac output (more blood pumped per minute). Later you can use the postexercise method to determine whether your aerobic workout is elevating your heart rate above the target level.

3

Behavioural Change and Motivational Techniques

CHAPTER OBJECTIVES

By the end of this chapter, you should be able to:

1. Discuss the importance of psychosocial lifestyle factors such as locus of control, social support, and self-esteem in deciding on a fitness program.

2. Describe several techniques that researchers have demonstrated to be effective in helping people achieve their fitness goals.

3. List several means of improving the chances of maintaining a physical fitness program once one has been started.

4. Modify a physical fitness program in the face of obstacles so it need not be interrupted.

THE COMEDIAN HENNY Youngman tells of a man who told his psychiatrist, "Doc, I have a guilt complex," to which his doctor replied, "You ought to be ashamed of yourself!" We do not want to shame you into regularly engaging in physical activity. That would be dysfunctional, something like a physical education instructor who makes physical activity so distasteful that students are repelled by exercise for the remainder of their lives. Instead, we want you to appreciate the benefits of being physically fit and then to decide for yourself whether to engage in regular exercise. If you decide to do that, we can show you how to begin a program and to continue participating in it over an extended period of time.

PSYCHOSOCIAL FACTORS TO CONSIDER

To plan an exercise program, you need to know something about yourself: your motivations, your perceptions of the amount of control you have over your life, the degree to which you associate with other people, and the confidence you have in yourself. This chapter makes the importance of this information clear.

Locus of Control

Some people believe they can control events in their lives. This construct is called one's **locus of control**. People who believe this construct possess an internal locus of control, or *internality*. People who do not believe in the construct possess an external locus of control, or *externality*.

Externals believe that the course of their lives is a matter of luck, fate, or chance or of the actions of powerful others. This is more than merely an academic distinction. If you do not believe you control events in your life, you are apt to adopt a laissez-faire attitude. Relative to physical fitness, you might believe that whether you are in good shape is a function of luck or of genetic makeup. There is no sense in engaging in an exercise program if you do not control your fitness level.

Internals believe that what they get is, for the most part, a result of what they do. Therefore, internals will probably learn a good deal about exercise and physical fitness and plan a program in which they can participate. An internal locus of control is very important if you are serious about becoming physically fit and maintaining that level of fitness.

Complete Lab Activity 3.1: Locus of Control Assessment at the end of this chapter to determine your locus of control. If you score as an external, make a list of the parts of your life that you influence. Then read that list daily to change your focus. In addition, take some measures before beginning an exercise program (for example, your pulse rate and weight) and measure those variables again after engaging in exercise for several weeks. The change will reinforce the notion that you can influence your body rather than resigning yourself to being a victim of your habits or of your genetic makeup.

Social Isolation

We all need to interact with other people. Researchers have found that the social support we have actually helps prevent us from getting ill and enhances the quality of our lives. Conversely, not having significant others with whom to share our joys and sorrows causes ill health or **social isolation**. Refer to Lab Activity 3.2: Alienation Test at the end of this chapter for a social isolation scale that will help you determine whether this is a problem for you.

If you find you need to improve your social network, structure your fitness program accordingly. Consider joining an exercise club, a health spa, the YMCA, or the Jewish Community Centre. You might meet people there with whom you can become friendly. Participation in organized sports (at levels suited to your skill and experience) can also provide an opportunity to meet people. Playing in leagues and tournaments (team as well as individual) is another avenue for alleviating social isolation. You should not ignore your social self when structuring your fitness program. To do so is to endanger your health and wellness.

Self-Esteem

What you think of yourself, no matter whether that perception is accurate, influences your fitness, health, and wellness. If you do not think highly of yourself, you might not believe you can become fit. You may lack confidence, see yourself as genetically inferior, or think you have so far to go that beginning a fitness program is futile.

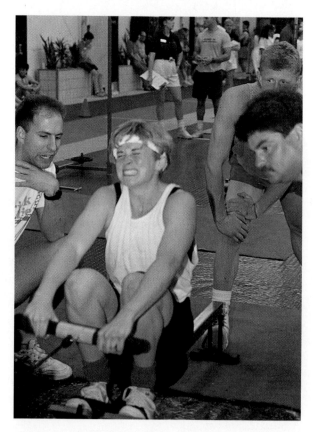

Having friends who encourage you can be an important part of achieving your fitness goals.

DIVERSITY ISSUES

Locus of Control and Exercise

Believing you have control of your exercise behaviour (an internal locus of control) is crucial to becoming physically fit and maintaining an adequate level of fitness and wellness. If you do not believe you can control your exercise behaviour (an external locus of control), you will believe that whether you develop a high level of fitness and/or achieve a high level of wellness is a matter of luck, chance, or some other factor outside of your own influence. Therefore, you will not plan a fitness program or join a health club or organize friends in sports or fitness activities.

This is the case with too many low-income people. Studies have shown that people of lower socioeconomic status possess external loci of control and feelings of powerlessness regarding their lives. They do not believe they control their lives, their health, or their wellness. Given their daily struggle to survive and to provide for their families, it is not surprising that they pay little attention to becoming physically fit and maintaining adequate levels of fitness, health, and wellness. They cannot afford to join a health club or hire a personal fitness trainer or purchase exercise videos for a VCR/DVD player they do not own.

Still, everyone can take charge of their fitness and wellness behaviours. To do so need not cost money. Jogging around a school track is free. Doing isometric exercises does not require the purchase of weights or any other equipment. Stretching can be done at home at one's leisure.

Unfortunately, too many community health programs ignore the importance of being physically fit. They are often focused on encouraging immunizations or removing lead-based paint or identifying pregnant women in need of prenatal care. These certainly are important goals, but they are not the only valid goals for low-income people. These individuals also need to, and can be taught to, develop and maintain a life of physical fitness and wellness for themselves and for their children. To do less—to withhold fitness and wellness information from low-income families, to refrain from motivating them to engage in fitness activities, to ignore the benefits fitness and wellness activities could provide them—is to discriminate against a significant segment of our citizens. This simply cannot be tolerated. ✦

In particular, what you think of your body, your bodily self-esteem—sometimes called **body cathexis**—will affect your health and fitness. Lab Activity 3.3: Body Self-Esteem Assessment at the end of this chapter contains a scale to help you determine your bodily self-esteem.

There may be parts of your body with which you are satisfied and parts with which you are dissatisfied. Be proud of those parts about which you scored 4 or 5 in Lab Activity 3.3. And do not fret about those parts of your body for which you scored a 1 or 2. You can improve them, at least many of them, and thereby feel better about yourself. For example, if you are dissatisfied with your waist, you can do exercises to strengthen the muscles in your waist. We discuss these in Chapter 6 on muscular strength and endurance. There are even useful strategies for those body parts you assigned a 1 or 2 value that cannot be changed, such as your nose. These are body parts about which you need to become more accepting. One effective way of doing this is to recognize that things could be worse. Volunteering for an organization that caters to the needs of the physically challenged or the socioeconomically disadvantaged can help you put your concern about your nose, for example, in proper perspective.

STRATEGIES FOR ACHIEVING YOUR FITNESS GOALS

There is a good deal of research identifying effective ways of achieving your fitness goals. Before the appropriate techniques can be applied, however, you must first identify the goals.

Goal-Setting

In determining your fitness goals, it's important to set realistic goals and to assess your progress periodically.

Be Realistic Jorge was playing tennis with a friend one pleasant summer day. The sun was out; the birds were chirping; the water in the creek alongside the tennis court was gently caressing the rocks as it moved downstream.

Locus of control The degree to which you believe you are in control of events in your life.

Social isolation The lack of other people with whom to discuss important matters relevant to your life.

Body cathexis Physical self-esteem; how highly you regard your physical self.

You couldn't ask for a better day, that is, unless you were Jorge. His game was off. "Enough is enough," Jorge thought when he netted still another backhand. Before anyone realized what was happening, he hurled his tennis racquet over the fence, above the trees beyond, and into the middle of the creek. When last seen, the racquet was heading downstream, never again to be used.

Some of you may know a Jorge or even be one. The problem is in being realistic. Some of us are has-been athletes expecting to perform at the level we could when we were younger and practised daily. Others of us are never-beens with grand delusions and dreams that will never be fulfilled. Do not fall into either trap when setting your fitness goals. Be realistic in what you can attain and how long it will take you to attain it. If your goals are unobtainable, you will become frustrated and give up on physical fitness altogether.

In fact, it is wise in the beginning to set goals that are easy to achieve. In that way, when you do attain them, you will reinforce fitness behaviour and be more likely to achieve subsequent goals.

Periodically Assess Once you decide on your fitness goals, periodically assess how you are meeting those goals. If you conclude that you are making progress in an appropriate amount of time, keep doing what you are doing. If your assessment indicates problems meeting your goals, it is time to make adjustments. Maybe you need to exercise longer, more intensely, or more

frequently. Without periodically assessing your program, you will not identify needed changes to help you achieve your fitness goals.

Behavioural Change Techniques

Among the more effective techniques you can employ in meeting your fitness goals are the use of social support, contracting, reminder systems, self-monitoring, gradual programming, tailoring, chaining, and covert techniques.

Social Support This is just another way of saying that you need other people to encourage and help you. It is much easier to adopt a habit of regular exercise, or any habit for that matter, if you are encouraged by others. If you can get someone else to exercise with you, to ask you daily whether you have exercised, or to buy you a piece of exercise clothing or equipment periodically, you will be more apt to stick with your regimen. To begin, make a list of people you think would be willing to assist you and discuss with them how they can help.

Contracting One way to use social support is to develop a contract to achieve a certain exercise goal and to have it witnessed by someone else. If that person then helps you periodically to assess your progress, you will be more likely to be successful. Figure 3.1 shows a sample contract. It identifies the *behaviour goal*, the *date* when

Figure 3.1 ✦ Fitness Contract

I _____ desire to improve my physical fitness
　　　　(your name)

because _____ .
　　　　　　　　　　　　　(the reason)

I have decided I intend to _____
　　　　　　　　　　　　　　　　　　　(your goal)

by _____ . If I achieve this goal, I will reward myself
　　　　(date)

by _____ . If I do not achieve my
　　　　　　　　(the reward)

goal, I will punish myself by _____ .
　　　　　　　　　　　　　　　　　(the punishment)

_____　　　_____
　　　(your signature)　　　　　　　　　(today's date)

_____　　　_____
　　　(witness signature)　　　　　　　　(today's date)

it should be achieved (and assessed), and the *reward* for achieving the goal as well as the *punishment* for not achieving it. Rewards can be going to the movies, buying something you have wanted for a long time, or taking a night off from schoolwork. Punishments might include not watching television for a week or not eating your favourite snack for several days. Although rewards are more effective than punishments in controlling behaviour, punishments have a place as well. And although contracts have been found to work best when there is a witness, they can also be effective if you merely contract with yourself.

Reminder Systems One way to remember things is to make a note of them. Reminder notes will help you remember to exercise, especially if you leave the notes in places where you cannot miss them—for example, on refrigerator doors or bathroom mirrors. You can also use notes in appointment books and calendars as reminders.

Self-Monitoring Researchers have found that people who monitor their physical activity sessions on a regular basis are more likely to maintain their exercise program than people who do not monitor their activity. Taking five minutes (or less) each day or two to record the type and duration of the activity performed seems to help people stick to their exercise schedule and therefore reach their fitness goals. People also find it helpful to make a note of progress made (for example, jogging for 15 minutes to jogging for 20 minutes without stopping).

Gradual Programming Too often, people who have never exercised regularly or who have not done so for some time expect to be able to run a couple of kilometres in under four minutes. Less obvious, but no less unrealistic for many people, is the goal of exercising every other day when they have been sedentary for years or of exercising intensely when they have not done so for a while. Giving up the sedentary life *cold turkey* may be extremely difficult. If it is, do not fret. Instead, use a graduated plan in which you start slowly and gradually increase both frequency and intensity. In fact, to prevent injury, fitness experts recommend graduated plans even for those who are already highly fit. For example, runners are warned not to increase their distance by more than 10 percent a week, and weight trainers not to increase the weight they lift by more than 5 percent. Researchers have found that significant health gains emerge when sedentary people simply start to engage in moderate physical activity, and these gains increase as the exerciser gradually increases his or her exercise frequency and duration (Blair, 1996). A reasonable shorter-term goal for people who are starting an exercise program is to walk at a strong pace three days per week for a total of 20 minutes (all at once or in 10-minute bouts).

A suitable *longer-term* goal is to engage in moderate physical activity, such as walking at a strong pace, five or more days each week for a total of 30 minutes on each of these days (either all at once or in 10-to-15-minute bouts). At this level and duration, people experience the health benefits of exercise (listed in Chapter 1).

Tailoring No two people are alike. This is not the most provocative of statements, yet we sometimes act as though we do not know this simple fact. When you adopt a wholesale exercise program designed for a group, without adjusting that program to your own needs and circumstances, you are increasing the likelihood that you will soon stop exercising regularly. Some people are free to exercise in the mornings, others in the evenings. Some people are in better physical condition than others. People vary in their choice of mealtimes. Some are more committed to exercise than others. We could go on and on, but the point is that any program of regular exercise must be tailored to the individual. We will present exercise activities in later chapters, but you must choose which ones to do, when, how frequently, and how intensely for your program to be successful.

Chaining In chaining, one behaviour is linked to a previous one, and that to a previous one, and so on, like links in a chain. You can use chaining to help you achieve your fitness goals. To adopt a behaviour, such as exercising regularly, you want to have as few links as possible between deciding to exercise and actually engaging in a fitness activity. To demonstrate, let us look at two people, U.R. Wrong and I.M. Right.

U.R. Wrong decides to exercise at about 5:30 in the afternoon. So U.R. rushes home and starts gathering exercise clothes. In one drawer are gym shorts and socks, in another a shirt, and under the bed in another room running shoes. Then U.R. looks for the car keys so as to drive to the track to jog. The track is 10 minutes away. On the way there, U.R. realizes the car needs gas and stops to get some. Finally, U.R. arrives at the track and is ready to exercise.

I.M. Right decides to exercise at the same time of day. However, I.M. prepares beforehand. All the clothes needed for later are left on the bed in the morning. I.M. decides to run around the neighbourhood instead of the track, so that all that is required at 5:30 is to come home, dress, step outside the front door, and exercise.

If we consider each behaviour needed to exercise as a link in a chain, we see that U.R. Wrong has many more links. The more links, the more difficult it is to exercise, and the more likely it is not to happen. The trick is to

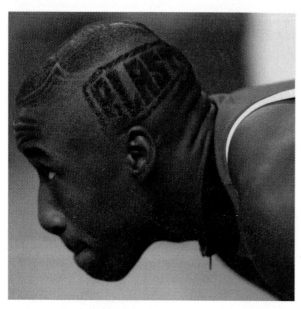

Research indicates that simply thinking about doing something can help you actually do it. That applies to exercising as well.

decrease the links for a behaviour you want to adopt and to increase the links for a behaviour you want to give up (for example, cigarette smoking).

Covert Techniques Some people are so inactive or busy that it is difficult for them to engage in regular exercise. Three *covert techniques* can help these people change behaviour without requiring them to do anything physically:

1. **Covert rehearsal** This procedure requires that you imagine yourself exercising regularly. Your image must be extremely vivid; that is, you must notice all the details (your outfit, the weather, the location), smell the atmosphere, feel the bodily sensations, and so on. Being able to imagine yourself exercising makes it more likely that you will actually exercise. You will have desensitized yourself to the image of you exercising so that seeing yourself exercising will not seem foreign to you.

2. **Covert modelling** For some of us, even imagining ourselves exercising is difficult. If that is the case with you, there is still hope. First, identify someone else you *can* envision exercising. Next, imagine as vividly as you can that person exercising. Once that image is clear in your mind, substitute yourself for that person. Model the image of you exercising after the image of that person exercising. After a while, it will be easier for you to think of yourself as a potentially regular exerciser, and you will be more likely actually to become one.

3. **Covert reinforcement** With this technique, you imagine yourself exercising and then reward yourself for it with another image. Usually, a pleasant image is used as a reward (a day at the beach, a calm lake) and is allowed to surface and be focused on only after the goal image is successfully accomplished.

MAINTAINING YOUR FITNESS PROGRAM

Once you have begun a regular program of exercise, the trick is to maintain it. In addition to the methods already described, here are additional suggestions for keeping at it.

Material Reinforcement

Behaviour that is rewarded tends to be repeated. Consequently, if you want to exercise regularly, reward yourself when you do. Material rewards can take many forms. For example, you might treat yourself to a movie. Or you might buy yourself an article of clothing you have been eyeing for some time.

Social Reinforcement

Peer group pressure need not be limited to negative influences. We can use such pressure to encourage and reward desirable behaviour. Take a moment to list five people whose opinions you value. Then enlist them as social reinforcers to inquire about your exercise behaviour and to pat you on the back if you report exercising regularly. After a while, exercise will become part of your lifestyle, and you will no longer need to be rewarded for continuing.

Joining a Group

One of the reasons Weight Watchers is so effective in helping people lose weight is that it employs group support and positive peer pressure. It is often easier to accomplish your goals if you are working with others. You can join a health club, a local YMCA, or a Jewish Community Centre. Or you can organize a group of friends to exercise together at a predetermined time. You can even enroll in an exercise class at a local university or community college or in a community program. Any group involvement will increase the likelihood of your maintaining a fitness program.

◼ Boasting

Many people, while they are students, have two tests returned the same day, one on which they did well and the other on which they did not. They complain about the poor grade for days while ignoring the test on which they did well. Many of us react this way. We relive negative experiences by repeatedly thinking about them, by being embarrassed about them over and over again, or by feeling inadequate in other ways. For positive experiences, such as getting an A on a test, we exhibit false modesty and say, "It was nothing." We would do better to learn from our mistakes and let them go and to relive our positive experiences and even boast about them. Of course, you do not want to be obnoxious or to be perceived as conceited. Yet, if you run five kilometres daily and someone asks how far you usually run, rather than say, "Only five kilometres," you might say, "I'm proud to say that I run five kilometres regularly." Boasting in this way will help reinforce your exercise behaviour.

◼ Self-Monitoring

It is helpful to know that your fitness program is having a positive effect, that it is moving you toward your goal. Remember not to expect immediate, dramatic results. Assuming your exercise goal is realistic, accept small gains. Do not expect more rapid change than is warranted by the general effects of exercise and training on the body. Eventually, with persistence, you will attain your goal. When you see slow but steady progress toward your goal, you will be encouraged to maintain the program.

◼ Making It Fun

If the fitness program you designed is not fun, you selected the wrong activities. If it is not fun at least most of the time, you will not continue it for very long. We present so many options in this book that you should be able to find activities that accomplish your goals while providing enjoyment. All you need to do is be selective. Think about your choices carefully, and seek help from others when that is necessary.

*E*XERCISING UNDER DIFFICULT CIRCUMSTANCES

If you maintain a fitness program long enough, you will undoubtedly encounter obstacles. We have selected five such obstacles to demonstrate how, if you are serious about training, your program need not be interrupted. These obstacles are travelling, being confined to a limited space, being injured, being busy, and having visitors.

WELLNESS HEROES

Simon Whitfield

From the time he was 14, Canadian triathlete Simon Whitfield dreamed of Olympic gold. It was a dream on which he focused unwaveringly for the next eight years. When he got to the Sydney Olympics in 2000, he was ranked 21st in the world, and not expected even to medal. In one of the most dramatic contests of those games, Whitfield came from behind, having crashed in the cycling portion of the race, to win Canada's first gold medal of the 2000 games in the last stretches of the 10-kilometre run.

Winning the gold medal at Sydney changed Whitfield's life considerably, in a number of ways. For one thing, for the first time in years, he felt his motivation sagging. How do you motivate yourself once you've accomplished your ultimate dream? Many athletes experience feeling somewhat at a loss after winning an Olympic medal. Whitfield admits to a touch of this angst: "I was really worried after the Olympics that I wouldn't get the goosebumps anymore."

However, after a little time off and watching his former training partner win a few Ironman competitions, Whitfield began to get his second wind. He rediscovered his love of racing and set new goals for himself. In January 2002, he began training again for Olympic competition. Since his gold medal win in 2000, Whitfield has won two World Cups, and placed sixth at the World Championships, his best placing ever for that event, and won gold at the Commonwealth Games in Manchester in 2002. Currently, he's ranked sixth in the world.

As part of his busy schedule, Whitfield gives motivational speeches at schools and businesses. One tactic he recommends for people who wish to achieve excellence is that they surround themselves with excellence. That is, they should find a person from whom they can learn, and just soak up everything that person can teach them.

Sources: Based on Stefan Timms, "Moving Forward: Whitfield Focused on 2002 Season," *TriCafe*, March 14, 2002. Available at **www.trainright.com/triathlongold/tricafe/news/2002/03142002movingforwardwhitfieldfocused.htm**. Accessed March 12, 2003; Commonwealth Games Association of Canada Web site, "Team Canada 2002 Profiles," available at **http://www.commonwealthgames.ca/eng/manchester/profiles/SimonWhitfield.htm**. Accessed March 12, 2003. IMG Canada Athletic Representatives. ✦

Travelling

If you travel often, you should consider that when you develop your program. For example, rather than joining a local health club, you would be wise to join one with facilities throughout the country so you can exercise when you are in other cities. YMCAs, Jewish Community Centres, and some nationally franchised health clubs have facilities throughout Canada and the United States. In addition, select activities that take regular travel into account. You would be better off jogging, for example, than playing tennis. Jogging involves little in the way of equipment or facilities and does not require a partner. So, if you travel often, consider equipment, facilities, and dependence on other people in formulating your exercise program.

Being Confined to a Limited Space

If you sometimes are confined to a limited space (for example, if you are a student studying for final examinations and seldom leaving your dormitory room), you need not abandon your physical fitness program. If you have access to an exercise room, you might be fortunate enough to have treadmills, stair steppers, ski machines, stationary bikes, or rowers at your disposal. But you can still exercise without ever leaving your office or room. For example, you can run around the room, which can fill your need for cardiorespiratory endurance. If you do, be sure not to run in one place because that might cause too much strain on your legs and knees. Alternatively, you can purchase a jump rope and use it in your room. You can even do some of the flexibility exercises described in Chapter 7 or perform isometric muscular strength activities.

Isometric contractions involve exerting a force that is equal to, or less than, that required to move an object. Therefore, the object does not move, there is no movement in the joint, and there is no change in the length of the muscle. For example, if you push against a wall, that is an isometric contraction. You can also do isotonic activities. **Isotonic contractions** consist of movement at the joint and changes in the length of the muscle. For example, if you lift weights, you are engaged in isotonic contractions. It needn't be a barbell or other weight-lifting equipment that you use. Lifting any object of sufficient weight to offer resistance will suffice. You might also be able to find someone else who also feels confined to exercise with you. For example, rather than pushing against a wall, you might be able to push against each other and thereby create the resistance you require (see Figure 3.2).

Figure 3.2 ✦ Improving Muscular Strength with a Partner

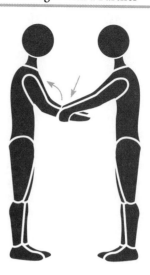

Being Injured

If you exercise long enough, you will inevitably experience an injury of some sort. As with any other obstacle, you can always use such an injury as an excuse not to exercise. On the other hand, you can almost always find a way to exercise around the injury. For example, a leg injury may preclude jogging but not swimming, and a shoulder injury may eliminate a regular racquetball game but not jogging. For most injuries, common sense will dictate what you can and cannot do. For more serious fitness injuries, however, consult a professional for advice. By doing so, you might prevent further damage or prolonged recovery.

Being Busy

"I don't have time to exercise. I'm too busy," sounds like a battle cry from some people. Yet when even busy schedules are dissected, there is always enough time for participation in fitness activities. The problem is that people decide to use this time for other activities, such as watching television, partying, or talking on the telephone. It may make sense to use your time in this way. But that is your decision to make, and as with all decisions, you can change it if you so choose.

It seems self-destructive to say you value health and fitness but to take a long lunch instead of a short lunch and a short workout or to meet your friends at the local watering hole instead of exercising. You can find time to exercise if you really value health and

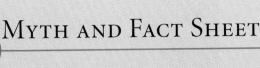

MYTH AND FACT SHEET

Myth	Fact
1. Everyone should develop an internal locus of control, because people really can control all aspects of their lives.	1. Although most people can take charge of more parts of their lives than they believe they can, that does not mean that we all can take control of all aspects of our lives. There are parts of all of our lives that are simply beyond our control. However, we can always take control of our feelings and reactions. In other words, we are neither masters nor victims of our futures. We participate in developing our lives and can decide to become and remain physically fit and achieve high-level wellness if we choose to.
2. The best way to become fit is simply to make up your mind that you will do it.	2. Motivation is certainly an important factor in developing fitness. However, it is usually not enough by itself. It is similar to people deciding to diet or to give up smoking cigarettes. Their intentions are honourable and may serve them well for a time, but all too frequently they revert to the behaviour they were trying to avoid. Chapter 3 provides you with many behavioural change techniques that should accompany your motivation to be fit. In this way, you will be maximizing the probability of your achieving that goal.
3. The reason people do not achieve their fitness goals is because they do not work long enough.	3. Even if you are motivated to achieve a fitness goal, you may not be successful. You may use all of the behavioural change techniques outlined in this book and come up short. In this case, you may have selected an unrealistic or unobtainable goal. Try as you might, you will not achieve that goal. Therefore, the first thing you should do in deciding on your fitness goal is to determine whether you think you are likely to achieve that goal. If not, choose a more realistic goal. Perhaps you can work your way up to that other goal after achieving more obtainable ones first.
4. When trying to change a behaviour, it is best to work at changing by yourself so you do not embarrass yourself in front of other people.	4. In fact, the opposite is true. It is best to involve other people to help you change a behaviour because they can provide you with the support and peer pressure to encourage you to be successful. Unfortunately, studies show that people hesitate to join health and fitness clubs because the ads for these clubs usually show members with fantastic bodies, in brightly coloured leotards, engaged in strenuous exercises. People think they will be embarrassed by not being able to lift as much weight, run as fast on the treadmill, or look as good in spandex. As a result, they refrain from joining a club. That is unfortunate because exercising with other people is often the best way to develop recommended levels of fitness and wellness.

fitness. In fact, exercise can rejuvenate you, make you more efficient, and provide just the break you need, both physically and mentally.

We do not mean to imply that no adjustments are necessary during particularly busy times. The operative word here, however, is *adjustment*. With the proper adjustment, you can maintain your program and resume your normal activities when the busy period passes.

Isometric contraction Force applied to an immovable object that does not result in muscle shortening.

Isotonic contraction Shortening of the muscle in the positive phase and lengthening during the negative phase of an action.

Having Visitors

Suppose someone comes to stay with you. What happens to your fitness program? Although visits from friends or relatives can encourage fitness, especially if they also exercise regularly, such visits usually interfere with your exercise program. There are several strategies you can use to maintain training during visits. If visitors are regular exercisers, there is no problem. Just exercise at the same time they do. If your visitors do not exercise regularly, help them organize short trips they can take while you exercise. Sightseeing trips are ideal. If relatives or friends are nearby, perhaps they can entertain your visitors while you exercise. What is required is some ingenuity, not interruption of your training.

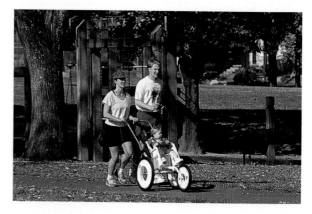

Maintaining a fitness program is possible, even in the face of obstacles. This couple is using a special stroller to take their baby on a jog.

SUMMARY

Psychosocial Factors to Consider

To plan a fitness program, you need to know certain things about yourself. These include your locus of control, the degree to which you feel socially isolated, and your level of self-esteem (in particular, your bodily self-esteem).

Locus of control is your perception of the amount of control you exert over events in your life. If you believe you have a great deal of control, you have an internal locus of control. If you believe you have little control, you have an external locus of control.

People who are socially isolated are susceptible to illness and disease. Fitness programs can be organized to respond to social needs as well as to physical ones.

What you think of yourself and your body has significant influence on your health and wellness. Body cathexis is the esteem in which you hold your body and bodily functions. Fitness programs can improve self-esteem while they improve more traditional fitness components.

Strategies for Achieving Your Fitness Goals

Among the more effective strategies for achieving your fitness goals are goal-setting and behaviour-change techniques. When you are determining fitness goals, be realistic about what is possible and periodically assess your progress toward meeting your goals. Behavioural change techniques that can be used to help you achieve your fitness goals include developing social support, contracting with yourself and others, using reminder systems, self-monitoring, programming gradually, tailoring, chaining, and practising the covert techniques of rehearsal, modelling, and reinforcement.

Maintaining Your Fitness Program

Strategies to use to maintain your fitness program include getting material and social reinforcement, joining a group, boasting, self-monitoring, and making your program fun.

Exercising Under Difficult Circumstances

Periodically, you will face obstacles to maintaining your fitness program. Among these are travelling, being confined to a limited space, being injured, being busy, and having visitors. In spite of these and other obstacles, adjustments can prevent interruption of your program. All that is required is a little ingenuity and determination to continue exercising.

STUDY QUESTIONS

1. Wesley would like to start an exercise program and wants your advice. He tells you that he wants to train for a five-kilometre road race that is taking place in six months' time. What advice do you give him about how to start his exercise program and how to maintain it so that he reaches his ultimate goal of being able to complete a five-kilometre run?

2. Would internals or externals be more likely to maintain an exercise program? Explain your answer.

3. Explain the difference between isometric and isotonic exercise.

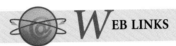

WEB LINKS

Health Canada
www.hc-sc.gc.ca

Merck: Physical Activity
www.merck.com/disease/arthritis/wellbeing/exercise.html

REFERENCES

Blair, S.N. "How Much Physical Activity Should We Do? The Case for Moderate Amounts and Intensities of Physical Activity." *Research Quarterly for Exercise and Sport* 67, 2 (1996): 193–205.

Lab Activity 3.1

Locus of Control Assessment

INSTRUCTIONS: *For each pair of statements, circle the item that best describes your beliefs.*

1. a. Grades are a function of the amount of work students do.

   b. Grades depend on the kindness of the instructor.

2. a. Promotions are earned by hard work.

   b. Promotions are a result of being in the right place at the right time.

3. a. Meeting someone to love is a matter of luck.

   b. Meeting someone to love depends on going out often in order to meet many people.

4. a. Living a long life is a function of heredity.

   b. Living a long life is a function of adopting healthy habits.

5. a. Being overweight is determined by the number of fat cells you were born with or developed early in life.

   b. Being overweight depends on what and how much food you eat.

6. a. People who exercise regularly set up their schedules to do so.

   b. Some people simply don't have the time for regular exercise.

7. a. Winning at poker depends on betting correctly.

   b. Winning at poker is a matter of being lucky.

8. a. Staying married depends on working at the marriage.

   b. Marital breakup is a matter of being unlucky in choosing the wrong marriage partner.

9. a. Citizens can have some influence on their governments.

   b. Citizens can do nothing to affect governmental functioning.

10. a. Those skilled at sports are born well-coordinated.

    b. Those skilled at sports work hard learning the skills.

11. a. People with close friends are lucky to have met people with whom to be intimate.

    b. Developing close friendships takes hard work.

(continued)

Lab Activity 3.1 *(continued)*
Locus of Control Assessment

12. a. Your future depends on whom you meet and on chance.

    b. Your future is up to you.

13. a. Most people are so sure of their opinions that their minds cannot be changed.

    b. A logical argument can convince most people.

14. a. People decide the direction of their lives.

    b. For the most part, we have little control over our futures.

15. a. People who do not like you simply do not understand you.

    b. You can be liked by anyone you choose to like you.

16. a. You can make your life a happy one.

    b. Happiness is a matter of fate.

17. a. You evaluate feedback and make decisions based on it.

    b. You tend to be easily influenced by others.

18. a. If voters studied candidates' records, they could elect honest politicians.

    b. Politics and politicians are corrupt by nature.

19. a. Parents, teachers, and bosses have a great deal to say about your happiness and self-satisfaction.

    b. Whether you are happy depends on you.

20. a. Air pollution can be controlled if citizens get angry about it.

    b. Air pollution is an inevitable result of technological progress.

To determine your locus of control, give yourself one point for each listed response:

ITEM	RESPONSE	ITEM	RESPONSE	ITEM	RESPONSE
1	a	8	a	15	b
2	a	9	a	16	a
3	b	10	b	17	a
4	b	11	b	18	a
5	b	12	b	19	b
6	a	13	b	20	a
7	a	14	a		

Scores of 10 or above indicate you believe you are generally in control of events that affect your life (an internal locus of control). Scores below 10 indicate you believe you generally do not have control of events that affect your life (an external locus of control).

Lab Activity 3.2

Alienation Test

INSTRUCTIONS: *In the boxes below, record how you feel about each sentence according to the following scale. Then, turn the page and calculate your results on various components of alienation.*

5 = I agree strongly   2 = I disagree

4 = I agree   1 = I disagree strongly

3 = I am neutral, or I don't know

_____ **1.** I don't understand the way people behave nowadays.

_____ **2.** I don't want what most people seem to want.

_____ **3.** The future of humankind looks pretty hopeless.

_____ **4.** Most people act as if the end justifies the means.

_____ **5.** I don't get much satisfaction from my work (or schoolwork).

_____ **6.** It's a lonely life for more and more people nowadays.

_____ **7.** Things don't make much sense to me anymore.

_____ **8.** My values are different from society's values.

_____ **9.** There is little room for personal choice anymore.

_____ **10.** There just aren't any definite rules to live by today.

_____ **11.** I wish I could feel more involved in my job (or schoolwork).

_____ **12.** I wish people would be a lot kinder than they are.

_____ **13.** I feel confused about the world a lot.

_____ **14.** Most people don't have the same priorities that I do.

_____ **15.** You can only get ahead if you get some lucky breaks.

_____ **16.** It seems that right and wrong are pretty ambivalent nowadays.

_____ **17.** Sometimes I just feel like a robot at work (or school).

_____ **18.** Sometimes I feel all alone in the world.

_____ **19.** I don't know what the purpose of life is anymore.

(continued)

Lab Activity 3.2 *(continued)*
Alienation Test

_____ **20.** I don't identify with my culture's values.

_____ **21.** There are so many decisions to make that I could just scream.

_____ **22.** It seems as if you have to play dirty to win.

_____ **23.** I don't have much opportunity to be creative.

_____ **24.** I don't get to go out with friends much anymore.

_____ **25.** Life has become less and less meaningful to me.

_____ **26.** Everybody seems to have a different idea of success than I have.

_____ **27.** It is (or would be) scary to be responsible for a child nowadays.

_____ **28.** It often seems that it's the nice people who lose.

_____ **29.** It's frustrating if you really care about the quality of your work.

_____ **30.** I don't see my family as much as I'd like to.

✦ **Alienation Test Results:**

Your Scores

Meaninglessness:

To obtain your score, add up your answers to Questions 1, 7, 13, 19, and 25:

(1) _____ + (7) _____ + (13) _____ + (19) _____ + (25) _____ = _____

Cultural Estrangement:

To obtain your score, add up your answers to Questions 2, 8, 14, 20, and 26:

(2) _____ + (8) _____ + (14) _____ + (20) _____ + (26) _____ = _____

Powerlessness:

To obtain your score, add up your answers to Questions 3, 9, 15, 21, and 27:

(3) _____ + (9) _____ + (15) _____ + (21) _____ + (27) _____ = _____

Normlessness:

To obtain your score, add up your answers to Questions 4, 10, 16, 22, and 28:

(4) _____ + (10) _____ + (16) _____ + (22) _____ + (28) _____ = _____

Estrangement from Work:

To obtain your score, add up your answers to Questions 5, 11, 17, 23, and 29:

(5) _____ + (11) _____ + (17) _____ + (23) _____ + (29) _____ = _____

Social Isolation:

To obtain your score, add up your answers to Questions 6, 12, 18, 24, and 30:

(6) _____ + (12) _____ + (18) _____ + (24) _____ + (30) _____ = _____

Scores should range between 5 and 25. Scores from 5 to 10 could be considered "low," from 10 to 15 "low average," from 15 to 20 "high average," and from 20 to 25 "high."

Source: Adapted from "Alienation Test." Available at **http://www.ship.edu/~cgboeree/alientest.html**. Accessed March 12, 2003. Reprinted with permission of Dr. C. George Boeree.

(continued)

Lab Activity 3.3

Body Self-Esteem Assessment

INSTRUCTIONS: *Using the scale, place the number alongside each body part or body function that represents your feelings about that part of yourself.*

- ✦ **Scale**

  1 = Have strong feelings and wish to change

  2 = Do not like, but can tolerate

  3 = Have no particular feelings one way or the other

  4 = Am satisfied

  5 = Would not change and consider myself fortunate

- ✦ **Body Part or Function**

_____ hair	_____ appetite	_____ shoulder width
_____ hands	_____ fingers	_____ energy level
_____ nose	_____ waist	_____ shape of head
_____ wrists	_____ ears	_____ body build
_____ back	_____ weight	_____ ankles
_____ chin	_____ profile	_____ height
_____ neck	_____ chest	_____ eyes
_____ arms	_____ lips	_____ skin texture
_____ hips	_____ teeth	_____ forehead
_____ legs	_____ voice	_____ health
_____ feet	_____ posture	_____ face
_____ knees	_____ facial complexion	

(continued)

Lab Activity 3.3 *(continued)*
Body Self-Esteem Assessment

✦ **Scoring**

Now add up the point values you assigned and divide the total by 35. Your score should fall between 1 and 5. If your score is below 2.5, you do not hold your body in high esteem. If your score is above 2.5, you do think well of your body. In particular, look at those items you assigned a 1 or a 2. Those are the parts of your body or bodily functions that you think are most in need of improvement. Concentrate on making those parts or functions better and you will think better of your body.

Principles of Exercise

CHAPTER OBJECTIVES

By the end of this chapter, you should be able to:

1. Identify the key components of a complete fitness program.

2. Apply the progressive resistance exercise (PRE) principle to your specific workout program.

3. Design formal warm-up and cool-down sessions for your exercise program.

4. Identify your target heart rate range, and determine whether your exercise program is intense enough to elevate and maintain your heart rate within that range.

5. Evaluate various exercise programs in terms of their effectiveness in developing aerobic fitness, muscular strength, muscular endurance, flexibility and in lowering body fat and improving lean body mass.

FOR THE PAST year, I have seen Maya in the university gymnasium almost every time I work out. It doesn't seem to matter what time I choose to exercise, she is also there exercising. Finally, I couldn't resist asking her about her exercise habits and was not surprised to learn that she trains seven times a week for 2 to 3 hours each session in a combination of formal aerobic classes, weight training, jogging, and stationary cycling. Nor was I surprised to hear that she has recovered from a number of overuse injuries, is tired most of the time, and suffers from aching muscles and sore knees.

Although Maya is doing a lot of things correctly, she obviously is overdoing the training and does not thoroughly understand the basic principles of exercise such as the PRE principle, cross-training, alternation between light and heavy workouts, and other key concepts that protect the body from injury and ensure safe progression to higher levels of fitness.

You may know someone like Maya. Her situation is a common one that can be avoided through the application of the exercise principles discussed in this chapter. Once you decide to begin a fitness program, you are ready to master the principles that will help you achieve a higher level of aerobic (cardiorespiratory) fitness; increase muscular strength, muscular endurance, and flexibility; and help you lose or maintain body weight and fat. It is important to keep in mind that participation in an exercise program or a sport is no guarantee that your fitness level will improve unless you apply the exercise principles discussed in this chapter to your routine.

THE IDEAL EXERCISE PROGRAM

The following principles can be applied to most exercise choices to develop the five key components of health-related fitness: (1) cardiorespiratory endurance, (2) body composition (fat, muscle, and bone), (3) flexibility, (4) muscular strength, and (5) muscular endurance. Programs that imzprove these components also provide the health benefits discussed in Chapter 1. Because motor skill–related areas such as agility, explosive power, balance, coordination, and speed are important to competitive athletes but have very little to do with health-related fitness, these components are not addressed in this chapter.

Cardiorespiratory Endurance

Cardiorespiratory function, or aerobic fitness, is the most important health-related fitness component and should be the foundation of your complete program. You should choose at least one aerobic exercise activity that requires 20–30 minutes of continuous, uninterrupted exercise. Walking (6 kilometres per hour or faster), jogging, running, cycling, lap swimming, aerobic dance, aerobic exercise, and conditioning classes all are excellent aerobic choices. If you choose the sports approach to aerobic fitness, you may want to consider handball (singles), soccer, rugby, lacrosse, hockey, or full-court basketball. These activities can help prevent heart disease and other disorders and can also contribute heavily to fat and weight loss or maintenance.

Body Composition

Aerobic exercise burns more calories than do other exercises. Activities such as walking, jogging, cycling, and lap swimming allow you to exercise for longer periods of time (20–60+ min) than activities requiring a higher intensity such as sprinting and full-court basketball. The key to fat loss through exercise is volume, not intensity. The longer you can continue to exercise, the more calories you burn and the more your fat cells shrink. To reduce body fat, lower your weight, and improve your appearance, you need only three ingredients: (1) a reduced caloric intake to put yourself into a negative daily calorie balance, (2) daily aerobic exercise to burn calories and tone the body, and (3) flexibility, strength, and endurance training to add muscle mass and eliminate skin sagging. These ingredients are discussed in detail in Chapter 6.

Flexibility, Muscular Strength, and Muscular Endurance

Improved flexibility may help reduce the incidence of both home and exercise-related injuries and allow you to perform various activities more efficiently and effectively.

Strength training will increase the strength and the size of your muscles. The additional muscle mass also elevates metabolic rate (calories burned at rest over a 24-hour period) and assists you in losing fat and maintaining body weight. And by improving the ratio of muscle mass to body fat, you can exercise longer and more intensely and efficiently.

Improved muscular endurance enables you to exercise for longer periods of time and is critical to participants in sports requiring short, all-out efforts such as sprinting, football, field hockey, and soccer. Depending on the design of your weight-training program (see Chapter 6), you will develop muscular endurance and strength simultaneously.

For the adult population and the elderly, strength and endurance training is even more important. Studies report a number of significant findings among the elderly who engage in weight training that have implications for improved quality of life. In fact, as mentioned in Chapter 2, the mandate of the Centre for Physical Activity and Ageing at the University of Western Ontario is to investigate the interrelationships of physical activity and aging and to develop strategies to promote the independence of older adults. Years of study and published research, combined with community outreach programs through the Centre, support and endorse the important role of regular exercise in improving posture, strength, balance, and reaction time within an aging population. To ensure the positive benefits of exercise for the elderly, the Centre recommends that any exercise program be performed at least three times per week; moreover, it should include general aerobic exercise (ideally, weight-bearing to prevent or alleviate problems associated with reductions in bone density), strengthening, postural and balance exercise, and flexibility and relaxation exercises (Newsletter of the Centre for Physical Activity and Aging). The point is, you are never too old to improve muscular strength and endurance. The loss of lean muscle tissue that occurs with aging among the sedentary population can be prevented, and additional muscle tissue can actually be added. Even as few as two strength-training workouts per week can produce positive results.

Now complete Lab Activity 4.1: Choosing and Committing to an Exercise Program at the end of this chapter, keeping in mind the importance of the five key components of health-related fitness discussed in this section.

FITNESS CONCEPTS

This section discusses in detail the specific components of a proper exercise program. Study them carefully so you can apply each concept to your specific exercise choice.

◼ Begin with a Preconditioning Program

It requires a minimum of 6–8 weeks to improve your aerobic fitness. Attempts to move quickly from one fitness level to another should be avoided in the early stages of your program. *Too much too soon* can produce muscle soreness, increase the chances of soft-tissue injury (see Chapter 12), and cause you to quit long before results are noticeable.

The first 2–3 weeks of your new program should be considered a **preconditioning period** during which you progress very slowly and enjoy each workout session. Although preconditioning will help reduce residual muscle soreness, you can expect some delayed soreness following an exercise session that involves unconditioned muscles. The time between the exercise session and the highest soreness level is somewhat dependent on your age—the older you are, the longer it takes to experience the soreness. Even with use of a preconditioning period, maximum-effort fitness tests may result in severe muscle soreness the following day.

◼ Apply the Progressive Resistance Exercise (PRE) Principle

The **progressive resistance exercise (PRE) principle** is simple to understand and has fascinating implications when correctly applied. If you gradually overload one of the body's systems (muscular, circulatory, or respiratory), it will develop additional capacity. When you repeatedly perform more strenuous exercise, the body repairs itself through elaborate cellular changes to prepare for more challenging exercise demands.

Application of the PRE principle produces dramatic changes in the heart and also in the circulatory system. Regular exercise places stress on the heart, causing it to become larger and stronger and improving **stroke volume** (by pumping more blood each beat). A trained heart muscle with improved **cardiac output** pumps considerably more blood per beat and per minute, allowing the heart to slow down, beat fewer times per minute, and rest longer between beats. As the heart

muscle adapts to the stress of exercise, the arteries that supply it also enlarge.

Although everyone starts at a different conditioning level, we can generalize about what happens to your body when you begin an exercise program (see Figure 4.1). You start the program at a certain functioning, or conditioning, level (level A in Figure 4.1). During and immediately after your first workout, this conditioning level temporarily declines to point B. You are now actually in worse shape, in terms of physical capacity to exercise, than you were before the workout. During the recovery phase, however, tissue will rebuild beyond your original level of conditioning to level C. You are now able to perform more work than you could before you began your exercise program, but with no more effort. You are also in better physical condition 24 hours later than you were before you completed your first workout. Repetition of this simple process will lead to continued improvement of conditioning levels—E, G, then I—provided you follow certain basic guidelines:

1. Keep exercise sufficiently strenuous to cause an initial decrease in the conditioning level; the depth of the valley (A to B) and the corresponding increase (B to C) in Figure 4.1 is in proportion to the intensity and duration of your workout.

2. Allow sufficient time for recovery; improvement will not occur and conditioning will suffer if your second workout is performed before the recovery phase is complete (48 hours for strength training and 18–24 hours for aerobic and other workouts). Failure to follow this principle of recuperation can lead to overuse injuries and reduce the benefits of your workout.

3. Conduct your next workout within 24–48 hours; a greater time lapse will cause your conditioning level to decline.

Preconditioning period A period of several weeks taken to prepare the body gradually for maximum effort testing or engagement in a vigorous activity or sport.

Progressive resistance exercise (PRE) principle The theory of gradually increasing the amount of resistance to be overcome and/or the number of repetitions in each workout.

Stroke volume The amount of blood ejected per beat.

Cardiac output The volume of blood pumped by the heart per minute.

DIVERSITY ISSUES

Income Level and Physical Activity Level

The majority of people in Canada are now aware that exercise is a crucial component to maintaining health. They also realize that physical inactivity is a serious threat to the health of the nation. Yet some groups in our society, such as individuals in the lower-income groups, engage in exercise considerably less often than others.

The association between income level and physical inactivity makes maintaining physical health difficult for the lower-income population. The Canadian Fitness and Lifestyle Research Institute (CFLRI) warns that over half of Canadian children and youth are at risk due to high levels of inactivity. Only 33 percent of all Canadian adults whose family income level is less than $60 000 per year exercise for at least one hour per week. When household incomes rise above $60 000, the percentage of active adults rises to 45 percent. Lower income levels are definitely associated with more sedentary lifestyles in Canada.

A number of factors contribute to the exercise habits of lower-income families. A higher school dropout rate in this group immediately eliminates both the required and the voluntary school exercise programs. For inner-city residents, opportunities are virtually eliminated simply because there is no affordable place to exercise. For those who do not drop out, after-school hours are often needed to work and help supplement family income. Regardless of whether low-income families live in urban or rural settings, experts realize that it is difficult to influence these individuals to practise good health habits such as regular exercise and proper nutrition when they are fighting for their economic lives.

Making school and recreational facilities available at hours when low-income youths are less likely to be working is one way to improve the situation. The 2000 Physical Activity Monitor conducted by the Canadian Fitness and Lifestyle Research Institute revealed that inexpensive activities that, with proper supervision, can take place during the day or evening are among the most popular activities for adolescents. Included in this list are walking, social dancing, basketball, swimming, and tobogganing. ✦

Figure 4.1 ✦ Concept of Work Hypertrophy: (A) pre-exercise functioning level; (B) functioning level following exercise; (C) elevated functioning level following recovery; (E) elevated functioning level at the proper point to resume exercise; (G) and (I) elevated functioning levels following additional workout and rest periods.

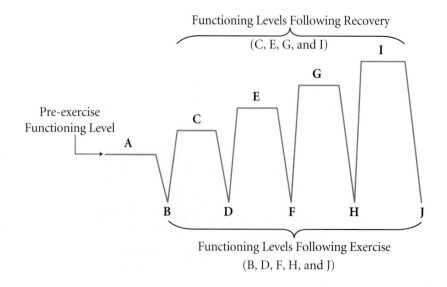

MYTH AND FACT SHEET

Myth	Fact
1. You can achieve aerobic development in half the time by doubling the workout intensity.	1. Short, high-intensity workouts will improve anaerobic, not aerobic, fitness. There are no shortcuts to aerobic development.
2. More of a good thing results in added health benefits.	2. Health fitness levels for life can be achieved by following the concepts described in this text. Going too far beyond the FIT (frequency–intensity–time) limits increases the risk of injury. Those persons who exercise beyond the health fitness level usually are seeking conditioning for athletic competition rather than health.
3. You should wear a hat when exercising.	3. Although hats are extremely popular in tennis, baseball, and some other activities, their value depends on the type you choose. Hats help keep the sun off the face, reduce glare, and allow you to see better. One with an open top (visor) should be used in hot, humid weather because considerable heat loss and cooling occurs through the head. In cold weather, a full hat is recommended to prevent heat loss.
4. Because the main source of energy (fuel) in aerobic exercise is fat, this is the best type of activity for weight and fat loss.	4. A calorie is a calorie is a calorie. To lose weight, your caloric intake must be less than your caloric expenditure, regardless of the type of fuel used. As the intensity of a workout increases from a resting state (when two-thirds of energy used comes from stored fat) to low or moderate aerobic activity (when fat is still the main fuel) to more intense, anaerobic activity, the percentage of fat used decreases and glycogen (stored glucose) provides much more fuel. After exercise ceases, regardless of the fuel used (fat or glucose), the internal calorie count is what matters. If you burn up more calories than you consume on a particular day, you will lose weight. The main advantage of aerobic activity (walking, slow jogging, cycling, dancing, swimming laps) for weight and body-fat loss is that you are likely to continue exercising for longer periods of time when the intensity is low and therefore will burn more total calories each workout. You also receive considerable health benefits that anaerobic exercise does not provide.

If you apply this concept to any training program, improved conditioning is guaranteed. Even strength training (see Chapter 6) uses this approach to acquire muscle mass and increase strength and endurance.

The resistance principle also applies to the skeletal system. Gradual stress to the bones stimulates the accumulation of calcium and other minerals. In the adult years, **osteoporosis** can occur. When you walk, jog, run, or perform other aerobic exercise, the force of your feet hitting the ground sends an important signal to your body to maintain bone density. At this point, more of the calcium consumed in your diet reaches the orthopedic system. Other key factors that are also important in the prevention and treatment of osteoporosis are discussed in Chapter 14.

Osteoporosis An abnormal decalcification of bones causing loss of bone density.

WELLNESS HEROES

Gordie Howe

No professional athlete has ever maintained as high a level of fitness for as long a period of time as hockey Hall of Famer Gordie Howe. Howe could do it all—he was big, strong, fast, smart, and cool. For 32 seasons, he dominated the sport, knocking in 801 goals over 20-plus seasons in the National Hockey League (NHL) and then 174 more in seven seasons in the World Hockey Association (WHA), where he helped his team win two championships and won an MVP award at the age of 46. Howe was an NHL All-Star selection 23 times before being elected to the Hall of Fame in 1972. He came out of retirement in 1973 to play seven more seasons with the WHA and achieve a father–son feat that may never be topped—league MVP in the same year his son Mark was named Rookie of the Year.

"Mr. Hockey" knew a lot about the principles of conditioning and remained a highly fit player until retirement at the age of 53. His longevity and achievements during his later years in professional hockey may never be surpassed. Gordie Howe is truly one of Canada's greatest wellness heroes. ✦

Exercise Five Times a Week for 30 Minutes at Your Target Heart Rate (THR)

Although results can be attained without lengthy workouts, there are no shortcuts. Ten-second contractions, mechanical devices, steam baths, 3-minute slimnastic programs, and other such approaches range from slightly effective to worthless.

To receive the health-related benefits of exercise, you must apply the FIT principle:

Frequency	5 or more days per week
Intensity	At or above your target heart rate
Time	30 minutes of exercise (continuously or in 10-to-15-minute bouts)

Frequency of exercise is the key to the success of your program. Exercising five times per week rather than undergoing one hard workout per week will greatly increase the chances of meeting your training objectives. Frequency is also strongly related to weight and fat loss, cardiovascular development, and disease prevention. One 30-minute session will not transform you into a lean, mean, muscle machine, but 5 sessions weekly for 6–12 months will do wonders. Regularity is also a critical factor in changing the way your body handles fats (cholesterol and triglycerides).

Intensity (work per unit of time) is the aspect of your training that determines whether you are receiving any cardiorespiratory (heart–lung) benefits. Researchers have developed simple formulas to determine how much your heart rate must increase during exercise and how long you need to keep it elevated (20–30 minutes) to improve cardiovascular fitness (other health benefits can be obtained at lower intensity levels, as discussed in chapters 1 and 4). In the early stages of your newly started program, you will need to work up to 20–30 minutes of continuous activity slowly, over 4–6 weeks, rather than attempt to maintain such a high intensity in early workout sessions. To locate your THR, complete Lab Activity 4.2: Finding Your Target Heart Rate at the end of this chapter.

Time (the duration of your workout) is the final aspect of the complete cardiorespiratory exercise session. Exercise duration is affected by intensity. Obviously, you cannot sprint at near-maximum effort for 20 minutes. If aerobic conditioning is your goal, the session should maintain your THR for 20–30 minutes. If the purpose of your program is cosmetic—to lose weight and fat and to improve your appearance—duration is the key. In general, the longer you exercise, the more calories you burn and the more fat you use as fuel. If weight loss is your primary objective, keep in mind that walking 5 kilometres burns only slightly fewer calories than running 5 kilometres. The longer you walk or run, the more calories you use. Thus, you might want to slow down your walking, pedaling, running, rope jumping, and so on and exercise longer. To exercise longer, it is important to stay near the lower portion of your THR range. Providing your THR is reached, you are not only burning a high number of calories but improving your cardiovascular system as well.

Running or walking 5 kilometres on each of two successive days also burns more calories than one 10-kilometre run. This is due to the extra 60–150 calories burned because of metabolic rate increases (calories burned while the body is at rest) following the exercise period. In other words, two short exercise sessions burn more calories than one long session, because the metabolic rate will become, and remain, elevated for several hours after each session. This extra calorie usage after exercise ceases is called **afterburn**. If you walk or run too far in one day and are unable to exercise the next day, you will eliminate one afterburn period and forfeit 60–150 calories. Late afternoon, when metabolic rates begin to slow in most people, may be one of the best times to exercise. You then burn calories while exercising and activate a faster metabolic rate for 2–4 hours at a time in the day when metabolic rate normally slows down.

If you follow the FIT principle, there is solid evidence that you will receive considerable health benefits from your exercise program. The benefits of physical activity follow a dose–response gradient (that is, the higher the dose, the greater the benefits). At a recent conference entitled "Communicating Physical Activity and Health Messages—Science into Practice" in Whistler, B.C., researchers agreed that the most sedentary people benefit from moderate increases in activity, that moderately active people benefit from increased activity, and that the most active people benefit from staying active. What remains unclear is whether the dose–response relationship is maintained at levels that far exceed the FIT principle, or if it evens off at the inherent optimal level for each person. In one study, men who exceeded the levels of the FIT principle were found to have greater levels of the protective HDL cholesterol, less body fat, lower triglyceride levels, and a better ratio of "good" to "bad" cholesterol. And the more both men and women exercised, the more benefits they received. The study also recommended that cardiorespiratory endurance activity be supplemented with strength-developing exercises at least twice per week. *Canada's Physical Activity Guide to Healthy Active Living* incorporates these findings and advocates exercise duration goals based on intensity level. If someone should engage in exercise requiring light effort, such as light walking, a pickup game of volleyball, or easy gardening, according to the *Guide* he or she would need to participate for 60 minutes every day to get the health benefits of physical activity. However, if someone should engage in exercise requiring vigorous effort, such as aerobics, hockey, or jogging, according to the *Guide* he or she would need to participate for 20–30 minutes four days a week to get health benefits. The overall message within the pages of the *Guide* is "The more active you are, the more benefits you will get."

Unfortunately, over 65 percent of all Canadians are not physically active enough to promote good health. Making the change from being sedentary to physically active facilitates improvements in an individual's heart health, stress level, and overall quality of life.

◼ Apply the Principle of Specificity

The effect of training is unique to an activity or sport. Football or field hockey players who have just completed seasons, for example, will find that they are not capable of meeting the physical demands of wrestling or basketball. The scientific basis for this is that training occurs, in part, within the muscles themselves and that training is specific to the energy system being used. Thus, complete training transfer, regardless of the closeness of the activities, is not possible.

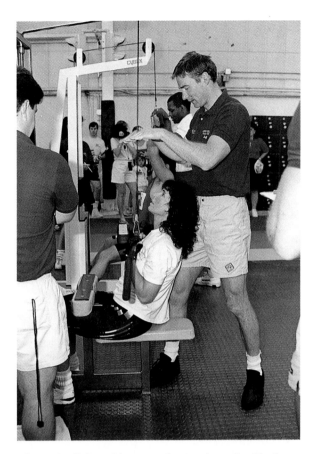

Alternating light and heavy workouts reduces the risk of injury and gives the muscles time to recover.

Training a particular muscle group is referred to as **neuromuscular specificity**; training one of the energy systems is called **metabolic specificity**. If your main training objective is to improve aerobic fitness, you must include activities such as jogging, running, cycling, aerobic dancing, and distance swimming. Although gains in cardiorespiratory fitness will occur from each of these activities, a specific activity that closely simulates the movement of the sport for which you are training provides the most transfer. In other words, swimming is the preferred training method to improve distance swimming, running is the preferred training method for 10-K races, and so on.

Afterburn The period of time following exercise when resting metabolism remains elevated.

Neuromuscular specificity Training a specific muscle group.

Metabolic specificity Training a specific energy system (citric acid cycle or glycolysis cycle).

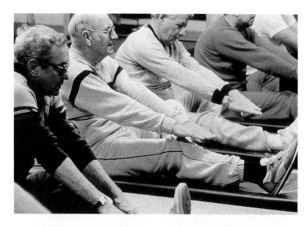

Warming up muscles improves performance and prevents injuries.

Alternate Light and Heavy Workouts

The body responds best to training programs that alternate light and heavy workouts. This approach reduces the risk of injury, provides several emotionally relaxing workouts each week, and allows the body time to recover. In other words, it helps you receive maximum benefits from a fitness program. Thus, you should consider (1) never training extremely hard on consecutive days, (2) training hard no more than three times a week, (3) scheduling one extra-hard, all-out workout once a week, and (4) knowing your body and allowing it to direct you (if pain continues or worsens or if you get heavy-legged, stop regardless of whether it is a light- or heavy-workout day). The PRE principle is applied by increasing the volume and/or intensity on the heavy-workout days.

Warm Up Properly Before Each Workout

A **warm-up** is almost universally used at the beginning of an exercise or activity session to improve performance and prevent injury. The theory behind the warm-up is that muscular contractions are dependent on temperature. Because increased muscle temperature improves work capacity and a warm-up increases muscle temperature, it is assumed that one is necessary. The amount of knee fluid is also increased with a warm-up; oxygen intake is improved; and the amount of oxygen needed for exercise is reduced. Nerve messages also travel faster at higher temperatures.

Suggestions that can be drawn from the findings of well-controlled studies on the warm-up include the following:

1. Warm up for 10–15 minutes prior to the actual workout or exercise session. A longer period is needed in a cold environment to allow the body to reach the desired temperature prior to activity.

2. Warm up until you begin to sweat. The main purpose of a warm-up is to elevate core temperature by 1 to 2 degrees before engaging in stretching exercises or explosive muscular movements; you will generally reach this point at the same time your warm-up routine causes sweating.

3. Let only a few minutes elapse from completion of the warm-up until the start of activity.

4. Remember that warm-up will not cause early fatigue or hinder performance.

Warm-up methods fall into four categories:

1. **Formal** This involves the skill or act that will be used in competition or in your workout, such as running before a 100-metre dash, jogging before a 5-kilometre run, or shooting a basketball and jumping before a basketball game.

2. **Informal** This involves a general warm-up, such as calisthenics or other activity unrelated to the workout routine to follow.

3. **Passive** This involves applying heat to various body parts.

4. **Overload** This involves simulating the activity for which the warm-up is being used by increasing the load or resistance, such as swinging two bats before hitting a baseball.

Each of these methods has been shown by some researchers to be helpful and by other researchers to be of little value. Formal warm-up appears superior to informal procedures. When body temperature is elevated and sweating occurs, your muscles are ready for a brief stretching or flexibility session (see Chapter 7).

How long you decide to engage in warm-up activities is also important. The temperature of your muscles will rise in about 5 minutes and continue to rise for 25–30 minutes. If you stop exercising and become inactive, your muscle temperature will decline significantly, and you may need an additional warm-up period. The best advice is to use a 10- to 15-minute warm-up period that ends in an all-out effort and causes you to perspire. You should plan to complete your warm-up period about 5 minutes before an exercise session or competition begins. Find the magic combination for you and your activity and stay with it.

Cool Down Properly at the End of Each Workout

The justification for a **cool-down** period following a vigorous workout is quite simple. Blood returns to the heart through a system of vessels called *veins*. The blood is pushed along by heart contractions, and the veins' milking action is assisted by muscle contractions during exercise. Veins contract, or squeeze, and move the blood forward against gravity while valves prevent the blood from backing up. If you stop exercising suddenly, this milking action will stop, and blood return will drop quickly and may cause blood pooling (blood remaining in the same area) in the legs, leading to shock or deep breathing, which may in turn lower carbon dioxide levels and produce muscle cramps.

At this point, blood pressure also can drop precipitously and cause trouble. The body compensates for the unexpected drop in pressure by secreting as much as 100 times the normal amount of **norepinephrine**. This high level of norepinephrine can cause cardiac problems for some individuals during the recovery phase of vigorous exercise, such as a marathon or a triathlon.

Postexercise peril can occur in some individuals immediately after very strenuous exercise—particularly the elderly, the nonfit, and those who fail to use a cool-down period. The least desirable postexercise behaviour is standing. Lying down flat is acceptable; the preferred activity, however, is walking or jogging for 4–5 minutes (light exercise).

You should also cool down following a long aerobic exercise session. A general routine might consist of walking or jogging 150 metres to 1.5 kilometres at a pace of 3–4 minutes per 150 metres, each 150 metres slower than the previous one. The ideal cool-down routine should take place in the same environment as the workout (except in extremely hot or cold weather), last at least 5 minutes, and be followed by a brief stretching period.

Dress Appropriately for Ease of Movement and Heat Regulation

What you wear depends on your exercise program and the weather. The general rule is to have good shoes and to wear as little clothing as the weather permits.

Shoes To avoid injuries, quality shoes are essential for most aerobic activities. The primary criteria are fit, comfort, and quality. Most activities require a specialized shoe, and although they often look identical, the various styles affect individuals differently. Specialty stores are more likely to provide sound advice about the best shoe for your aerobic goals. Because fit is so important, wear the same style of socks you use for exercising when you are selecting a shoe.

Clothes For indoor and warm-weather outdoor exercise, wear the least clothing possible. The cooling process requires air to pass over the skin for evaporation; clothing must allow this process to take place. Some individuals mistakenly feel they will lose weight by wearing multiple layers of clothes to increase fluid loss. It is the total calories expended, however, not the total sweat count, that determines weight and fat loss.

When you are exercising outside during the winter, do not either overdress or underdress. Like summer clothing, winter attire must allow the skin to breathe. Windbreakers and other nylon garments are therefore not recommended. Combining a polypropylene shirt with a wool sweater, a hat, and gloves is usually sufficient for protection down to temperatures below 0° C (32° F). Under extremely cold conditions, however, frostbite is a real danger, particularly to exposed skin. The skin can be protected, but only to a degree, with creams and jellies. Men, for example, must protect the penis and testicles from frostbite; nylon shorts are of little value, and frostbite can occur without warning. Table 12.4 provides additional information on the prevention of hypothermia and heat-related disorders.

Warm-up The preparation of the body for vigorous activity through stretching, calisthenics, running, and specific sport movements designed to raise core temperature.

Cool-down The use of 3–10 minutes of very light exercise movements at the end of a vigorous workout designed to cool the body slowly to near-normal core temperature.

Norepinephrine An end product of some of the secretions of the adrenal gland; influences nervous system activity, constricts blood vessels, and increases blood pressure.

Postexercise peril Illness, dizziness, nausea, and sudden death following vigorous exercise, particularly when a cool-down period is not used.

Take Special Precautions When Exercising Outdoors

Weather conditions are not your only concern when you exercise outside. Pollution, particularly lack of clean air, is indeed a danger worth paying attention to. Although the benefits of exercise overshadow the dangers of unclean air, workouts during smog alerts and in high traffic areas should be avoided. Motor vehicles and even bicycles can present life-threatening situations to runners and others who exercise outside. Cars and bicycles should be given the right-of-way no matter what you or the law indicates. It is also advisable to run or walk toward traffic and to wear reflective gear at night. Do not be aggressive, because you are no match for a vehicle that weighs a thousand kilograms.

Dogs tend to have considerable bark and little bite, but the exceptions can produce disaster. Because dogs are extremely territorial, it is wise to avoid crossing property lines. For the occasional dog that comes after you, the best action is to stop, face the dog, and assume a passive posture before slowly backing away. As you vacate the property, the animal generally becomes less aggressive.

Exercising at any time outdoors has the potential for danger, particularly at night. It is wise to anticipate dangerous situations and take care to exercise with others, avoid outside exercise at night, ignore taunts, and remain alert at all times.

Choose Soft Surfaces Whenever Possible

Although exercise involves some risk of injury (see Chapter 12), choice of surface can reduce the risk. Generally, the harder the surface, the greater the injury potential. A surface that is too soft or uneven also increases the risk of certain types of exercise injuries. A soft, uneven surface, such as a beach, can cause ankle and knee injuries. Dirt and gravel paths and trails covered with wood chips are best for walking and running, but the isolated nature of most trails increases the chances of assault. Public park fitness courses usually provide relatively safe, soft places to exercise. Exercising on concrete floors, sidewalks, hard tennis courts, and gymnasium floors should be avoided whenever possible. Daily activity on such surfaces is almost certain to produce injury.

> **Cross-training** The practice of alternating exercise choices throughout the week to avoid overuse injuries from repetitive movements.

Use Cross-Training in the Aerobic Component of Your Program

Repetitive motion syndrome can produce both injury and loss of interest in exercise. Daily step classes or 8-kilometre runs, for example, both involve the same motion, movement, muscles, and joints over and over and are almost certain to result in injury over time. More and more individuals use **cross-training** and avoid these dangers by varying their exercise choices weekly. Runners may choose to ride a stationary cycle or swim once or twice a week. Aerobic dancers cycle, walk, swim, or play racquet sports. Such an approach provides a more complete workout and eliminates exercise boredom and burnout.

Use a Maintenance Approach After Reaching Your Desired Level of Fitness

It is possible to alter your exercise program to maintain the level of conditioning you have acquired. Considerable strength, for example, can be maintained by completing one or two hard weight-training workouts weekly. Maintaining your cardiorespiratory endurance may require two to three workouts weekly. During times when you are unable to exercise daily, you may choose to alter your routine by increasing the intensity and duration of the workouts you complete.

Monitor Your Progress Carefully

Records can be a source of motivation in addition to aiding in the prevention of injury. Keeping records of resting heart rate, kilometres walked or run, laps swum, weight lifted, and workouts completed can provide the needed incentive to continue an exercise program.

Recordkeeping also helps you apply the PRE principle to guarantee continued improvement. It is difficult to improve and work harder today when you are not aware of the intensity and duration of your previous workouts.

If an overuse injury occurs, a perusal of records can aid in determining its cause and help you set a course toward recovery. Unfortunately, records can also lead to compulsive behaviour known as *negative addiction*. To the addicted, records are made to be broken, more is better, and the record rather than the fitness benefits becomes the goal. Such individuals experience frequent injury intermixed with emotional stress in attempting to maintain or break records.

The daily log in Table 4.1 can help you apply many of the exercise concepts discussed in this chapter. The log information should include the time spent in aerobic

Table 4.1 ✦ Daily Exercise Log

Name _____

Weight _____   **Starting date** _____

Date _____   Time of day _____

Cardiorespiratory Activities: _____

Weight Training:

Exercises	Starting Weight	Repetitions	Sets
_____	_____	_____	_____
_____	_____	_____	_____
_____	_____	_____	_____
_____	_____	_____	_____
_____	_____	_____	_____
_____	_____	_____	_____
_____	_____	_____	_____
_____	_____	_____	_____
_____	_____	_____	_____

Intensity:

Heart rate _____   Repetitions _____   Rest interval _____

Distance covered _____   Pace _____

Duration:

Total exercise time _____

Positive impressions of the workout:

_____

_____

_____

_____

Unusual feelings or problems during workout:

_____

_____

_____

_____

activity, the distance covered, and rest intervals between repetitions, if applicable. Your log should also note weather conditions, water temperature, heart rate, positive impressions, particular problems that indicate the possibility of future injury, number and type of activities completed, and (for weight training) the weight and number of repetitions for each exercise. It is also important to monitor your aerobic exercise choices periodically.

MAKING THE RIGHT EXERCISE CHOICES

The ideal, complete exercise program should have four components: aerobics, muscular strength, muscular endurance, and flexibility. The aerobic component will provide the health-related benefits in addition to controlling and maintaining body weight and fat. A sound weight-training program will: improve muscle tone, strength, and endurance; prevent the loss of lean muscle mass; add muscle mass; and help control body weight and fat by increasing metabolism. Flexibility training will help maintain and improve your range of motion and prevent joint stiffness.

▪ Choosing an Aerobic Program

It is important to select a program that is effective in developing the cardiorespiratory system, and is compatible with your training objectives, amount of time available, and interests. Table 4.2 compares aerobic exercise choices on the basis of the characteristics of the ideal program. Study this table carefully before making your selection. It is also a good idea to sample different approaches to help you find activities you enjoy for use in cross-training later.

If you are interested in the sports approach to aerobic fitness, study Table 4.3 before making your selections. As you are now aware, the term **aerobic** means "with oxygen" and describes extended vigorous exercise that stimulates heart and lung activity enough to produce a

training effect. This occurs when your target heart rate is reached and maintained for 20 minutes or more. Many sports are more anaerobic than aerobic and fail to improve heart–lung endurance or provide the health benefits you desire.

Anaerobic means "without oxygen" and describes short, all-out exercise efforts such as the 100-, 200-, or 400-metre dash and sports such as football and baseball. Anaerobic metabolism is the immediate energy source of all muscle work at the beginning of any type of exercise. This energy source, called *adenosine triphosphate* (ATP), is formed in the muscles primarily through the metabolization of carbohydrates. Every muscle needs ATP to perform its work. The process is anaerobic because ATP is metabolized without the need for oxygen. For short sprints and all-out efforts, the heart and lungs cannot deliver atmospheric oxygen to the muscles fast enough; anaerobic energy sources therefore must provide the fuel. The very instant the amount of oxygen breathed in is not enough to supply active muscles, **oxygen debt** occurs and you begin to breathe heavily. After you stop exercising, oxygen debt is repaid and normal breathing returns. Unfortunately, anaerobic activities cannot be sustained for long periods of time, burn fewer calories, and fail to provide some important health benefits. It is difficult to improve your aerobic fitness through mere participation in a sport, and we recommend that you supplement such participation with a minimum of two aerobic workouts weekly.

Aerobic exercises should produce some changes within 3–4 weeks.

▪ Choosing Muscular Strength and Endurance Programs

Chapter 6 describes numerous choices for increasing your muscular strength and endurance effectively. Your choice of workout routine depends on your training objectives, which also help you decide between free weights and the other types of exercise equipment.

▪ Selecting an Appropriate Flexibility Training Program

Although a simple, static stretching routine is the wisest choice for effectively improving your flexibility, specific exercise choices depend on your objectives, including that of the particular activity for which you are training. The detailed information in Chapter 7 will help you make the right decision. In less than 10 minutes daily, you can maintain and even improve range of motion in your major joints.

Aerobics Activity performed in the presence of oxygen, using fat as the major source of fuel.

Anaerobics High-intensity activity, such as sprinting, that is performed in the absence of oxygen, using glucose as the major source of fuel.

Oxygen debt The difference between the exact amount of oxygen needed for an exercise task and the amount actually taken in.

Table 4.2 ✦ Evaluation of Exercise Programs

Characteristics of Ideal Program	Aerobic Exercise and Dance	Anaerobics	Calisthenics	Cycling	Rope Jumping	Running Programs	Sports[a]	Walking	Swimming (laps)	Weight Training
Easily adaptable to individual's exercise tolerance	P	Y	Y	Y	Y	Y	P	Y	Y	Y
Applies the progressive resistance principle	Y	Y	Y	Y	Y	Y	P	Y	Y	Y
Provides for self-evaluation	Y	Y	P	Y	Y	Y	P	Y	Y	Y
Practical for use throughout life	Y	N	N	Y	Y	Y	P	Y	Y	Y
Scientifically developed	Y	Y	P	Y	Y	Y	U	Y	Y	Y
Involves minimum time	Y	P	N	Y	Y	Y	N	Y	Y	Y
Involves little or no equipment	P	Y	Y	N	Y	Y	N	Y	Y	N
Performed easily at home	N	N	Y	Y	Y	Y	N	Y	Y	N
Widely publicized	Y	N	N	Y	Y	Y	Y	Y	Y	Y
Accepted and valued	Y	P	N	Y	Y	Y	P	Y	Y	Y
Challenging	Y	Y	N	Y	Y	Y	Y	Y	Y	Y
Firms body	Y	Y	Y	Y	Y	P	P	Y	Y	Y
Develops flexibility[b]	Y	N	Y	N	Y	Y	Y	N	P	N
Develops muscular endurance	Y	Y	Y	Y	Y	Y	Y	Y	Y	Y
Develops cardio-vascular endurance: Prevents heart disease	Y	N	Y	Y	Y	Y	Y	P	Y	P
Develops strength	P	P	Y	P	P	Y	Y	P	P	Y
High caloric expenditure: Weight loss	Y	P	P	Y	Y	P	Y	Y	Y	N

Note: Y=yes, P=partially, N=no provision, U=unknown (referring to meeting ideal characteristics).

[a]The value of the sports approach depends on the activity and the level of competition.

[b]Flexibility can be improved only if the complete range of movement is performed in each exercise, applying static pressure at the extreme range of motion before returning to starting position.

Source: Adapted from John Unitas and George B. Dintiman, *Improving Health and Fitness in the Athlete* (Englewood Cliffs, NJ: Prentice-Hall, 1979), p. 180.

Table 4.3 ✦ Ratings of Sports

Sport	Type	Cardiovascular	Caloric Expenditure	Legs	Abdomen	Arms/ Shoulder	Age range Recommended
Archery	Anaerobic	L	L	L	L	L	Ages 10 and up
Backpacking	50% aerobic	M-H	H	H	M	L	All ages
Badminton	40% aerobic	M-H	H	H	L	M	Ages 7 and up
Baseball/softball	Anaerobic	L	L	M	L	L	All ages
Basketball	25% aerobic	M	H	H	L	L	Ages 7 to 60
Bicycling (competitive)	Aerobic	H	H	H	L	M	All ages
Bowling	Anaerobic	L	L	L	L	L	All ages
Dance (aerobic)	Aerobic	M-H	M-H	M	M	M	All ages
Canoeing/rowing							
Recreational	Anaerobic	L	M	L	L	M	Ages 12 and up
Competitive	Aerobic	H	H	M	M	H	Ages 12 to 40
Fencing	Anaerobic	L-M	M	M	L	M	Ages 12 and up
Field hockey	40% aerobic	M-H	M-H	H	L	M	Ages 7 and up
Golf (motor cart)	Anaerobic	L	L	L	L	L	All ages
Walking	Aerobic	L	M	M	L	L	All ages
Handball/racquetball/							
squash (singles)	40% aerobic	M-H	H	H	L	H	All ages
Hiking	Aerobic	L-M	M	H	L	L	All ages
Hunting	Aerobic	L-M	M	M	L	L	All ages
Ice/rollerskating							
Speed	Anaerobic	L-M	M	H	L	L	Under 50
Figure	Aerobic	L-M	H	H	M	M	All ages
Jogging	Aerobic	M-H	H	H	L	L	Ages 7 and up
Lacrosse	40% aerobic	M-H	H	H	M	M	Under 45
Orienteering	50% aerobic	M-H	H	H	M	L	All ages
Rugby	60% aerobic	H	H	H	L	H	Under 45
Skiing (cross-country)	Aerobic	H	H	H	H	H	Under 65
Skin and scuba diving	Aerobic	M	M	M	M	L	All ages
Soccer	50% aerobic	H	H	H	L	H	Under 55
Surfing	Anaerobic	L	M	H	M	L	Ages 7 and up
Swimming	Aerobic	M	H	M	L	H	Ages 7 and up
Tennis (singles)	40% aerobic	M	M	H	L	L	All ages
Touch football	Anaerobic	L	L-M	H	L	L	Under 55
Volleyball	Anaerobic	L	L	M-H	L	M	All ages
Walking	Aerobic	L-M	M	H	L	L	All ages
Water-skiing	Anaerobic	L-M	M	H	L	M	All ages
Weight training	Anaerobic	L	L	H	H	H	All ages
Wrestling	30% aerobic	M	H	H	H	H	Under 45

Note: H=high; M=medium; L=low.

BEHAVIOURAL CHANGE AND MOTIVATIONAL STRATEGIES

There are many things that might interfere with your application of sound exercise principles. Here are some typical barriers (roadblocks) and strategies for overcoming them.

Roadblock	Behavioural Change Strategy
Exercise just isn't fun anymore, and you no longer look forward to your afternoon workout session. Even if you do get into the workout, there is no motivation to put forth much effort.	You may be experiencing some of the emotional and physical effects of overtraining or exercising too often. To renew your interest: 1. Change aerobic activities every other day as a cross-training technique. If you are jogging or using STEP daily, for example, substitute cycling, lap swimming, aerobic dance, or a sports activity two to three times weekly. 2. Change the time you exercise. Try early mornings, noon, or just before bedtime to see if your mood improves. 3. Apply the light–heavy concept discussed in this chapter and avoid two consecutive workouts of the same level of difficulty. 4. Add one or two fun workouts weekly, and exercise with a group of friends.
Your muscles are sore the following morning, making your day unpleasant, as sitting, standing, and moving around on the job is somewhat painful.	A number of factors may be causing the problem. You may be: exercising untrained muscles; training much too hard; not consuming enough fluids before, during, and after your workout; or stretching improperly or not at all. Try some of these remedies for at least one week: 1. Hydrate 15–30 minutes before your workout by drinking three or four 230-millilitre glasses of water. 2. Record the amount of water and other fluids you consume daily, making certain to drink at least eight glasses of water. 3. Alternate light- and heavy-workout days. 4. Warm up for a longer period of time than you normally do, then stretch carefully for at least 10 minutes. 5. At the end of your workout, cool down properly and end with a mild 5-minute stretching session.
Although you have been exercising daily for a month, you don't seem to be losing weight and fat.	To lose body fat and weight, you need to change your exercise emphasis and reduce your caloric intake. Don't give up. Be certain you: 1. Monitor both your exercise sessions and your food intake by keeping accurate records of total exercise volume and daily calories consumed. 2. Increase the duration of your workout and exercise every day. If you are walking, try to walk continuously for at least one hour. Reduce the intensity of your workout and continue exercising longer each workout. 3. Schedule your workout about two hours before mealtime or two hours after your evening meal to help control hunger and the temptation to overeat or snack.
List other roadblocks you are experiencing that seem to be reducing the effectiveness of your program and limiting your success. 1. _____ 2. _____ 3. _____	Now list behavioural change strategies that can help you overcome the roadblocks you listed. If you need to, refer to Chapter 3 for behavioural change and motivational strategies. 1. _____ 2. _____ 3. _____

SUMMARY

The Ideal Exercise Program

A complete exercise program should bring about improvement in five key health-related fitness areas: cardiorespiratory endurance, body composition, muscular strength, muscular endurance, and flexibility. Aerobic exercise is the most important component and should form the foundation of the ideal program. The principles of exercise must be applied specifically to your workout choice to guarantee continued improvement.

Fitness Concepts

A preconditioning period may be necessary before beginning a new exercise program, particularly if you have previously been inactive. This 3-to-4-week period will prepare you for more vigorous workouts and allow you to reach and maintain your THR for 20–30 minutes safely.

The PRE principle can easily be adapted to aerobic, muscular strength and endurance, and flexibility training to ensure steady progress and improvement in these areas. To train for a specific sport or activity, you must apply the principle of specificity by using movements and exercises that closely simulate those performed in the sport. Using a warm-up and cool-down period, applying FIT to your aerobic workout, alternating light- and heavy-workout days, dressing appropriately for the weather, monitoring your progress with recordkeeping, and cross-training will improve the benefits of each workout, keep you emotionally and physically healthy, and eliminate boredom and overtraining.

Making the Right Exercise Choices

It is important to select aerobic activities you enjoy that are also effective and that meet your training objectives. The sports approach to aerobic fitness requires special care in selecting activities, such as soccer, rugby, and field hockey that are primarily aerobic in nature. Anaerobic activity choices will provide very little in the way of health-related benefits. Two to three additional workouts weekly in an aerobic activity are also recommended.

STUDY QUESTIONS

1. List the components of an ideal exercise program, and explain how each contributes to the health of an individual.

2. Using the concept of work hypertrophy, describe what happens to the body when beginning an exercise program.

3. Identify the components of the FIT principle and explain how they are used to optimize health-related benefits of exercise.

4. Why is a proper cool-down an important way to end each workout?

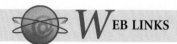

WEB LINKS

Health Information and Weblinks Page
www1.sympatico.ca/Contents/health

Canadian Society of Exercise Physiology
www.csep.ca

REFERENCES

Canadian Fitness and Lifestyle Research Institute, 2000. *2000 Physical Activity Monitor.* **www.cflri.ca/**

"Director's Report." Newsletter of the Centre for Physical Activity and Aging, University of Western Ontario, London, December 1998.

Haskell, W.L. "Physical Activity and Health: Existing Data and Current Issues." *Communicating Physical Activity and Health Messages—Science into Practice.* Whistler, B.C., Canada (December 9–11, 2001).

U.S. Department of Health and Human Services. *Physical Activity and Health: A Report of the Surgeon General.* Atlanta: U.S. Department of Health and Human Services, Centers for Disease Control and Prevention, National Center for Chronic Disease Prevention and Health Promotion, 1996.

Wee, C.C. "Physical Activity Counseling in Primary Care: The Challenge of Effecting Behavioral Change." *JAMA 286,* 6 (2001): 718–719.

Lab Activity 4.1

Choosing and Committing to an Exercise Program

INSTRUCTIONS: *This Lab will assist you in identifying specific times, dates, and places to exercise in activities you enjoy that also produce significant health benefits.*

1. Determine the best time and days for you to exercise. Prepare a schedule of your daily routine Monday through Sunday. Include your class, study, work, mealtime, church, and other activities.

	Monday	Tuesday	Wednesday	Thursday	Friday	Saturday	Sunday
7–8		shower		shower			
8–9	workout	class	workout	class	workout		shower
9–10	workout	↓	chapel	↓	chapel	Shower	church
10–11	shower	chapel	class	Chapel		brunch	↓
11–12	lunch	class	shower	class	shower	work	↓
12–1	homework	snack	lunch	snack	lunch		lunch
1–2		class	homework	class	homework	↓	
2–3		lunch	↓	lunch	↓	homework	
3–4		homework	work	homework	work		
4–5	↓					↓	
5–6	supper	↓		↓		supper	supper
6–7	class	futsal		futsal			
7–8							
8–9		↓	↓	↓	↓		
9–10	↓						

Now choose a block of time (at least 1 hour, ideally 1.5 hours) on three separate days, avoiding two days in succession. You may want to exercise early in the morning (which has been shown to boost metabolic and energy levels), keep exercise as a reward at the end of the day, or take advantage of a lull between classes to break up your day. Whatever your choice, force yourself to adhere to the schedule for at least a month.

Weekly exercise days and time __M, W, F approx 8 - 9am__
__T, R 7-9 pm__

(continued)

Lab Activity 4.1 *(continued)*
Choosing and Committing to an Exercise Program

2. List the three most important outcomes you expect from your exercise program.

   a. Stay in shape

   b. lose weight

   c. look better

3. Determine the type of exercise you are most likely to enjoy. Review Table 4.3 and select several different activities you can try in your newly chosen exercise time slot that develop a moderate to high level of cardiorespiratory fitness. You may want to use the sports approach and play tennis, handball, racquetball, squash, badminton, basketball, soccer, or some other sport that is convenient and enjoyable for you; or you might prefer to take an aerobic approach and join an exercise class, walk, cycle, or swim. Each of these activities and many others can provide significant health benefits over time. Try several activities until you discover a cardiorespiratory workout you really enjoy. If your schedule allows, consider using two weight-training workout sessions per week for 20–30 minutes following your cardiorespiratory exercise. Go to the university weight room and ask for help in setting up a program that meets your needs. Make certain your exercise choices are capable of producing the desired outcomes you identified in Step 2.

4. Keep a record of each workout using a form like the one in Table 4.1. By monitoring your progress and recording your feelings, you are more likely to avoid overuse and other injuries and remain motivated enough to stay with your program. After a month, you should begin to feel better and have more energy.

5. Sign the exercise contract on the next page to confirm your commitment to one month of regular exercise 3–4 days per week.

✦ Contract to Increase My Physical Activity Level

During the next 4 weeks, from _____ to _____, I hereby agree to work as hard as possible at achieving the following:

1. Physical activity goals for increasing my energy use during occupational time:

   a. I will park my car or leave public transportation and walk _____ additional minutes per day.

   b. I will spend _____ minutes daily standing instead of sitting while I work.

   c. I will walk up _____ flights of stairs each working day.

   d. I will walk around my work area _____ minutes every day.

   e. I will spend _____ minutes during each coffee break standing instead of sitting.

   f. I will spend _____ minutes during each lunch break walking outdoors.

2. Physical activity goals for increasing my energy use during recreational time:

   a. I will spend _____ minutes daily doing stretching activities to increase my flexibility.

   b. I will spend _____ minutes at least three times per week doing aerobic activities to improve my endurance.

   c. I will spend _____ minutes at least three times per week doing strength activities.

   d. I will spend _____ minutes Saturday and Sunday in active recreational activities.

3. By increasing my activity levels in the work and recreational periods listed above, I will use up _____ more calories per week.

4. My rewards and consequences:

   a. I will reward myself daily with one of the following when I achieve my daily goals in increased activity.

   1) _____   4) _____

   2) _____   5) _____

   3) _____   6) _____

   b. When I do *not* achieve my daily goals I agree to do the following:

   1) _____   2) _____

   c. I will reward myself every week with one of the following when I achieve my weekly exercise goals:

   1) _____   4) _____

   2) _____   5) _____

   3) _____   6) _____

(continued)

Lab Activity 4.1 *(continued)*
Choosing and Committing to an Exercise Program

      d. When I do *not* achieve my weekly goals I agree to do the following:

        1) _____   2) _____

I agree to follow this contract until my goals are reached.

Signed _____ Date _____

Witnessed _____

Name _Ang Chafey_

Date _06/02/06_

Lab Activity 4.2

Finding Your Target Heart Rate (THR)

INSTRUCTIONS: *The target heart rate (THR) is the range of heart rate that will produce training effects on the heart if it is maintained for a sufficient length of time (usually 20–30 minutes) at least three times per week. This is commonly known as aerobic exercise. The purpose of this Lab is to determine your THR or exercise benefit zone (EBZ).*

1. Determine your resting heart rate (RHR). This is the lowest heart rate you experience at any time during your waking hours—day or evening. Check it several times during the day when you feel really relaxed. (Refer to Steps 1 and 2 of Lab Activity 2.2 for specific instructions on finding your RHR.)

2. Use the formula below to compute your 60 percent, 70 percent, and 85 percent target heart rates. This is the zone you should stay in during aerobic exercise.

60% THR*	70% THR	85% THR*
220	220	220
Subtract age − 21	− 21	− 21
Subtract RHR − 80	− 80	− 80
× 0.60	× 0.70	× 0.85
+ RHR	+ RHR	+ RHR
= 151.4	= 163.3	= 181.15

*A 60 percent THR would be regarded as the minimum target heart rate to achieve a cardiorespiratory training effect; a THR of 85 percent would be regarded as the maximum target heart rate for optimal cardiorespiratory training without adverse effects.

5

Exploring Cardiorespiratory Fitness

CHAPTER OBJECTIVES

By the end of this chapter, you should be able to:

1. Give alternative names for cardiorespiratory endurance.

2. List benefits to be derived from participating in a cardiorespiratory conditioning program.

3. Describe maximal oxygen uptake (VO_2) and show different ways of expressing it.

4. Assess your VO_2 and determine your cardiorespiratory fitness.

5. Explain guidelines for safely beginning and progressing in an aerobic fitness program.

6. Develop your own cardiorespiratory conditioning program.

RECENTLY, TWO WOMEN were shopping in a department store. Ms. Green, a professional, 40-year-old, single female, was purchasing exercise clothing and accidentally bumped into Mrs. Taylor, a 45-year-old, lower-income woman, who was purchasing clothing for her grandchildren. As the two women struck up a conversation, Ms. Green explained that she had just enrolled in the new pool aerobics class at the local health club. She asked Mrs. Taylor if she had considered joining the class because pool aerobics is very popular and is a great form of exercise. Mrs. Taylor responded, "Well, you know, I'm so busy cleaning houses that I just don't have the time or the energy to join an exercise class!"

Unfortunately, the cardiorespiratory exercise boom has not reached all segments of the Canadian population for various reasons. Many obstacles, such as increased time demands, may make exercise seem impossible. As your time management skills improve, finding time to exercise will not be as difficult as it may seem. Also, many people mistakenly believe, as Mrs. Taylor does, that participating in an exercise class will make them more fatigued. In reality, the opposite is true. Improved cardiorespiratory fitness often increases your energy level. Many other benefits are to be derived from participating in an aerobic conditioning program.

BENEFITS OF CARDIORESPIRATORY FITNESS

Cardiorespiratory fitness or endurance is referred to by many names, including aerobic power, **maximal oxygen consumption (VO$_2$)**, physical fitness, and **aerobic metabolism. Cardiorespiratory endurance** is the ability of the heart, blood vessels, and lungs to deliver oxygen to the exercising muscles in amounts sufficient to meet the demands of the exercise load. **Endurance** is the ability to perform prolonged bouts of exercise without experiencing fatigue or exhaustion. As your cardiorespiratory endurance level increases, so does your ability to engage in sustained physical activity. By the end of several months of cardiorespiratory activities, you will be able to exercise for long periods without experiencing prolonged fatigue.

As their bodies adapt to an aerobic conditioning program, many individuals report feeling more alert and less fatigued throughout the day. A high level of cardiorespiratory endurance also can help postpone or delay several chronic diseases, such as heart disease and high blood pressure. Recent research has even shown that people with high levels of cardiorespiratory endurance are less susceptible to cancer. Because heart disease, high blood pressure, and cancer are among the leading causes of death in Canada, it is especially important for you to maintain a healthy cardiorespiratory system.

Let us examine the physiological benefits (see Table 5.1) to be derived from participating in a cardiorespiratory endurance conditioning program. Although the list presented in Table 5.1 may seem overwhelming at first glance, all these physiological changes can be reduced to one primary benefit—increased aerobic power. What effect do all these changes have on level of performance? All the changes that occur to the heart, blood, blood vessels, and lungs, which make up the **cardiorespiratory system**, increase the amount of blood that is delivered to the muscles. Also, these benefits make exercise feel easier at workloads below maximum and increase your ability to perform at maximal exercise intensity. The changes that occur in the muscles, bones, and joints combine to improve the efficiency of your body's physical movements and/or to increase your ability to extract oxygen from the bloodstream. Thus, both exercise duration and exercise intensity increase. In short, the total amount of work that you are able to do increases as a result of cardiorespiratory adaptations from an aerobic conditioning program.

In the remainder of this chapter, we explore aerobic exercise choices and discuss the differences in oxygen uptake and utilization for various sports. We will also discuss guidelines for beginning and safely progressing in an aerobic conditioning program and conclude with some sample starter programs for aerobic activities. You will then have the opportunity to design your own aerobic exercise program.

Table 5.1 ✦ Physiological Benefits of Increased Cardiorespiratory Endurance Following Participation in an Aerobic Training Program

HEART, BLOOD VESSELS, AND LUNGS	MUSCLES, BONES, AND JOINTS
Lower resting heart rate	Increased bone strength and density
Lower submaximal exercise heart rate	Increased thickness of cartilage, tendons, and ligaments
Increased maximal cardiac output	Increased oxygen consumed by muscles
Increased stroke volume	Increased number of mitochondria
Decreased recovery time	Increased size of mitochondria
Increased strength of heart muscle	Increased concentration of oxidative enzymes
Decreased resting blood pressure in hypertensives	Increased muscle glycogen stores
Increased number of capillaries in muscles	Increased ATP and phosphocreatine stores
Increased total blood volume	Increased ability to burn fat for energy
Increased hemoglobin (carries oxygen to muscles)	Decreased body-fat percentage
Increased vital capacity (lung capacity)	Increased muscular endurance
Decreased blood lipids:	Increased flexibility
Increased high-density lipoprotein (HDL) cholesterol	
Decreased low-density lipoprotein (LDL) cholesterol	
Decreased triglycerides (fats)	

ANAEROBIC ENERGY SYSTEMS

The major energy systems in the body are the anaerobic and aerobic metabolism systems. The energy that is released when food is broken down in the body is used to manufacture a substance called **adenosine triphosphate (ATP)**, the primary energy molecule of the body. ATP is either stored in small amounts in the muscles or manufactured through the process of metabolism.

The immediate energy system is composed of ATP and *creatine phosphate (CP)* stored in the muscles. Because much larger amounts of CP than ATP are stored in the muscles, the body can quickly produce more ATP through the immediate energy system by adding free phosphates to the *adenosine diphosphate (ADP)* molecule. This anaerobic energy system is generally used for high-intensity activities that last less than 30 seconds.

The lactic acid system is a second source of energy for anaerobic activities. It provides energy for high-intensity activities lasting from 30 seconds to two or three minutes. Events that require a combination of speed and power over a short time typically rely heavily on the lactic acid energy system.

OVERVIEW AND ANALYSIS OF AEROBIC EXERCISE CHOICES

Only aerobic activities will increase your level of cardiorespiratory endurance. Fortunately, there are numerous aerobic choices available, including walking, jogging/running, swimming, bicycling, aerobic dancing and step aerobics, water aerobics, rope skipping, cross-country skiing and stepping.

Nearly all aerobic sports will lead to the same benefits with respect to increased aerobic power, so it makes little difference whether you choose to walk, jog, or ride a bike. When you choose a conditioning program, however, you must realize that the larger the amount of muscle mass used in an activity, the greater will be your level of endurance, especially during the initial phase of the conditioning program. For example, if you walk for 45 minutes, you will probably not become fatigued as quickly as if you play tennis for 45 minutes. The muscles that grip the tennis racquet tire more quickly because you place a high energy demand on a very small muscle mass. In contrast, your leg muscles, as used in walking, are a much larger group, are more accustomed to this activity, and so will not fatigue as quickly. For this reason, you will find that your endurance is greater when you engage in activities such as swimming, walking, and jogging/running than when you perform activities that rely primarily on the arms. Remember that in the initial

phase of a conditioning program, you can expect to fatigue sooner when small muscle groups are used.

Regardless of how exciting a new aerobic conditioning program may be, eventually boredom might creep in. Therefore, we recommend that you participate in a variety of aerobic activities in order to maintain cardiorespiratory fitness. The greater the diversity in your program, the greater the likelihood that you will maintain a lifetime of physical fitness. Also, whenever possible, exercise with a partner or with a group of people. The benefits of exercising with other people are discussed elsewhere in this book, but a major benefit is that exercising with a partner or a group increases the likelihood you will stay with your conditioning program.

MAXIMAL OXYGEN CONSUMPTION (VO₂)

"Cardiorespiratory endurance" is often used interchangeably with "VO₂," or maximal oxygen uptake. When a person is tested either in a laboratory or in the field, the highest level of oxygen uptake achieved is called the VO₂, which actually represents the volume of oxygen consumed by the muscles.

Maximal oxygen consumption (VO₂) The optimal capacity of the heart to pump blood, of the lungs to fill with larger volumes of air, and of the muscle cells to use the oxygen and remove waste products that are produced during the process of aerobic metabolism.

Aerobic metabolism The process of breaking down energy nutrients such as carbohydrates and fats in the presence of oxygen in order to yield energy in the form of ATP.

Cardiorespiratory endurance The ability of the heart, blood vessels, and lungs to deliver oxygen to the exercising muscles in amounts sufficient to meet the demands of the workload.

Endurance The ability to work a long time without experiencing fatigue or exhaustion.

Cardiorespiratory system Joint functioning of the respiratory system (the lungs and airway passages) and the circulatory system (the heart and blood vessels).

Adenosine triphosphate (ATP) The basic chemical used by a muscle to provide energy for muscle contractions.

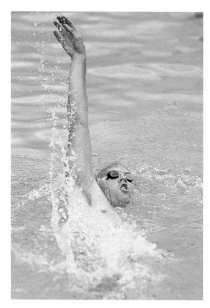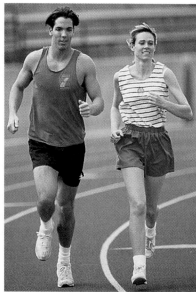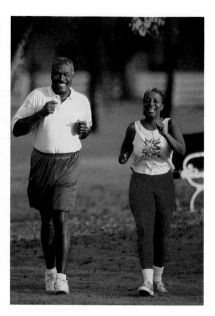

Endurance is greater when you exercise by using large muscle groups, such as swimming, jogging, or walking.

The VO_2 is regarded as the single best indicator of cardiorespiratory endurance or aerobic fitness. However, some caution needs to be observed in equating maximal oxygen uptake directly with cardiorespiratory endurance; VO_2 is rather like a gas gauge in a car in that it tells you how much gas you have to consume, but it does not tell you how efficient the engine is. Thus, we should view VO_2 as the potential for performance, but not the only factor in cardiorespiratory fitness.

A high VO_2 indicates a large capacity of the heart to pump blood, of the lungs to fill with larger volumes of air, and of the muscle cells to use the oxygen and remove the waste products that are produced during the process of aerobic metabolism. The two primary factors influencing maximal aerobic power are (1) the ability of the cardiorespiratory system to deliver oxygen to the muscles and (2) the ability of the muscles to extract oxygen from the blood.

Oxygen is used in the process of aerobic metabolism. When you exercise for prolonged periods of time, vast quantities of energy are needed by the muscles. Foodstuffs stored in the muscles, such as fats and **glycogen** (the stored form of carbohydrate in the muscles), are broken down continuously in order to provide ATP, which is used by the muscles to provide energy for contractions. The greater the quantity of ATP available, the greater your work capacity is.

As long as adequate amounts of oxygen are delivered to the muscles, the process of breaking down glycogen proceeds aerobically (in the presence of oxygen). When you reach peak VO_2, however, you are no longer able to supply adequate amounts of oxygen to the muscles solely through aerobic metabolism, and for a short period of time, glycogen is additionally broken down anaerobically (in the absence of oxygen). You can only exercise for a brief period of time when energy is provided through **anaerobic metabolism**. Fat is the major energy source used for sustained physical activity, and it cannot be burned through anaerobic processes. Thus, the higher your level of aerobic fitness, the more fat you can burn during an exercise session.

Oxygen uptake is influenced by factors such as age, sex, genetic background, and physical training. Typically, as you get older, your maximal level of aerobic power declines. After age 30, sedentary individuals experience a decrease in VO_2 of about 1 percent per year. The rate of decline is much slower among active individuals. Also, men tend to have a higher level of aerobic power than women of similar ages. This is primarily due to men's larger body size and greater amount of lean muscle tissue.

Some people are born with a genetic predisposition to be elite endurance athletes. They inherit larger and stronger hearts, greater lung capacity, better blood supply in their muscles, larger quantities of red blood cells, and higher percentages of slow-twitch muscle fibres, which are found in greater percentages in the muscles used in aerobic exercise. These muscle fibres contain energy foodstuffs and enzymes that enhance aerobic metabolism and promote exercise of longer duration. As shown in Table 5.1, aerobic training also leads to many of these same changes. Thus, even if you are not born an elite marathon runner, you can become a pretty good one by engaging in a prolonged aerobic conditioning program.

WELLNESS HEROES

Michael Smith

Michael Smith epitomizes the completeness of an athlete seeking to be the best that he can be in his chosen sport: the decathlon. Born in the small town of Kenora, Ontario, in Canada's centennial year, Michael excelled in a variety of high school sports including football and basketball, as well as in track and field. In fact, at the end of Grade 12, he was offered several football scholarships to American universities. Still, it was the lure of the demanding ten track and field disciplines—100-metre run, long jump, shot put, high jump, 400-metre run, 110-metre hurdles, discus, pole vault, javelin, and the 1500-metre run—collectively called the decathlon that enticed the talented Canadian.

At first, Michael trained in the meagre (by the standards of elite, competitive sport) facilities of the Kenora recreation centre. Eventually, he moved to Toronto to take advantage of his talents and of the high quality coaching and facilities available there. By the mid- to late 1980s, he had become successful in national and international junior decathlon competitions. In 1988, he placed 14th in the event at the Seoul Olympic Games. The high hopes of a media-driven nation were placed on him, and he had high expectations of himself. In World Championship events, he won a silver in 1991 and a bronze in 1995. However, a veteran of three consecutive Olympics, Smith withdrew from the 1992 Games because of injuries and then placed 13th at the Atlanta Games in 1996. The latter performance was labelled a great "disappointment" by the expectant Canadian media.

The 102 kg, 196 cm athlete avoided the temptation of taking banned substances in an international arena plagued by substance abuse. Smith was ranked number one in Canada and among the top 10 in the world from 1989 to 1998, and as high as 5th in the world (1996) during his career in the decathlon. Moreover, he is a two-time winner of the prestigious Jack W. Davies trophy (1989 and 1991) as Canada's outstanding track and field athlete. In 1999, the three-time Canadian Olympic Team member joined CBC Sports as an athletics analyst. Michael Smith's longstanding commitment to his exacting sport and his persistence on the national and international track and field scene mark him as a significant Canadian Wellness Hero. ✦

Sources: **http://cgi.canoe.ca/AthcanAthletes/msmith.html** (Athletics Canada Web site); **http://cgi.canoe.ca/97Worlds/aug1_buffery2.html** (Toronto Sun media report on Smith during the 1997 World Championships in Athens); Jill Le Clair, *Sport and Physical Activity in the 90s* (Toronto: Thomson Educational Publishing, 1992), p. 312; **http://cbc.ca** (CBC 2001, On-Air Hosts); **http://finsandskins.com** (Fins and Skins Worldwide, 2001, Celebrity Profiles).

The VO$_2$max, or aerobic power, of an individual is expressed in volume (in litres) per unit of time (in minutes). Scores ranging from three to four litres per minute are common for the average healthy individual who exercises three to four times per week. Highly trained endurance athletes, however, may have a VO$_2$max ranging from five to six litres per minute. Usually, the greater the amount of muscle mass used in a sport, the higher the maximal oxygen uptake obtained through training. Thus, people who engage in activities such as running, cross-country skiing, and cycling often have the highest measured VO$_2$max.

There are several ways of expressing the maximal oxygen uptake. When expressed in units of litres per minute (**absolute VO$_2$**), it is often difficult to compare the actual fitness level of one individual to another. The reason is that the larger the body size, the higher the oxygen uptake, regardless of the level of fitness. Expressing **VO$_2$ relative** to a person's body weight allows individuals of different sizes to be compared. Hence, a smaller individual may have a lower VO$_2$ when it is expressed in units of litres per minute, but when it is expressed in units of millilitres oxygen per kilogram of body weight per minute (mL/kg × min^{-1}), the smaller person may actually have a much higher level of cardiorespiratory fitness.

Let us use an example to illustrate this point. Antony weighs 75 kg and has a maximal oxygen uptake of 4.2

Glycogen The stored form of carbohydrate in the muscles and liver.

Anaerobic metabolism The process of breaking down carbohydrates (glucose or glycogen) in the absence of oxygen in order to yield energy in the form of ATP.

Absolute VO$_2$ Expressing the volume of oxygen consumption in the units of litres of oxygen consumed per minute (L/min).

Relative VO$_2$ Expressing the volume of oxygen consumption in the units of millilitres of oxygen per kilogram of body weight per minute (mL/kg × min^{-1}).

Diversity Issues

Gender Differences

It was not until 1929 that Canadian women were legally pronounced "people" and not until well into the 1900s that women's participation in intense physical activity was considered "safe." History is full of accounts of sex discrimination on the basis of faulty political thinking and/or ignorance about human anatomy and physiology. Not only is women's participation in physical activity and sport safe, encouraged, and physically advisable, but also it sends powerful messages to other women and men alike.

Physical activity is one way of exercising our country's principles of choice, equality, and greatness. Taking ownership of and pride in our bodies through the lifestyle choice of exercise is a right every Canadian has the power to fulfill regardless of sex. Unfortunately, some people still think that exercise makes women less feminine and that weight training makes them too masculine.

Women are equally as skilled as men and capable of performing well in any type of exercise. In fact, in some fitness areas, women are superior to men. Women have greater buoyancy than men because of a higher proportion of fatty tissue, which is advantageous in swimming because they require less energy to stay afloat. They are more flexible than men, as is evidenced in their ability to perform dance and aerobic routines. Even sedentary women can be as flexible as active men and remain so throughout life. Women have a definite edge in the areas of grace and beauty of movement, which is important in competitive gymnastics and dance. Women have as great a physical skill learning rate and capacity as men, and only in the areas of strength and endurance do women have some catching up to do. In fact, women's finishing times in marathons are coming closer to men's every year.

Although women's bodies do not respond to training at the same rate as men's, women have a tremendous capacity for improving their muscular strength, muscular endurance, flexibility, body composition, and aerobic fitness levels. ✦

litres per minute. Miranda weighs 59.1 kg and also has a maximal oxygen uptake of 4.2 litres per minute. Who is more fit? Antony's maximal oxygen uptake expressed in relative units is determined by:

$$\frac{4200 \ (1000 \ \text{mL} = 1 \ \text{L})}{75 \ \text{kg}} = 56 \ \text{mL/kg of body weight}$$

Miranda's maximal oxygen uptake expressed in relative units is determined by:

$$\frac{4200 \ (1000 \ \text{mL} = 1 \ \text{L})}{59.1 \ \text{kg}} = 71.1 \ \text{mL/kg of body weight}$$

Were you surprised? What a big difference between their levels of fitness when you express their maximal oxygen consumption relative to their body weight. Apparently, Miranda has a much higher level of fitness even though she has a much smaller body size than Antony. Normally, active university-age females have average maximal oxygen uptake values of 38 to 42 mL/kg $\times$ min^{-1}, compared to a value of 44 to 50 mL/kg $\times$ min^{-1} for university-age males.

The most accurate method of measuring maximal oxygen uptake is through direct gas analysis in a laboratory setting. This procedure involves the use of computerized equipment, such as a treadmill or a bicycle ergometer, and a mouthpiece, which is cumbersome. This procedure is quite sophisticated and the equipment is expensive. Thus, indirect methods of assessing the VO$_2$ in healthy individuals are often used.

Several field tests are used to measure aerobic power indirectly. The most commonly used field tests are the 4.8-kilometre walking test, the 12-minute run test, the 12-minute swimming test, and the YMCA bicycle test. If you have been involved in a physical conditioning program, you may elect to complete the 12-minute run test (Lab Activity 5.2). If you are just beginning your aerobic exercise program, however, you should assess your maximal oxygen uptake by completing the 4.8-kilometre walking test in Lab Activity 5.1: Assessing Your Level of Aerobic Fitness at the end of this chapter.

The 4.8-kilometre walking test is an excellent means of assessing cardiorespiratory endurance with a low risk of injury for someone who is just beginning an exercise program. Once you complete Lab Activity 5.1, use Table 5.2 to determine your fitness classification according to gender and age. If you are in the Poor or Fair fitness category, begin with the sample walking program presented later in this chapter. If you are in the Good or Excellent fitness category, begin with the sample jogging/running program also presented later in this chapter.

Table 5.2 ✦ Cardiorespiratory Fitness Classification for Women and Men According to Maximal Oxygen Uptake (in mL/kg × min^{-1})

		FITNESS CLASSIFICATION			
GENDER	AGE	*Fair*	*Average*	*Good*	*Excellent*
Women	<30	24–30	31–37	38–48	>49
	30s	20–27	28–33	34–44	>45
	40s	17–23	24–30	31–41	>42
Men	<30	25–33	34–42	43–52	>53
	30s	23–30	31–38	39–48	>49
	40s	20–26	27–35	36–44	>45

HOW TO BEGIN AND PROGRESS IN AN AEROBIC FITNESS PROGRAM SAFELY

You should be aware of several concepts and conditions in order to minimize risk of injury when you begin an aerobic fitness program.

1. **Total work concept** The total amount of work you do each week is important when you are attempting to increase cardiorespiratory fitness and change body composition. Total work is usually calculated in units of calories (kilocalories) per week. Total work is assessed by quantifying the frequency, intensity, and duration of your exercise sessions. For instance, if you burn 300 kilocalories per 30-minute exercise session, four times per week, your total energy expenditure is 1200 calories per week. The next week, however, you might exercise three times per week for 45 minutes at the same exercise intensity and burn 400 kilocalories per session. Your total expenditure would still be 1200 calories. Thus, if your schedule fluctuates constantly, you might still maintain your exercise schedule and meet your energy expenditure goals by manipulating exercise intensity, frequency, or duration. By the way, there are 3500 kilocalories in 454 grams of fat.

2. **Shin splints** Exercisers who engage in hard-impact, high-intensity exercise for extended periods of time are at risk of developing *shin splints*. This condition is an inflammation of the muscle and its skin-like sheath (fascia) on the inner front side of the lower leg. Shin splints are believed to be caused by overuse, improper shoes, poor exercise technique, hard surfaces, and back defects. To avoid shin splints, use a variety of activities, especially water aerobics, and avoid chronic exercise on hard surfaces so that you will not overstress the lower extremities.

3. **Stitch-in-the-side phenomenon** Adequate breathing while running is essential for maintaining sufficient oxygen to exercising muscles. Diaphragmatic breathing (underneath the abdomen muscles) often results in the pain associated with the *stitch-in-the-side* phenomenon. The cause of this condition is unknown, but it is believed to be associated with an inability of the diaphragm muscles to use oxygen. If you do not use the diaphragm while breathing, the stitch-in-the-side phenomenon is less likely to occur. Expand your abdomen rather than your chest. Breathing should be rhythmic and closely associated with your exercise pace. Most exercise physiologists recommend that you take a deep breath every two to four strides.

4. **Blisters** These can be very painful and are often debilitating. Friction develops at the point of contact between your foot and the running surface and initially causes hot spots. If this friction is not minimized, fluid will eventually develop between the layers of skin at the point of contact and swelling will occur, leading to a blister. To prevent blisters from developing, wear two pairs of cotton socks, especially when you are doing hard-impact exercises for long periods of time. Also, if you place a bandage at the point of contact before the exercise session, the skin is protected, and blisters are less likely to develop. If a blister ruptures, you should treat it as an open wound and keep it sterile.

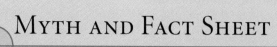

MYTH AND FACT SHEET

Myth	Fact
1. Most Canadians are getting enough aerobic exercise to reduce their risk of heart disease.	1. To a large extent, heart disease remains a national crisis. More than 60 percent of adults do not achieve the recommended amount of regular physical activity, and 25 percent of adults are not active at all. Even more distressing is that nearly half of young people (ages 12–21) are not vigorously active on a regular basis.
2. It is not as important for younger individuals to stretch before exercising.	2. Whatever your age, being flexible helps you use your muscles more effectively and efficiently. When you have complete range of motion, you tend to perform better in your workout activity, with a decreased risk of muscle injury. Other benefits of stretching include less muscle fatigue, less soreness after exercise, better posture, and reduced risk of lower-back pain.
3. You should exercise every day in order to increase your level of cardiorespiratory fitness.	3. When you begin an exercise program, you should *not* exercise every day because you will increase the risk of getting injured. It is best to exercise on alternate days to allow adequate time for recovery. After you reach your maximal level of aerobic fitness, you can exercise daily because your risk of injury will be lower after a long period of training.
4. You are more likely to stick with an exercise program if you maintain the same exercise program each workout.	4. Many individuals find that their motivation tends to decrease when engaging in the same routine for weeks or months. Cross-training is an attractive option to help put the pizzazz back in your workout. Switching activities once or twice a week may provide the variety you need to stay motivated over the long haul. Cross-training can also help you prevent injuries caused by overtraining. By alternating high- and low-impact activities or routines that involve different parts of your body, you give overstressed muscles a chance to heal without interrupting your training.

5. **Muscle soreness** Often, **delayed-onset muscle soreness (DOMS)** occurs within 12–24 hours after a high-intensity exercise session. During the initial phases of an exercise program, DOMS is most likely to occur. Most physiologists believe the cause is related to minute tears in the muscle fibres and connective tissue. After a few days, the pain subsides. You may take aspirin or another painkiller, such as acetaminophen, to relieve the pain. Gentle stretching after the workout, mild-intensity exercise, and light massage may also help decrease the pain.

6. **Heat illness symptoms** Most heat problems arise because of inadequate fluid intake and/or improper heat dissipation. As you begin exercising, your body temperature increases greatly because of the increased rate of metabolism. Normally, the body temperature is regulated by sweating. As the sweat evaporates from your body, your body cools, and its inner temperature decreases. When you do not drink enough fluids before and during exercise, especially in hot, humid or hot, dry weather, the sweating mechanism becomes less effective and your inner-body temperature remains elevated. Also, when you do not wear proper exercise clothing, the sweating mechanism becomes ineffective, and the core temperature remains elevated.

As your core temperature rises, symptoms such as muscle cramps, excessive fatigue, nausea, dizziness, light-headedness, headaches, diminished coordination, and cotton mouth or dry lips may develop. You may have any combination of these symptoms when heat illness occurs. As **heat exhaustion (heat prostration)** develops, your rate of sweating increases, and you develop cold, clammy skin. As it intensifies, you may lose consciousness, and suddenly sweating will cease. If the skin becomes hot and dry and your pulse becomes rapid and strong, you may have suffered **heat stroke**.

If any of these symptoms occur while you are exercising, stop immediately, get out of the sun, and begin removing layers of clothing. Also, drink as much fluid as you can tolerate, and elevate your feet. Begin cooling your body by using cold, wet towels; place ice on your body in more severe cases. Heat illness is extremely dangerous, and you should see a physician if it occurs.

7. **Prevention, rest, ice, compression, and elevation (PRICE)** Avoidance of injury is crucial as you begin your conditioning program. PRICE is the acronym for the recommended steps to follow in the immediate treatment of an injury. We recommend isolating the injured extremity instead of trying to walk it off in order to avoid creating a more serious condition. Ice the injured area using a wrapped cold-pack or ice wrapped in a light towel. Ice three times per day using a 10–10–10 formula; that is, apply the ice pack for 10 minutes, take if off for 10 minutes, then apply it for 10 minutes. This will help decrease pain and minimize swelling. Leaving ice on an injured area longer than 10 minutes may result in the body treating the cold as heat, thereby increasing swelling. Compressing the injury with a bandage and elevating the injured part above the level of the heart and head also help reduce swelling. Protect your body at all times by warming up before, and cooling down after, each exercise session. Also, remember that pain is your body's mechanism for letting you know that something is wrong, so *do not ignore it or try to push through it*. Stop and investigate the problem in order to minimize the risk of developing a more serious condition.

SAMPLE STARTER PROGRAMS

Sample Walking Program

In recent years, walking has become one of the most popular of all aerobic activities. One reason for its popularity is that it does not require any specialized skills and is both safe and painless when some basic guidelines are followed. You can walk almost anywhere, at any time, and at little cost. Many people choose walking over activities like jogging because it puts less stress on the hips, knees, and ankles and results in a reduced risk of orthopedic injuries. Also, exercisers have found walking to be an excellent means of reducing body weight and lowering body fat percentage.

Many people feel that because they have been walking all their lives, they do not need instructions on how to begin a walking program. Any successful walking program depends, however, on your understanding of a few basic guidelines and principles. The basic principles of beginning an exercise program were covered earlier, so we will limit our discussion here to special considerations for the beginning and the advanced walker.

Duration During the initial phase of a walking program, you should walk 10–15 minutes at a pace that is comfortable to you. After one or two weeks, you can advance to 30-minute sessions. Continue walking for 30 minutes per session for at least four weeks in order to decrease your risk of injury and to minimize fatigue. After approximately six weeks, you can increase the exercise period to 45 minutes. The more advanced walkers typically progress to 60-minute walking sessions.

Intensity The first step in regulating exercise intensity is to *forget* the familiar saying "No pain, no gain." Calculate your target heart rate (THR); begin your walking program at 50–60 percent of that rate. Once you advance to 30-minute walking sessions, you can increase your exercise intensity to 60–65 percent of your THR. As you advance to 45- to 60-minute exercise sessions, remember to stay within your THR.

It is best to use your THR as a measure of intensity rather than using a particular walking speed. That will give you the best measure of the cardiorespiratory benefits of your workout. During the initial phase of your walking program, check your exercise heart rate every five minutes. Use a 10-second pulse count while walking, multiplying the result by 6 to determine your heart rate per minute. At the end of your exercise session, if you have walked at a comfortable pace, your heart rate should drop below 100 beats per minute following a ten-minute cool-down period.

A great way of monitoring exercise intensity while walking without actually counting your pulse is to use the talk test. Any time you are walking with a partner, if your breathing rate is so fast that you cannot carry on a conversation with that person, you are probably walking too fast. Beginning to feel winded is an instant indication that you should slow the pace down.

Delayed onset muscle soreness (DOMS) Muscle soreness that typically occurs 12–24 hours after a high-intensity exercise session.

Heat exhaustion (heat prostration) Collapse due to loss of fluid and salts caused by oversweating.

Heat stroke Severe, sustained rise in fever due to the failure of the body heat–regulating mechanism after a prolonged period of elevated temperature.

If you are walking alone, a simple test to monitor exercise intensity is to take one inward breath for every three strides and one outward breath for the following three strides. If you are inhaling and exhaling every two strides, you are probably exercising above your THR and should slow down. Remember, exercise intensity is inversely related to exercise duration. If your exercise heart rate is too high, you will tire more quickly and exercise for shorter periods of time, and you will also increase your risk of getting injured. Exercise should be fun and relaxing; it is not meant to cause pain.

Frequency At the beginning of your exercise program, you should walk every other day up to a maximum of 3–4 days per week. After the first six weeks, you can increase your frequency to 4–5 days per week. Limit your exercise frequency to a maximum of 5 days per week in order to allow a few days for recovery, thereby minimizing your risk of injury.

Caloric Cost When you begin your walking program, choose some premeasured distance, whether on a track, a cross-country trail, or a treadmill. This will enable you to calculate the number of calories burned as an estimate of the total amount of work you have completed. Table 5.3 shows one method of determining the energy cost of walking in units of kilocalories per minute. To use this table, find the approximate speed you walk in kilometres per hour. Next, locate your approximate body weight. The figure at the intersection represents an estimate of kilocalories used per minute. Multiply this figure by the number of minutes you exercise to get the total number of kilocalories used.

For example, Jennifer weighs 64 kilograms and walks at a speed of 5.6 kilometres per hour for 45 minutes:

$$3.9 \text{ (kcal/min)} \times 45 \text{ (min)} = 176 \text{ calories}$$

Her total caloric expenditure based on this table is approximately 176 kilocalories per exercise session.

Rate of Progression Do not get discouraged if you do not see immediate progress, especially if you have not been exercising on a regular basis. During the initial phases of a walking program, gradually increase the distance that you walk at a slow pace for a few weeks, and then increase the speed that you walk. This will give your body time to adjust to your new training program and reduce your chances of injury. It is best to increase your exercise time by no more than 10 percent per week. Most people will use 90–150 calories per session during a 30-minute walk covering 2.5 kilometres. When you reach this level, you are ready to move on to a more advanced phase of walking.

Advanced walkers typically use 200–350 calories per session by manipulating their exercise intensity and duration. Once you reach an advanced level of walking, you may choose to begin a walk/jog/run program. Many people enjoy just walking, however, reaping many fitness benefits with little risk of injury.

As you begin your walking program, try to:

1. Maintain good postural alignment to avoid tension in the neck, back, and shoulders.

2. Hold your head high to help maintain good posture.

Table 5.3 ✦ Energy Costs of Walking (kcal/min)

| BODY WEIGHT (kg) | KILOMETRES PER HOUR | | | | | | |
	3.2	4.0	4.8	5.6	6.4	7.2	8.0
50	2.1	2.4	2.8	3.1	4.1	5.2	6.6
54	2.3	2.6	3.0	3.4	4.4	5.6	7.2
59	2.5	2.9	3.2	3.6	4.8	6.1	7.8
64	2.7	3.1	3.5	3.9	5.2	6.6	8.4
68	2.8	3.3	3.7	4.2	5.6	7.0	9.0
73	3.0	3.5	4.0	4.5	5.9	7.5	9.6
77	3.2	3.7	4.2	4.8	6.3	8.0	10.2
82	3.4	4.0	4.5	5.0	6.7	8.4	10.8
86	3.6	4.2	4.7	5.3	7.0	8.9	11.4
91	3.8	4.4	5.0	5.6	7.4	9.4	12.0
95	4.0	4.6	5.2	5.9	7.8	9.9	12.6
100	4.2	4.8	5.5	6.2	8.2	10.3	13.2

Source: Adapted from *Fitness Leader's Handbook,* 2nd Edition (p. 133), B. D. Franks and E. T. Howley, Champaign, IL: Human Kinetics Publishers. Copyright 1998 by B. Don Franks and Edward T. Howley. Reprinted by permission.

3. Use full, deep, abdominal breathing to enhance relaxation and monitor your walking pace.

4. Hold your arms in a relaxed position with the elbows flexed at a 90-degree angle.

5. Form a slightly clenched, relaxed fist with your hands.

6. Swing your arms naturally back and forth to add power to each stride.

7. Begin each stride with a slight forward lean of your body at the ankles.

8. Make contact on the outer edge of your heel as your foot contacts the surface.

9. Roll your foot smoothly forward on impacting the surface, with most of your body weight distributed along the outer edge of the foot, transferring the weight to the ball of the foot and on to the toes for the pushoff.

10. Walk at a pace of 4.8–5.6 kilometres per hour for a comfortable workout.

11. Walk at a pace of 6 kilometres per hour for a vigorous workout.

12. Walk faster than 6.4 kilometres per hour if you are an advanced walker.

13. Walk on dirt trails or grass for a more comfortable workout than if you walked on concrete sidewalks.

14. Be cautious when walking on uneven surfaces such as grass or dirt because of the increased risk of ankle sprains.

15. Walk in shoes with a comfortable fit, a cushioned sole, and good arch support.

16. Wear loose-fitting clothing to allow freedom of movement and dissipation of heat.

17. Wear several layers of clothing in cold weather to slow down the rate of heat loss.

18. Wear a cap in cold weather to avoid heat loss through the scalp.

19. Wear cotton socks to avoid getting blisters and to absorb perspiration.

20. Warm up before, and cool down after, each walking session.

Sample Jogging/Running Program

Once you complete an advanced walking program, you may be ready for a jogging program. Some people find walking so enjoyable that it is their exercise of choice. If you are not excessively overweight and do not have any orthopedic problems, however, you may decide to increase your exercise intensity and begin jogging. If you have any congenital heart defects or metabolic and/or cardiorespiratory diseases, consult a physician before beginning a jogging program.

For purposes of changing body composition, increasing muscular endurance, and improving cardiorespiratory endurance, jogging is one of the most effective activities. The energy costs of running are greater than those of walking the same distance (see Tables 5.3 and 5.4). Thus, if you have reached a moderate to high level of fitness and want to increase your caloric expenditure but are unable to increase the amount of time you exercise, you should increase the exercise intensity by jogging instead of walking.

Table 5.4 ✦ Energy Costs of Jogging and Running (kcal/min)

BODY WEIGHT (kg)	KILOMETRES PER HOUR							
	4.8	6.4	8.0	9.7	11.3	12.9	14.5	16.1
50	4.7	5.9	7.2	8.5	9.8	11.1	12.3	13.6
54	5.1	6.4	7.9	9.3	10.6	12.1	13.4	14.8
59	5.5	7.0	8.6	10.1	11.5	13.1	14.6	16.1
64	5.9	7.5	9.2	10.8	12.4	14.1	15.7	17.3
68	6.4	8.1	9.9	11.6	13.3	15.1	16.8	18.5
73	6.8	8.6	10.5	12.4	14.2	16.1	17.9	19.8
77	7.2	9.1	11.2	13.1	15.1	17.1	19.1	21.0
82	7.6	9.7	11.8	13.9	15.9	18.1	20.2	22.2
86	8.1	10.2	12.5	14.7	16.8	19.1	21.3	23.5
91	8.5	10.8	13.2	15.4	17.1	20.1	22.4	24.7
95	8.9	11.3	13.8	16.2	18.6	21.1	23.5	25.9
100	9.3	11.8	14.5	17.0	19.5	22.2	24.7	27.2

Source: Adapted from *Fitness Leader's Handbook*, 2nd Edition (p. 134), B. D. Franks and E. T. Howley, Champaign, IL: Human Kinetics Publishers. Copyright 1998 by B. Don Franks and Edward T. Howley. Reprinted by permission.

Complete the most advanced level of a walking program before you begin a jogging program. This will allow adequate time for the development of your cardiorespiratory system and the strengthening of your ligaments and tendons to reduce the risk of injury. There are many options in beginning a jogging program depending on your initial level of fitness and prior exercise experience. Here are a few guidelines for jogging.

Duration In the initial phase of a jogging program, exercise for 15–30 minutes. During the session, alternate brief periods of slow jogging (approximately 8–10 km/h) with intervals of walking. Gradually increase the amount of time spent jogging and decrease walking time until you reach a level of fitness in which you can jog continuously for 30 minutes within your THR. As you reach an advanced level of running, exercise sessions may last as long as 60 minutes. Most people jog 3–5 kilometres per exercise session during the first 10 weeks of a jogging/ running program. When you can jog 5 kilometres comfortably within 27–30 minutes, you are probably ready to advance to a running program. More advanced runners can cover 8 kilometres per session within 35–40 minutes.

Intensity An important factor in a jogging/running program is monitoring your exercise heart rate. During the initial phase of your program, stay in the 60–75 percent THR zone. As you reach a higher level of fitness, you may increase exercise intensity to 70–85 percent. Remember that as your exercise intensity increases, you tend to exercise less because of an earlier onset of fatigue. Keep your THR in the moderate range in order to reap the double benefits of improving cardiorespiratory fitness and increasing the percentage of fat calories used. You will see changes in body-fat percentage more quickly by exercising at a moderate intensity (60–75 percent THR zone).

Frequency The optimal frequency for jogging is every other day. If you want to exercise every day, use walking as a form of exercise on alternate days in order to decrease the amount of stress on your hips and the joints of the legs and feet. Even runners who participate in road races seldom exercise seven days per week. They recognize the need to allow a rest period between workouts. If you want to increase total work done on a weekly basis, it is better to increase exercise duration gradually and to maintain a moderate exercise intensity with a frequency of 4–5 days per week instead of jogging 7 days per week.

Caloric Cost Table 5.4 shows one method of estimating the energy costs of jogging and running, expressed in units of kilocalories per minute. Let us consider the differences between walking and running for the same time periods.

If Joseph weighs 68 kilograms and jogs at 11.3 kilometres per hour for 45 minutes, he will burn 13.3 kilocalories per minute. His total energy expenditure is:

$$13.3 \ (\text{kcal/min}) \times 45 \ (\text{min}) = 599 \ \text{kcal}$$

If Carlos weighs 68 kilograms and jogs at 4.8 kilometres per hour for 45 minutes, he will burn 6.4 kilocalories per minute. His total energy expenditure is:

$$6.4 \ (\text{kcal/min}) \times 45 \ (\text{min}) = 288 \ \text{kcal}$$

These two young men, with similar body weights and exercise durations, but with different exercise intensities, had vastly different caloric expenditures. Joseph burned more than twice as many calories as Carlos did. And because Joseph was moving at a faster pace, he covered more distance and had a higher caloric expenditure.

Another explanation for the difference in their energy expenditures is that the caloric costs of walking a certain distance and running the same distance are not the same. Walking at speeds slower than 5.6 kilometres per hour requires approximately half the energy cost of running at speeds greater than 9.7 kilometres per hour. That is because more energy is required to lift the body from the ground when you are running than when you are moving the body forward on a horizontal plane as you do when you are walking. If a person walks at speeds of 8 kilometres per hour, the energy cost of walking and running is similar. That is because his or her exercise heart rate will probably be nearly as high walking at 8 kilometres per hour as it is when running at 9.7 kilometres per hour. Thus, the caloric costs are similar for walking at fast speeds and jogging at relatively slow speeds. Remember that walking at slow speeds expends half the calories as does jogging the same distance at faster speeds, but walking at fast speeds can expend the same number of calories as jogging.

Rate of Progression During the initial phase of a jogging program, you should combine walking and jogging. If you maintain a constant walking interval of 60 seconds, you can increase the jogging intervals until you are doing more jogging than walking. Always be careful to use exercise heart rate (EHR) as your guide for determining the jogging/walking intervals. As your fitness level increases, you should be able to jog for longer periods of time while remaining within your THR zone. Most people use 350–750 kilocalories per session in a jogging/running program.

Concentrate on slow, steady progress. As long as you are constantly increasing the total amount of calories used from your weekly workouts, remaining within your THR zone, and having no problems with injuries, you are probably working out at a suitable level.

After the first two months of a jogging program, you may notice that you do not seem to be improving as much as you expected. During this time, you might easily become discouraged and bored with your training program. That is when you might consider changing the intensity and duration of your workouts or training for a short road race. Alternatively, you can change your exercise route so that the environment becomes more exciting. Try running with a partner or listening to music while you jog. By changing the environment and increasing the amount of visual or auditory stimulation during the workout, you will find that time seems to pass more quickly, and you become less focused internally on your body and more focused on external factors. This shift in your attention away from your body may enable you to exercise for longer periods of time without becoming bored.

Sample Swimming Program

Swimming Swimming is an excellent aerobic activity. Patients in cardiac rehabilitation programs and in physical therapy often use a pool as their primary means of aerobic conditioning because of the decreased stress on hips, knees, and ankles that exercising in water affords. In addition, the warmer water temperatures of a pool are therapeutic for arthritic patients. Further, because body weight is supported, obese persons have fewer injuries while exercising in water. As a consequence, a growing number of people are choosing aquatic exercises as their primary mode of fitness. Because the cardiorespiratory benefits derived from water exercises are similar to those derived from jogging and cycling, consider including water exercises as a part of your training program.

Water Exercises Water aerobics are highly touted by exercise physiologists because they have virtually no adverse effects on the muscles and the skeletal system and are safe for people of all ages regardless of health status.

For years, water exercises were avoided because it was believed the water provided insufficient resistance to stimulate cardiorespiratory endurance. In reality, water is nearly 1000 times more dense than air and thus creates greater resistance. This increased resistance provides a higher workload for the muscles. We now know that the resistance of the water is sufficient to challenge even the most elite athlete, and an increase in cardiorespiratory fitness can easily be experienced by participating in water exercises.

An added benefit is that this cushioned medium promotes a virtually injury-free environment. The density of water gives almost any object placed in it a certain buoyancy. Your body will weigh less in water

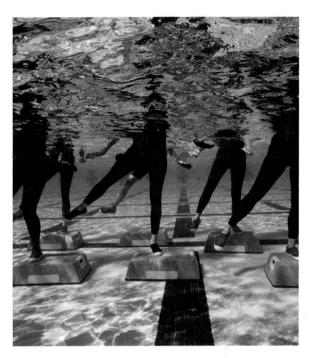

Water exercise places less stress on the body than many other exercises and is a great way for people of all ages to improve their cardiorespiratory fitness.

because of buoyancy, so less stress is placed on it when you exercise in water.

Obese people may especially enjoy exercising in water because it is much easier for them to dissipate heat. When you exercise, a great deal of heat is generated as a result of your metabolism. This heat is often difficult for an obese person to release because of the thick layer of fatty tissue underneath the skin. Heat is much easier to dissipate in water than it is in air, so the obese find exercising in water much more comfortable. One advantage water aerobics provides over jogging is that jogging does nothing to work the upper body, but water greatly increases strength and endurance in the upper body as well as the lower body. Here are guidelines to follow when you begin a water exercise program.

Duration Start at a comfortable level. This will vary depending on your initial level of fitness. If you are a swimmer but have been inactive for a long period of time, you may need to spend a few weeks walking across the width of the pool in chest-deep water until you can complete two 10-minute intervals at your EHR. Gradually alternate walking and jogging across the pool until you can complete four 5-minute intervals of jogging at your THR. As you progress, you can jog across the pool and swim back. Repeat this pattern until you can jog/swim for about 20–30 minutes. As your level of fitness increases, spend more time swimming and less time jogging until you can swim continuously for 20–30 minutes. Advanced swimmers can swim 30–45 minutes in each exercise session.

Intensity Research has shown that a person's maximal heart rate is approximately 10 beats lower in the water than it is on land. Thus, when women calculate their THR for water activities, use the formula 210 (rather than 220) minus your age to determine your maximal heart rate. From there, follow the standard formula for calculating your THR. During the initial phase of your swimming program, begin at a pace that keeps your heart rate at 50 percent of your THR zone. Gradually increase exercise duration and intensity as level of fitness increases, but be careful to remain within your heart rate zone.

Frequency As with other forms of aerobic exercise, you should swim 3–4 days per week. If you have trouble tolerating chlorinated pools, you can alternate swimming with other forms of aerobic exercise. You can also wear swimming goggles to protect your eyes from irritation.

Caloric Cost It is difficult to estimate the energy costs associated with swimming because there are vast differences between individuals in the efficiency of the stroke used. Table 5.5 shows the estimated caloric cost per kilometre of swimming the front crawl for men and women according to skill level. The values are expressed in units of kilocalories per kilometre. You may be surprised to find that the lower the skill level, the higher the energy expenditure for both men and women. That is because unskilled swimmers often fight the water and waste a lot of energy during each stroke. As the level of skill rises, however, the swimmer becomes more efficient and the caloric cost decreases. This might lead you to believe that less skilled swimmers will burn a lot more calories per workout than highly skilled swimmers will. This is not true. Less skilled swimmers exercise for a shorter period of time because they tire earlier than skilled swimmers do and will probably spend more time rest-

Table 5.5 ✦ Caloric Cost per Kilometre (kcal/km) of Swimming the Front Crawl for Men and Women, by Skill Level

SKILL LEVEL	WOMEN	MEN
Competitive	112	174
Skilled	162	224
Average	186	273
Unskilled	224	348
Poor	273	447

Source: Adapted from *Fitness Leader's Handbook,* 2nd Edition (p. 139), B. D. Franks and E. T. Howley, Champaign, IL: Human Kinetics Publishers. Copyright 1998 by B. Don Franks and Edward T. Howley. Reprinted by permission.

ing than actually swimming. For this reason, less skilled swimmers should use a combination of water exercises with swimming to increase their caloric expenditure.

Rate of Progression Unless you are a very good swimmer, you may become exhausted after swimming only one or two laps. Because continuous exercise is essential for improving cardiorespiratory fitness, begin with a walk/jog/swim program. As your level of aerobic conditioning increases and your swimming skills improve, you should be able to spend more time swimming and less time walking/jogging. It is not essential that you spend the entire workout actually swimming. You can easily achieve your EHR through other water exercises. As you begin your water aerobics program, follow these guidelines:

1. Always exercise in a supervised environment. It is possible to get muscle cramps in water, especially if you swim too soon after eating a meal. If you are exercising in chest-deep water, you could be in danger.

2. Exercise in water 5–8 centimetres above the waist. The depth of the water determines the amount of resistance experienced. When the water is too shallow, more stress is placed on the lower extremities. Conversely, when the water level is too high, buoyancy increases and less resistance results, making the exercises less effective.

3. Avoid excessive twisting in the water in order to minimize the risk of injury.

4. Wear cotton socks if the surface of the pool deck or bottom is rough to avoid scratching the soles of your feet.

5. Stand with your knees slightly bent, and avoid locking your joints.

6. Keep your arms in the water to generate more resistance. This helps raise the heart rate into the THR zone.

7. Cup your hands to increase the amount of resistance.

8. Use ankle weights to increase the intensity of lower-body workouts.

9. Use a stride stance (one foot forward, the other behind) to improve your balance in the water.

10. Use hand paddles, fins, pull buoys, and/or wrist weights to increase resistance.

11. Keep your pelvis tilted upward when you are doing lower-body exercises to help support the lower back.

12. Include warm-up exercises before and cool-down exercises after your water workout.

■ Sample Bicycling Program

Bicycling, or cycling, has become an increasingly popular aerobic activity especially for those who have joint problems or those who are overweight. For them, cycling is ideal because their weight is supported. Consequently, they can often exercise for longer periods of time. Today, stationary bikes are as popular as multispeed and mountain bikes are. Cycling has a high energy expenditure per minute and can result in tremendous increases in cardiorespiratory endurance and muscular strength and endurance.

Duration Each cycling session should last approximately 30–45 minutes. When you can cycle several kilometres within a 30-minute period, you have reached a high level of cardiorespiratory fitness.

Intensity When you are at the beginning of your cycling program, you may have to exercise below your THR in order to cycle 1.5–3 kilometres. After a few weeks of cycling this distance, however, you should be able to exercise at 60 percent of your THR zone. As you progress to cycling 5–8 kilometres, you may increase your exercise intensity to as high as 70–75 percent. Be careful to limit the intensity so that you can maintain your endurance. Once you reach a maximal level of fitness and can cycle 16–24 kilometres, you may increase your exercise intensity to 80 percent of your THR zone. A word of caution to those using stationary bikes: periodically check your resistance setting, because the workload tends to shift when you ride for long periods of time.

Frequency As with other forms of cardiorespiratory exercise, you should cycle 3–5 days per week. Bike on alternate days to allow adequate rest. During the first phase of a cycling program, bike a maximum of 3 days per week. Because cycling is not a familiar exercise to many people, they may experience more muscle soreness initially than they would with other activities such as walking.

Caloric Cost The type of bike you ride will affect the calories you expend. A person riding a multispeed bike can cover the same distance as a person riding a mountain bike and probably burn fewer calories, depending on which gear the bike is in. Thus, estimates of the caloric cost are approximations and may be less accurate than the estimates for activities such as walking and jogging.

Table 5.6 shows estimates for the caloric cost for cycling from 10 to 60 minutes for distances from 1.6 to 24 kilometres on a flat surface. To use the table, find the time closest to the number of minutes you cycle on the horizontal line. Then find the approximate distance in kilometres you cover on the vertical column. The number at the intersection represents an approximate caloric cost.

Table 5.6 ✦ Determining Caloric Cost for Bicycling

DISTANCE (KILOMETRES)	TIME (MIN)										
	10	15	20	25	30	35	40	45	50	55	60
1.6	.0705										
2.4	.0926	.0705									
3.2	.1367	.0860	.0705								
4.8		.1367	.0926	.0794	.0705						
6.4			.1367	.0970	.0860	.0771	.0705				
8.0			.2138	.1367	.0992	.0904	.0816	.0772	.0705		
9.7				.1940	.1367	.1036	.0926	.0860	.0794	.0750	.0705
11.3					.1786	.1367	.1080	.0948	.0882	.0838	.0794
12.9						.1720	.1367	.1102	.0970	.0904	.0860
14.5							.1675	.1367	.1124	.0992	.0926
16.1							.2138	.1631	.1367	.1124	.0992
17.7								.2050	.1609	.1367	.1146
19.3									.1940	.1587	.1367
21.0										.1852	.1565
22.5											.1786
24.0											.2138

Source: Adapted from Ivan Kusinitz and Morton Fine, *Your Guide to Getting Fit*, 2nd ed. (Mountain View, CA: Mayfield, 1991).

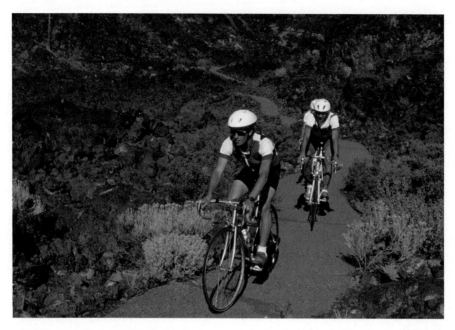

Begin a cycling exercise regimen by riding approximately 1–3 kilometres a session, increasing to 5–8 kilometres after several weeks.

For example, Anita weighs 84 kilograms and cycles 2.4 kilometres in 16 minutes. Her caloric expenditure is:

$$84 \text{ (kg)} \times 0.0705 \text{ (kcal/kg)} = 5.92 \times 16 \text{ min}$$
$$= 95 \text{ kcal expended}$$

Progressive Cycling Program Begin a cycling program by riding a few kilometres at a comfortable pace until your level of fitness increases to the point that you can train at the low end of your THR. Depending on your level of fitness, you may ride 1–3 kilometres per session for several weeks. Soon, you should be able to ride approximately 5–8 kilometres. Continue at this level for several weeks. Gradually add distance until you are able to cycle 16–24 kilometres each session. Depending on your rate of progression, you may be in a cycling program for six months or more before you can cycle continuously for 16–24 kilometres. Those who are very fit may need to ride faster than 20–24 kilometres per hour in order to reach their THR zone.

Rate of Progression As mentioned earlier, it is crucial to start at a comfortable pace in order to avoid injuries and extreme muscle soreness. It is better to increase the distance that you cycle instead of increasing your speed until you reach a high level of fitness. This will allow your body to adapt to this form of aerobic exercise. Do not be embarrassed to take rest periods during the early phases of your cycling program, and if you ride a multi-speed bike, switch gears periodically to lessen the resistance and make the ride a little easier. The key to a successful cycling program is to increase your total work gradually. Follow these guidelines when beginning your cycling program:

1. Adhere to all traffic rules and wear appropriate safety gear when you are cycling outdoors.

2. Adjust the seat height so that your knee has a slight bend when your foot is at the bottom of a pedal swing. This position gives you maximum power without creating stress on your spine.

3. Take precautions against saddle-soreness. Saddle-soreness occurs because of either chafing caused by friction on the skin of the buttocks or increased pressure on the genital area and the buttocks that causes pain and numbness. To avoid or minimize it, use corn starch or talcum powder. You may also consider purchasing a larger seat for the bicycle.

4. Wear cycling shorts padded by soft chamois sewn in the seat to increase the cushioning and reduce friction.

▪ Sample Rope-Skipping Program

On days when you cannot do outdoor aerobic activities or when you want to try a different form of aerobic conditioning, rope skipping is an excellent alternative. One factor that deters many exercisers from using this as their primary form of exercise is the amount of skill involved in turning and jumping. Because exercise needs to be continuous in order for you to achieve maximal cardiorespiratory benefits, you need to become proficient in jumping and turning. With practice, however, even a novice can become a good rope skipper.

It is important to purchase a rope of the correct length. The rope should be long enough to reach from armpit to armpit while it is passing under both feet. When the rope is too short, you are forced to jump in a humped position, and poor posture while exercising at high intensities causes increased strain on the back muscles. In addition, you need a good pair of exercise shoes because of the stress to the balls of your feet.

Duration Most beginners use an interval program consisting of brief periods of skipping followed by periods of rest. Unless you are already involved in a physical conditioning program, start with a beginning-level walking program to improve your level of fitness and strengthen your joints, tendons, and ligaments before you begin rope skipping. Because this exercise can cause fatigue in the arms, stretch before and after each session. Initially, the amount of time actually spent skipping may be small. As you continue exercising and your coordination improves, you will be able to increase the amount of time you spend skipping.

Intensity During the initial phase of a rope-skipping program, you may actually exercise at an intensity below your THR zone. Do not push too hard too soon. Rope skipping places constant stress on the bones in the feet and can cause trauma to them. As your level of fitness increases, you will be able to exercise at 65–75 percent of your THR. Avoid very high exercise intensities while rope skipping because of the stress to your hips, knees, ankles, and feet.

Rate of Progression Most beginners skip rope at 60 turns per minute. This is usually a comfortable pace that allows time for the beginner to develop coordination between turning and jumping. As you advance, you should be able to increase the number of turns to 70–100 per minute. Rope skipping can become boring, so, as your skill level increases, you may use tactics such as jumping on one foot or changing the direction of the rope to introduce variety into your program. If you have trouble with coordination, try jumping while you listen to music.

Frequency As with other forms of aerobic exercise, skip rope no more than three days per week on alternate days. Because a lot of stress is placed on the lower parts of the body, you may choose to alternate rope skipping with other forms of exercise to reduce the risk of injury. Water exercises are an especially good alternative because of the lack of stress to the joints.

Caloric Cost Table 5.7 shows the gross energy cost of rope skipping in units of kilocalories per minute. For example, Natasha weighs 50 kilograms and skips slowly for 20 minutes. Her estimated caloric expenditure is calculated as:

$$7.5 \text{ kcal/min} \times 20 \text{ min} = 150 \text{ kcal}$$

If Talinda also weighs 50 kilograms and skips at a fast pace for 20 minutes, her caloric expenditure would be:

$$9.2 \text{ kcal/min} \times 20 \text{ min} = 184 \text{ kcal}$$

Hence, these two women, who have the same body weight, would have different energy expenditures based on the speed of turning the rope.

Table 5.7 ✦ Gross Energy Cost of Rope Skipping (kcal/min)

BODY WEIGHT (kg)	SLOW SKIPPING	FAST SKIPPING
50	7.5	9.2
54	8.2	10.0
59	8.9	10.9
64	9.5	11.7
68	10.2	12.5
73	10.9	13.4
77	11.6	14.2
82	12.3	15.0
86	13.0	15.9
91	13.6	16.7
95	14.3	17.5
100	15.0	18.4

Source: Adapted from *Fitness Leader's Handbook*, 2nd Edition (p. 138), B. D. Franks and E. T. Howley, Champaign, IL: Human Kinetics Publishers. Copyright 1998 by B. Don Franks and Edward T. Howley. Reprinted by permission.

BEHAVIOURAL CHANGE AND MOTIVATIONAL STRATEGIES

Many factors might interfere with your ability to improve your cardiorespiratory fitness. Here are some barriers (roadblocks) and strategies for overcoming them.

Roadblock	Behavioural Change Strategy
You have been involved in an aerobic exercise program for four months and find that your motivation has decreased. You also have been walking the same exercise path for weeks and feel you need something new.	The simple answer is cross-training, which can help put the pizzazz back in your workout if you find your interest slipping after a few weeks or few months. Many regular exercisers use cross-training either to target different parts of their body or to add variety. Because it is an important motivation tool, it should be based on your individual needs and preferences. Some factors to consider when selecting activities are:

1. **Impact** Choose complementary workouts that provide different levels of impact in order to reduce risk of injury.
2. **Intensity** Alternate low- and higher-intensity workouts. You may consider a walking/cycling program.
3. **Location** Choose activities that take you to a variety of locations. Or alternate working out in a health club and a local public park.
4. **Weather** Consider choosing at least one indoor activity so that your workout schedule is not altered during periods of bad weather.
5. **Sociability** Find an activity in which you can participate with a partner. The buddy system is instrumental in increasing motivation for most individuals.
6. **Regularity** Always remember that it is okay to take a break from your workout routine periodically. You are more likely to enjoy yourself when your body and your mind are refreshed and relaxed.

Roadblock	Behavioural Change Strategy
You recently joined a health club but are dismayed because you find it difficult to gain access to the equipment. It seems as if "the regulars" have taken over and aren't too willing to accept a newcomer.	Health clubs are busy places, especially during peak hours (early mornings, noon, and early evenings). Most clubs post written rules for using the facility and the equipment. However, unwritten rules for behaviour simply boil down to one simple principle: Be considerate of others. Follow these guidelines in order to observe health club etiquette:

1. Put towels where they belong.
2. Use only one locker unless there are plenty available.
3. Limit your shower to five minutes tops when others are waiting.
4. Follow the flow of other exercisers when possible.
5. Be considerate of other individuals' time. Do not monopolize certain pieces of equipment. Remember, your favourite is probably theirs, too.
6. Don't interrupt exercisers while they are in the middle of a routine. Wait until they take a break.
7. Respect personal space. Learn to read other people. If someone obviously doesn't want to be disturbed, choose someone else to chat with.

Roadblock	Behavioural Change Strategy
You have been a regular aerobic excerciser for several years and find that exercise seems to consume your life. You have tried to decrease your time commitment but cannot seem to stop. Secretly, you fear that things are getting a little out of control.	It sounds as if you may be a victim of exercise addiction. If this is the case, consider seeking professional advice. Exercise addiction involves three classic characteristics: dependence, tolerance, and withdrawal. Signals of exercise addiction include: 1. Devoting less attention to interpersonal relationships. 2. Losing interest in work and other external issues relative to the gains made in your training program. 3. Exhibiting a pattern in which your feelings about your body and the euphoria from exercise become more important than anything else.
List other roadblocks preventing you from participating in a cardiorespiratory fitness program or factors hindering your progress in your current program. 1. _____ 2. _____ 3. _____	Now cite behavioural change strategies that can help you overcome these roadblocks. If you need to, refer to Chapter 3 for behavioural change and motivational strategies. 1. _____ 2. _____ 3. _____

Summary

Benefits of Cardiorespiratory Fitness

Many physiological benefits can be derived from participating in an aerobic fitness program, including a lower resting heart rate, a stronger heart, and a greater blood supply to exercising muscles. All these benefits will increase aerobic power and make exercise feel easier at workloads below maximum.

Anaerobic Energy Systems

The major energy systems in the body are the anaerobic and aerobic metabolism systems. The energy that is released when food is broken down in the body is used to manufacture adenosine triphosphate (ATP), which is either stored in small amounts in the muscles or manufactured through the process of metabolism.

The immediate energy system is composed of ATP and creatine phosphate (CP) stored in the muscles. This energy system is generally used for high-intensity activities that last less than 30 seconds. The lactic acid system is a second source of energy for anaerobic activities. It provides energy for high-intensity activities lasting from 30 seconds to two or three minutes.

Overview and Analysis of Aerobic Exercise Choices

Only aerobic exercises will increase your cardiorespiratory endurance. There are many options for aerobic activities, of which a number are not dependent on your having a high skill level. During the initial phase of your program, participate in activities that rely on large muscle groups to increase your endurance and minimize your risk of injury.

Maximal Oxygen Consumption (VO₂)

Cardiorespiratory endurance is synonymous with maximal oxygen consumption. The maximal oxygen uptake is influenced primarily by (1) the ability of the cardiorespiratory system to deliver oxygen to the muscles and (2) the ability of the muscles to extract oxygen from the blood. When comparing the fitness level of individuals, it is best to express the maximal oxygen uptake in units of $mL/kg \times min^{-1}$. Although the maximal oxygen uptake is best measured by gas analysis, field tests are often used to decrease the expense while still providing an accurate indication of aerobic fitness.

How to Begin and Progress in an Aerobic Fitness Program Safely

It is important to manipulate the exercise intensity, duration, and frequency to both (1) maintain the targeted amount of total work and (2) adjust to the schedule. If you have a busy week planned, you can easily manipulate these factors and still maintain your caloric expenditure. Avoid shin splints by wearing good running shoes, exercising on soft surfaces, and using a variety of aerobic exercise choices. Use the abdominal breathing technique to reduce the pain associated with the stitch-in-the-side phenomenon. Wear two pairs of cotton socks and place a bandage on hot spots to reduce blisters. When muscle soreness occurs, use light massage, static stretching, and light-intensity exercise to decrease pain and stiffness. Always maintain your level of hydration, and wear adequate clothing to avoid heat illness. Use PRICE as the immediate form of therapy for injuries.

Sample Starter Programs

Walking is one of the most popular aerobic activities because it does not require any specialized skills. When you start a walking program, begin walking 10–15 minutes per session at a comfortable pace at 50–60 percent of your THR 3–4 days per week. Gradually increase your rate of progression until you reach a distance of 8 kilometres. At this point, you may consider beginning a jogging program.

Complete the advanced walking program before beginning a jogging/running program. Gradually increase the amount of time spent jogging until you can jog continuously for 30–45 minutes. The average distance covered by more advanced runners is 8 kilometres per session within 35–40 minutes. During the initial phase, remain in the 65–75 percent THR zone. The optimal frequency is 3–4 days per week. Overuse can quickly result in injuries. To prevent injury, increase your distance before you increase your speed.

Swimming and water aerobics have increased in popularity because of the high rate of musculoskeletal injuries associated with other aerobic activities. The resistance in water is sufficient to elicit increased cardiorespiratory endurance while providing a virtually injury-free environment. If you are not a strong swimmer, begin with a walking program, and spend more time doing water exercises. As both your level of fitness and your swimming ability increase, you may make your total workout program one of swimming. The EHR is lower in water, so be careful to adjust for that.

Cycling is a great aerobic activity because your body weight is supported. Begin cycling a distance of 1–3 kilometres, even if you are exercising below your THR zone. Increase your intensity and duration until you can cycle 5–8 kilometres at 70–75 percent intensity. The type of bike used will affect caloric expenditure; thus, the caloric cost of cycling is difficult to estimate.

Rope skipping is too often avoided by aerobic exercisers because of the skill needed and the high amount of impact involved. Begin with brief periods of jumping followed by periods of rest. Complete a beginning walking program first in order to increase your level of fitness and decrease your risk of injury. Begin at 65–75 percent of your THR and exercise three days per week on alternate days. You may choose to participate concurrently in alternative aerobic activities, such as swimming, to experience a more rapid increase in cardiorespiratory fitness with little risk of injury.

STUDY QUESTIONS

1. Explain the different energy systems in the body as though you were explaining them to someone unfamiliar with body physiology.

2. Which variables do you "manipulate" in any exercise program? How do you manipulate them and for what reasons?

3. Larceny Wipsnade, a 37-year-old accountant and ex-university football player, is 12 kilograms over his ideal body weight. Larceny has done very little exercise since his football-playing days. Assuming that fat loss is Larceny's immediate exercise goal, outline a suitable 15-week starter exercise program for him.

4. Explain the concept of cardiorespiratory fitness in terms of your own cardiorespiratory level.

5. What does DOMS mean?

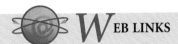 WEB LINKS

The Heart and Stroke Foundation of Ontario
www.hsfope.org

Health Canada's Heart Health
www.hc-sc.gc.ca/hppb/ahi/hearthealth/index.html

Heart and Stroke Foundation of Canada
ww1.heartandstroke.ca/

Health Canada's Healthy Heart Kit
**www.hc-sc.gc.ca/hppb/ahi/healthyheartkit/
healthyheartkit.htm**

Heart Information Network
www.heartinfo.org

Health Canada's Active Living Guides
**www.hc-sc.gc.ca/english/lifestyles/
physical_activity.html**

Health Canada's Cardiovascular Disease Division
www.hc-sc.gc.ca/hpb/lcdc/bcrdd/cardio/index.html

Lab Activity 5.1

Assessing Your Level of Aerobic Fitness by the 4.8-Kilometre Walking Test

INSTRUCTIONS: *This test is designed for older adults or for those who are just beginning an aerobic conditioning program. The time of the walk and the postexercise heart rate value are used to predict the subject's maximal oxygen consumption.*

✦ Step 1: Pretest Screening

1. If you are over age 35, seek the advice of your physician before taking this test.

2. Do not eat or drink anything except water for at least three hours before taking the test.

3. Avoid using any type of tobacco, including cigarettes and chewing tobacco, for at least three hours before taking this test.

4. Avoid heavy physical activity on the day of the test.

5. If you are on medication, report it to your instructor before you begin this test.

6. Wear loose-fitting clothes, such as shorts and a T-shirt, and running shoes.

✦ Step 2: Administration of the Test

1. Participants divide into two groups.

2. Each participant in the first group should choose a partner from the other group.

3. Those taking the test first complete a thorough warm-up session and slowly walk one lap around the track.

4. The partners maintain a scorecard that records time in minutes and seconds and keeps track of the number of laps walked.

5. The instructor explains the procedures (such as the fact that the faster the participants walk, the higher their level of cardiorespiratory fitness will be) and instructs the first group to begin.

6. The students walk the whole distance as fast as possible, and only walking is allowed.

7. As walkers complete each lap, the partners let them know how many laps remain and encourage them to maintain a steady pace.

8. The instructor calls out the time in minutes and seconds periodically.

9. The partners write the final time on the scorecard.

(continued)

Lab Activity 5.1 *(continued)*
Assessing Your Level of Aerobic Fitness by the 4.8-Kilometre Walking Test

10. The partners immediately take the walkers' 10-second heart rate. Instruct the walkers that the heart rate count should be completed within 15 seconds after the end of the walk. Any further time delay will result in an overestimation of the maximal oxygen consumption.

11. After all walkers in the first group have finished, the second group of walkers takes the test while the first group act as partners.

✦ **Step 3: Interpretation of the Results**

1. Tables A and B on pp. 113–114 contain the estimated maximal oxygen uptake (mL/kg $\times$ min^{-1}) for women and men ages 20–39 based on the test.

2. To use the tables, find the section that pertains to your age and sex. On the horizontal line across the top, find the amount of time (to the nearest minute) it took to walk the 4.8 kilometres. In the vertical column, find the point of intersection for your walking time and your postexercise heart rate (listed in the far left column). The number where the postexercise heart rate and the 4.8-kilometre time intersect is your maximal oxygen consumption expressed in mL/kg $\times$ min^{-1}. For example, a 34-year-old woman who walked the distance in 17 minutes and had a postexercise heart rate of 170 would have an estimated oxygen consumption of 17.3 mL/kg $\times$ min^{-1}.

3. Review Table 5.2 to obtain an estimate of your maximal aerobic power based on your performance in this test.

✦ **Step 4: Cardiorespiratory Endurance Record**

Name _____ Date _____

Age _____ Sex _____ Body weight _____

Walking time _____ Fitness category _____

Maximal VO$_2$ (mL/kg $\times$ min^{-1})

_____

Table A ✦ Estimated Maximal Oxygen Uptake (mL/kg × min⁻¹) for Women, 20 to 39 Years Old

HEART RATE	MINUTES PER KILOMETRE										
	10	*11*	*12*	*13*	*14*	*15*	*16*	*17*	*18*	*19*	*20*
Women (20–29)											
120	38.8	36.8	34.8	32.7	30.7	28.6	26.6	24.6	22.5	20.4	18.4
130	37.9	35.8	33.8	31.8	29.7	27.6	25.6	23.6	21.5	19.5	17.4
140	36.9	34.8	32.8	30.8	28.7	26.7	24.6	22.6	20.6	18.5	16.4
150	35.9	33.9	31.8	29.8	27.8	25.7	23.6	21.6	19.6	17.5	15.5
160	34.9	32.9	30.8	28.8	26.8	24.7	22.7	20.6	18.6	16.6	14.5
170	33.9	31.9	29.9	27.8	25.8	23.8	21.7	19.6	17.6	15.6	13.5
180	32.9	30.9	28.9	26.8	24.8	22.8	20.7	18.7	16.6	14.6	12.6
190	32.0	29.9	27.9	25.9	23.8	21.8	19.8	17.7	15.6	13.6	11.6
200	31.0	28.9	26.9	24.9	22.8	20.8	18.8	16.7	14.7	12.6	10.6
Women (30–39)											
120	36.4	34.4	32.3	30.3	28.3	26.2	24.2	22.1	20.1	18.1	16.0
130	35.4	33.4	31.3	29.3	27.3	25.3	23.2	21.1	19.1	17.1	15.0
140	34.4	32.4	30.4	28.3	26.3	24.3	22.2	20.2	18.1	16.1	14.1
150	33.4	31.4	29.4	27.4	25.3	23.3	21.3	19.2	17.1	15.1	13.1
160	32.5	30.4	28.4	26.4	24.3	22.3	20.3	18.2	16.2	14.1	12.1
170	31.5	29.4	27.4	25.4	23.4	21.3	19.3	17.3	15.2	13.1	11.1
180	30.5	28.5	26.4	24.4	22.4	20.3	18.3	16.3	14.2	12.2	10.1
190	29.6	27.5	25.5	23.4	21.4	19.4	17.3	15.3	13.3	11.2	9.1

Calculations assume a body weight of 56.7 kilograms for women. For each 6.8 kilograms beyond that, subtract 1 mL from the estimated maximal oxygen uptake given in the table.

Source: Adapted from *Fitness Leader's Handbook*, 2nd Edition (pp. 76–78), B. D. Franks and E. T. Howley, Champaign, IL: Human Kinetics Publishers. Copyright 1998 by B. Don Franks and Edward T. Howley. Reprinted by permission.

(continued)

Lab Activity 5.1 *(continued)*
Assessing Your Level of Aerobic Fitness by the 4.8-Kilometre Walking Test

Table B ✦ Estimated Maximal Oxygen Uptake (mL/kg × min^{-1}) for Men, 20 to 39 Years Old

	MINUTES PER KILOMETRE										
HEART RATE	10	11	12	13	14	15	16	17	18	19	20
Men (20–29)											
120	40.6	38.6	36.5	34.5	32.4	30.4	28.4	26.3	24.3	22.3	20.2
130	39.6	37.6	35.6	33.5	31.4	29.4	27.4	25.4	23.3	21.3	19.3
140	38.6	36.6	34.6	32.5	30.5	28.4	26.4	24.4	22.3	20.3	18.3
150	37.7	35.6	33.6	31.6	29.5	27.4	25.4	23.4	21.4	19.3	17.3
160	36.7	34.6	32.6	30.6	28.5	26.5	24.4	22.4	20.4	18.3	16.3
170	35.7	33.7	31.6	29.6	27.6	25.5	23.5	21.4	19.4	17.4	15.3
180	34.8	32.7	30.6	28.6	26.6	24.6	22.5	20.4	18.4	16.4	14.3
190	33.8	31.7	29.7	27.6	25.6	23.6	21.5	19.5	17.4	15.4	13.4
200	32.8	30.8	28.7	26.7	24.6	22.6	20.6	18.5	16.4	14.4	12.4
Men (30–39)											
120	38.2	36.1	34.1	32.1	30.0	28.0	25.9	23.9	21.9	19.8	17.8
130	37.2	35.2	33.1	31.1	29.1	27.0	24.9	22.9	20.9	18.8	16.8
140	36.3	34.2	32.1	30.1	28.1	26.0	24.0	21.9	19.9	17.9	15.8
150	35.3	33.2	31.2	29.1	27.1	25.1	23.0	20.9	18.9	16.9	14.9
160	34.3	32.3	30.2	28.1	26.1	24.1	22.0	20.0	17.9	15.9	13.9
170	33.3	31.3	29.2	27.2	25.1	23.1	21.1	19.0	16.9	14.9	12.9
180	32.3	30.3	28.3	26.2	24.1	22.1	20.1	17.6	16.0	13.9	11.9
190	31.3	29.3	27.3	25.2	23.2	21.1	19.1	17.1	15.0	13.0	10.9

Calculations assume a body weight of 77.1 kilograms for men. For each 6.8 kilograms beyond that, subtract 1 mL from the estimated maximal oxygen uptake given in the table.

Source: Adapted from *Fitness Leader's Handbook,* 2nd Edition (pp. 76–78), B. D. Franks and E. T. Howley, Champaign, IL: Human Kinetics Publishers. Copyright 1998 by B. Don Franks and Edward T. Howley. Reprinted by permission.

Lab Activity 5.2

Assessing Your Level of Aerobic Fitness by the 12-Minute Run Test

INSTRUCTIONS: *The objective of the test is to cover the greatest possible distance in a 12-minute period. It should be performed on a track or any other course that has been accurately measured.*

✦ **Step 1: Pretest Screening**

1. If you are over 35 years of age, seek the advice of your physician before taking this test.

2. Do not eat or drink anything except water for at least three hours before taking the test.

3. Avoid using any type of tobacco, including cigarettes and chewing tobacco, for at least three hours before taking the test.

4. Avoid heavy physical activity on the day of the test.

5. If you are on medication, report it to your instructor before you begin the test.

6. Wear loose-fitting clothes, such as shorts and a T-shirt, and running shoes.

✦ **Step 2: Administration of the Test**

1. Participants divide into two groups.

2. Each participant in the first group should choose a partner from the other group.

3. Those taking the test first complete a thorough warm-up session and slowly walk one lap around the track.

4. The partners maintain a scorecard that records the distance covered during the 12-minute period.

5. The instructor explains the procedures again and instructs the first group to begin.

6. As runners complete each lap, the partners let them know how much time remains and encourage them to maintain a steady pace.

7. The instructor uses a stopwatch or wristwatch to accurately mark off a 12-minute period.

8. The instructor calls out the time in minutes and seconds periodically.

9. The partners write the distance run in 12 minutes in fractions of a kilometre.

10. After all individuals in the first group have finished, the second group takes the test while the first group acts as partners.

(continued)

Lab Activity 5.2 *(continued)*
Assessing Your Level of Aerobic Fitness by the 12-Minute Run Test

✦ **Step 3: Interpreting the Results**

1. Table C contains five fitness classifications based on age and sex.

2. To use the table, find on the horizontal line the age of the individual and the distance covered in 12 minutes. Then locate on the vertical column the fitness category, according to sex.

3. For example, if you are an 18-year-old female and you covered 4 kilometres in 12 minutes, you are in the "high performance zone."

Table C ✦ Fitness Classification for Men and Women, Ages 17–50+

CLASSIFICATION (km)	MEN (AGE)			
	17–26	*27–39*	*40–49*	*50+*
High performance zone	2.88+	2.56+	2.40+	2.24+
Good fitness zone	2.48–2.86	2.32–2.54	2.24–2.38	2.00–2.22
Marginal zone	2.16–2.46	2.08–2.30	2.00–2.22	1.76–1.98
Low zone	<2.16	<2.08	<2.00	<1.76
	WOMEN (AGE)			
	17–26	*27–39*	*40–49*	*50+*
High performance zone	2.32+	2.16+	2.00+	1.84+
Good fitness zone	2.00–2.30	1.92–2.14	1.84–1.98	1.68–1.82
Marginal zone	1.84–1.98	1.68–1.90	1.60–1.82	1.52–1.66
Low zone	<1.84	<1.68	<1.60	<1.50

✦ **Step 4: Cardiorespiratory Endurance Record**

Name _____   Date _____

Age _____ Sex _____   Body weight _____

Distance covered _____   Fitness category _____

6

Improving Muscular Strength and Endurance

CHAPTER OBJECTIVES

By the end of this chapter, you should be able to:

1. Identify the factors that directly or indirectly affect muscular strength and endurance.

2. Cite the advantages of acquiring and maintaining adequate muscular strength and endurance throughout life.

3. Design a personalized strength-development program using weights that applies sound training principles and meets your fitness objectives.

4. Design a personalized muscular-endurance training program without weights that applies sound training principles and meets your fitness objectives.

5. Complete a strength and endurance routine using one of the methods described in this chapter.

6. Design a sound girth-control program to flatten your stomach.

ESTHER HAS BEEN interested in trying some form of strength training for years to firm her muscles and improve her appearance. She is also interested in it because she has heard that this type of training aids weight and fat loss. Some of her friends who use the weight room at the gym seem to have improved their bodies and are looking good. Esther wants to get started, too, but she has many questions and concerns. What type of program should she choose? How often should she work out? Should she use heavy or light weights? Will she add too much muscle and lose her femininity?

The answers to these and many more questions are provided in this chapter to help Esther and you implement sound strength-training programs designed to meet your personal objectives.

Although muscular strength and endurance are closely related, it is important to differentiate between the two. *Muscular strength* is the amount of force or weight a muscle or group of muscles can exert for one repetition. It is generally measured by a single maximal contraction. The amount of weight you can bench-press overhead one time, for example, measures the strength of the triceps muscle. You can measure the strength of other muscle groups the same way with specific tests (see Chapter 2). *Muscular endurance* is the capacity of a muscle group to complete an uninterrupted series of repetitions as often as possible with lighter weights. The total number of bench presses you can complete with one-half of your maximum weight on the barbell, for example, measures the endurance of the triceps and pectoralis muscles. Depending on the desired outcome, you can manipulate the training variables (choice of equipment and exercises, amount of resistance or weight, number of repetitions and sets, length of rest intervals) to make your program strength- or endurance-oriented or a balance of both.

This chapter addresses the key components in the development of strength and endurance, including importance, influencing factors, training principles, specific exercises, equipment, girth control, and other related concerns.

THE IMPORTANCE OF STRENGTH AND ENDURANCE

The improvement of muscular strength and endurance will affect almost every phase of your life. Some of the benefits, such as the loss of body fat and improved self-concept, have been overlooked in the past because of overemphasis on adding muscle mass and improving performance. A closer look at the true value of strength and endurance training makes it clear that a sound program can help to improve both physical and mental health. Begin by completing Lab Activity 6.1: Do You Need to Start a Strength-Training Program? to determine whether you need to begin a strength-training program.

■ The Management of Body Weight and Fat

Although strength training is generally associated with muscle-weight gain and not with body weight and fat loss, it is a critical part of a total weight-control program.

> **Basal metabolism** The minimum energy the body needs to support ongoing cellular activity when the body is at rest; work that goes on continuously without your awareness.

Unfortunately, metabolism slows with age and the amount of calories (cal) we consume does not. As a result, body weight and fat increase and the amount of lean muscle mass decreases.

Basal metabolism goes down about 3 percent per decade, mainly due to the loss of muscle mass. This occurs because inactive adults lose about 227 grams of muscle mass per year and gain about the same amount of fat. From age 20 to 60, a decrease in resting metabolism of 12 percent or more occurs and is a major contributor to weight and fat gain. The typical 60-year-old, for example, burns approximately 280 fewer calories daily at rest than that individual burned at age 20. This is equivalent to 457 grams of fat (= 3500 cal) every 12–13 days, nearly 1.4 kilograms per month, and about 16.8 kilograms per year. As you can see, even small decreases in metabolism produce large increases in body weight and fat. A 5 percent slowing of resting metabolism can add 2.7–4 kilograms of body fat in just one year depending on a person's weight and size at the time (see Chapters 8 and 9 for details on resting metabolism and weight loss). A comparison of two individuals identical in weight, one with 4.5 kilograms more muscle than the other, clearly shows that the resting metabolism is significantly higher in the more muscled individual. According to some experts, resting metabolism increases by approximately 30–40 calories per day for every 454 grams of muscle weight added. In other words, you burn enough extra calories at rest to lose 1.4–1.8 kilograms per year for every 454 grams of muscle mass you add.

Experts are fairly certain that by age 60, the amount of body fat you possess is directly related to the amount of time you spend exercising. The more active you are, the more lean you will be at any age. Thus, training with weights is crucial for both men and women as they age. Even as few as two weight-training sessions per week can significantly improve muscle mass and bone health. When you engage in weight training three times per week, the number of calories needed to maintain your weight increases by about 15 percent. The ideal exercise program for the management of body weight and fat throughout life would include aerobic exercise three to four times per week and three half-hour strength-training sessions every other day, coupled with sound nutrition.

■ Improved Appearance, Body Image, and Self-Concept

Muscular-strength and -endurance training can improve your physical appearance. By reducing your caloric intake, losing body fat and weight, improving muscle tone, and adding muscle weight, you will look and feel better.

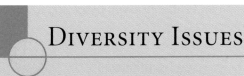

DIVERSITY ISSUES

Fitness, Strength, and Endurance for All Ages

In 1959, the Duke of Edinburgh delivered some disturbing news to members of the Canadian Medical Association (CMA). He suggested that Canadians of all ages had fitness deficiencies. This public berating seemed to prompt Canada to take action. With less than one-sixth of Canadians falling into the "physically fit" category, we had nowhere to go but up.

Two results of the Duke's comments were government initiatives such as Bill C-131 (*An Act to Encourage Fitness and Amateur Sport*) and the monumental conference between the CMA and the Canadian Association for Health, Physical Education, and Recreation in March 1961. The latter highlighted the importance of more research focusing on the currently unknown impacts of fitness on disease, well-being, growth, and development.

Today—in part due to government advocacy, the funding of physical fitness research agendas, and overall concern for our country's health—Canadians have a much better fitness profile than in the early 1960s. With over 13 million active on a regular basis, we have certainly become more aware of the importance of physical training, including strength and endurance training, for optimal health.

Strength training, particularly in its most popular form, weight training, has traditionally been a man's activity at all age levels. Unfortunately, boys, girls, men, and women are equally in need of this key aspect of a complete fitness program. Studies continue to indicate that elementary-school-aged children of both sexes are extremely weak in the upper body and the abdominal area.

For some time, it was thought that strength training for children was a dangerous idea—that isokinetic and isotonic exercises would be too taxing for their delicate skeletal frame and musculature. But numerous studies have demonstrated that moderate strength training can increase the muscular strength and endurance of children without increasing their risk of injury. It is necessary for the child, prior to participating in such a program, to receive proper explanations, demonstrations, and supervision by an adult qualified to develop and monitor low-to-moderate-intensity programs. ✦

Sources: American College of Sports Medicine. *ACSM's Guideline for Exercise Testing and Prescription,* 6th Edition. Philadelphia: Lippincott, Williams & Wilkins, 2000; V. G. Payne, J. R. Morrow, Jr., L. Johnson, and S. N. Dalton, "Resistance Training in Children and Youth: A Meta-analysis," *Research Quarterly for Exercise and Sport* 68, 1 (1997): 80–88.

When you lose weight too rapidly, particularly without exercise, your skin gives the appearance of not fitting your body very well. Sagging skin on the back of the arms, for example, is often an indication of either too rapid or too large an amount of weight loss. With reduced caloric intake, fat cells shrink, but the skin does not keep pace to provide a tight fit. One way to improve your appearance and help your skin fit better during and after weight loss is to include strength training as part of your total program. As fat cells shrink in the back of your arms, for example, strength training can enlarge the triceps muscle tissue and reduce sagging skin.

Keep in mind that these changes will not occur overnight. Depending on your age and current physical state, it may take 12 months or more of regular aerobic exercise, strength and endurance training, and dietary management of calories for you to decrease your total body fat significantly, add 2–6 kilograms of muscle weight, tone your entire body, give your skin sufficient time to rebound to a tight fit, and adjust to your new body. These changes will alter the way you both perceive yourself and feel others perceive you. Practically everyone who stays with a program experiences improved body image and self-concept that positively affects their personal and professional lives. Patience is necessary, however; proper nutrition and exercise, rather than diets, are meant to be lifetime activities.

▶ Increased Bone-Mineral Content

Recent studies suggest that regular strength training aids in optimal bone development by improving bone-mineral content. The use of strength training in addition to weight-bearing exercise, such as walking, jogging, racquet sports, and aerobic dance, may help women reach menopause with more bone-mineral mass, an important factor in the prevention or delay of osteoporosis (see Chapter 14).

Increased Strength and Endurance ▶ for Work and Daily Activities

Each of the training programs discussed in this chapter will effectively increase both muscular strength and endurance in the relatively short period of 8–12 weeks.

For example, if you are in the process of moving or helping a friend move, you will notice an improvement in your ability to lift furniture and other heavy objects without undue fatigue. Additional strength and endurance will also help you perform daily personal and work activities more efficiently and provide you with the extra strength needed to cope with unexpected emergencies in life.

Improved Performance in Sports and Recreational Activities

Children and adults often lack strength and endurance in the upper body (arms and shoulders) and in the abdominal area. Many studies also show that most women are weak in the arms and shoulders because they think strength training will cause a loss of femininity—a totally unfounded fear. It is important to recognize that individualized, safe weight-training programs can be designed for both sexes at all ages and that these programs will improve muscular strength and endurance in the upper body, stomach, lower back, and other areas with little or no health risk or change in femininity. Increased upper-body and abdominal strength and endurance also helps to improve physical appearance and self-concept. Weight training also helps children and young adults to perform better in a wide variety of sports such as tumbling, gymnastics, baseball, basketball, field hockey, touch football, and soccer. You will also notice a difference when you participate in an aerobic exercise or dance class, a conditioning class, or your favourite recreational activity. The additional

---

Muscle fibres Bundles of tissue composed of cells.

Myofibrils Thin protein filaments that interact and slide past one another during a muscle contraction.

Tendon The fibrous, inelastic band that attaches some muscles to the bones so that they move when the muscles contract.

Slow-twitch, oxidative muscle fibre Red muscle fibre used in aerobic activity that contracts and tires slowly.

Fast-twitch, glycolytic muscle fibre White muscle fibre used in anaerobic activity that contracts rapidly and explosively but tires quickly because it has a poor blood supply.

Fast-twitch, oxidative, glycolytic fibre An intermediate fibre that can be used in both anaerobic and aerobic activity.

---

strength and endurance will delay fatigue and make free movement easier.

Decreased Incidence of Sports- and Work-Related Injuries

Improved muscle strength surrounding the joints helps prevent injuries to your muscles, tendons, and ligaments. With regular training, bones and connective tissue become stronger and more dense. These changes make you less vulnerable to muscle strain, sprains, contusions, and tears (see Chapter 12 for more details). Even lower-back pain may be prevented by improved strength and flexibility in the abdominal and back extensor muscles.

Strength training is also an important part of recovery following certain injuries. A return to normal range of motion and strength following soft-tissue injuries occurs more rapidly and completely with rehabilitative strength training.

FACTORS AFFECTING MUSCULAR STRENGTH AND ENDURANCE

Muscle Structure

A cross-section of various parts of a muscle is shown in Figure 6.1. Each muscle contains bundles of tissue composed of cells known as **muscle fibres**. A muscle fibre is composed of contractile units called **myofibrils**.

The entire muscle, consisting of the bundles and the muscle fibres, is covered and bound together by layers of connective tissue that blend together to form **tendons** at either end of the muscle. When you contract your bicep, for example, the muscle shortens with the force moving through the tendon to the bones to bend the elbow.

Types of Muscle Fibre

The three types of muscle fibre contained in each muscle in the body can be classified by two factors: (1) the speed with which they contract and (2) their main energy system (see Figure 6.2). **Slow-twitch, oxidative fibre** is used primarily in aerobic endurance activities such as jogging, marathon running, and cycling. These fibres contract slowly but are also slow to fatigue because of their tremendous vascular supply. **Fast-twitch, glycolytic fibre** is used primarily for explosive anaerobic movements such as sprinting, jumping, and throwing. They contract explosively and tire rapidly. **Fast-twitch, oxidative, glycolytic fibre** has a speed of contraction faster than that of slow-twitch, oxidative fibre but slower than that of fast-twitch, glycolytic fibre, and fatigue occurs much more slowly than with the fast-twitch, glycolytic fibre.

Figure 6.1 ✦ The Structure of Muscle. The whole muscle (a) is composed of separate bundles of individual muscle fibres (b). Each fibre is composed of numerous myofibrils (c), each of which contains thin protein filaments (d) arranged so they can slide past one another to cause muscle shortening or lengthening. Various layers of connective tissue surround the muscle fibres, bundles, and whole muscles, which eventually bind together to form the tendon.

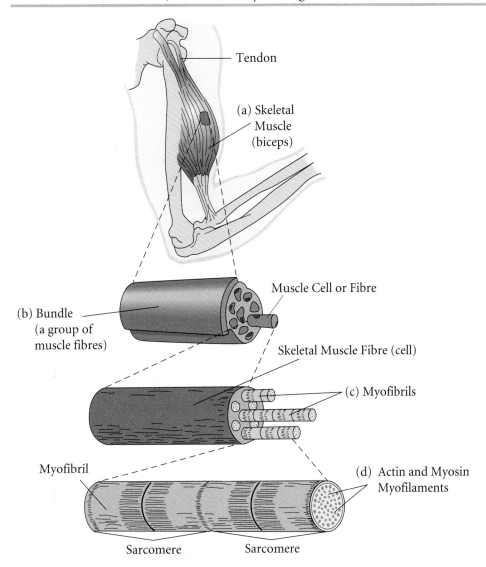

◼ How Muscles Become Larger and Stronger

The capability of a muscle or muscle group to generate force for one maximum repetition depends on such factors as size, type, number of muscle fibres activated, and ability of the nervous system to activate these fibres. Although your strength potential is limited by genetics and the number and size of fast-twitch fibres, everyone can improve strength with proper training. As training progresses, muscle cells will increase in size (particularly the fast-twitch fibres), the myofibrils in each cell may increase in number, and the connective tissue around muscle fibres and bundles of muscle may also thicken. These three factors will significantly increase the size of a muscle in 8–10 weeks. Women generally progress at almost the same rate as men do, and also experience significant increases in cell size after engaging in a sound weight-training program.

You can improve your muscular endurance by training both types of fast-twitch fibre by increasing the number of repetitions and by using lower weight. As training progresses, you will be capable of performing a greater number of repetitions for each exercise.

Figure 6.2 ✦ Muscle Fibre Types. SO is the slow-twitch, oxidative fibre; FOG is the fast-twitch, oxidative, glycolytic fibre; and FG is the fast-twitch, glycolytic fibre.

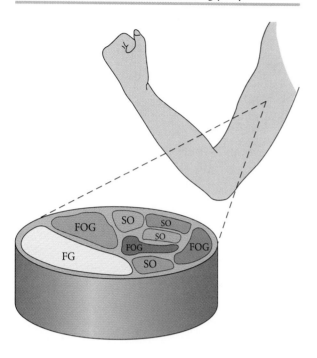

STRENGTH-TRAINING PRINCIPLES

The training principles discussed in this section will help you design a program to meet your specific needs. First, consult Table 6.1 and choose a primary training objective. This table allows you to approximate the weight and number of sets and repetitions needed to fit your training objectives. The following basic principles apply to any strength-training program:

1. Heavy weight and low repetitions (three to six) develop considerably more strength and muscle mass than endurance. Your starting weight for each exercise should be about 80 percent of your 1-RM (maximum amount of weight you can lift one time). For example, if your maximum lift on the bench press is 50 kilograms, your starting weight is 45 kilograms (50 × 0.80).

2. The closer you work to the 1-RM, the greater the strength gains. Unfortunately, the chance of injury increases with added weight, so this approach is somewhat impractical.

3. Heavy weight, a moderate number of repetitions (three to five), and multiple sets are more effective in adding muscle weight (mass).

4. Light weights and a high number of repetitions develop muscular endurance more than strength.

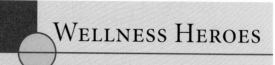

WELLNESS HEROES

David Patchell-Evans

At the age of eight, David Patchell-Evans lost his father to a chronic illness complicated by an accident. That loss magnified an already-determined personality. He decided that with his bike and a little conditioning, he would deliver newspapers in the hilly areas of Toronto and that not just one route, but three would be the most profitable.

Ten years later, in his first year at university, David seriously injured the whole right side of his body in a motorcycle accident. Temporarily paralyzed and with his body cantilevered to one side, he underwent rehabilitation over the next six months. During that time, he became intrigued by the exercise potential of the Nautilus equipment utilized in his physiotherapy recovery-work. He changed his academic goal from a business degree to one in kinesiology. To raise funds for his career goals, David set up his own snowplow business, often working all night while in full-time studies. Three years later, he opened his first fitness facility in London, Ontario, which he named #1 Nautilus and later renamed GoodLife Fitness Clubs. Within ten years, he had parlayed his fitness empire into some 42 clubs, the largest fitness chain in Canada, and become a multimillionaire in the process.

Shortly after his 32nd birthday, David was diagnosed with a potentially crippling form of rheumatoid arthritis. Armoured with a strong belief in the functional benefits of exercise, he worked hard on his personal fitness and mobility to alleviate the devastating effects of his condition. Even when advised by doctors not to exercise, he elected to follow his own lifestyle advice and maintained a very strong physical activity pattern.

Today, he is a five-time Canadian rowing champion, has competed in the Boston Marathon, and is a triathlete who works out regularly and favours mountain climbing and helicopter skiing for his vacations.

David currently runs 70 clubs and his business goal is to have 100 clubs by the year 2004 by opening new clubs and finding franchisees among his competitors. His philosophy is to make some sort of fitness routine available to all people, from manual labourers to home-care-givers to business executives, through convenient and accessible clubs. David Patchell-Evans is truly a person who practises the lifestyle he preaches, and his contribution to wellness in Canada is of paramount significance. ✦

Sources: Personal interview; "Bulking Up," *London Free Press,* March 22, 1999; Today's Health Club News. GoodLife rebranding. December 11, 2002.

Table 6.1 ✦ Strength- and Endurance-Training Objectives and Variable Control

DESIRED PHYSICAL OUTCOMES	VARIABLE CONTROL
Strength and power	Heavy weight (3-RM or 80% of 1-RM), low repetitions (6 or less), slow negative phase, multiple sets (3–5), moderate rest between each set and exercise (90 sec), use of maximum lift days
Muscular endurance	Light weight (10-RM), high repetitions (15–20), slow negative phase, multiple sets (2–3), minimum rest between each set and exercise (2 min decreasing to 30 sec)
Strength and endurance/general body development/improved athletic performance	Moderate weight (6-RM), moderate repetitions (6–9), slow negative phase, multiple sets (2–3), moderate rest between each set and exercise (1 min)
Muscle mass or bulk	Heavy weight (3- to 5-RM), low repetitions, multiple sets (5–10), minimum rest between sets and exercises (1 min), use of large number of different exercises for each muscle group and of periodization (2-to-3-week cycles that alter resistance, repetitions, and sets from low through moderate to high)
Speed and explosive power	Moderate weight (5-RM), low repetitions (3–5), explosive contractions, slow negative phase, use of Olympic power lifts
Rehabilitation from injury	Light weight and slow contractions performed without pain and to full range of motion, 6–10 repetitions, 3 sets, and use of exercises that activate supporting muscles of joints (ankle, wrist, knee, shoulder)

5. From a health standpoint, using 6-RM as the starting weight and progressing to nine repetitions is ideal for general body development and the improvement of muscular strength and endurance.

6. Regardless of your training objective, the final repetition in each set should result in complete muscle failure or the inability to perform even one more repetition.

◼ Types of Training

The three most commonly used strength- and endurance-training methods are isotonics, isokinetics, and isometrics, each with a number of variations and each requiring special equipment. During an *isotonic* contraction, such as the execution of an arm curl with free weights or Universal or Nautilus machines, the muscle shortens (**positive phase**) as the weight is brought toward the body and lengthens (**negative phase**) as it is returned to the starting position. Inertia helps move the weight during the positive phase, and the weight is slowly lowered under control during the negative phase. During an **isokinetic** arm curl with special equipment, the muscle also shortens and lengthens during the positive and negative phases; however, maximal resistance is provided throughout the full range of movement in both phases. Without the benefit of inertia or gravity to allow a weight

to drop, the routine would be considerably more difficult. In an *isometric* contraction, the exercised muscle contracts, but its overall length remains unchanged.

You are performing isotonic contractions when you use free weights or Universal, Nautilus, Cam II, Polaris, and other, similar equipment. New Life Cycle equipment has found a way to eliminate cheating and take full advantage of the negative phase of contraction. During the negative phase of each repetition, the weight automatically increases by 25 percent. It is also nearly impossible to drop the weight and cheat as you return

Positive phase of muscle contraction (concentric exercise) The phase of exercise when the muscle shortens rather than lengthens during muscular tension; the upward phase, or the phase of an exercise when weight is being lifted.

Negative phase of muscle contraction (eccentric exercise) The phase of exercise when a muscle lengthens rather than shortens during muscular tension; the downward phase, or the phase of an exercise when weight is being lowered.

Isokinetic A type of dynamic (concentric) muscular contraction that occurs at a constant velocity through the range of motion as controlled by an ergometer.

to the starting position in the negative phase or to use inertia to help during the positive phase.

The Mini-Gym uses the isokinetic, or accommodating resistance, principle designed to overload the muscle group maximally through the entire range of motion. The harder you pull, the harder the Mini-Gym resists your pull. Because there is no negative phase, strength gains are not as rapid as they are with other equipment.

Hydra Fitness and Eagle Performance systems combine the isotonic and isokinetic methods by automatically adjusting to the strength and speed of the individual.

Isometric exercises can be compared to weight-training movements in which the weight is so heavy that it cannot be moved. These exercises involve a steady muscle contraction against immovable resistance for 6–8 seconds. Strength gains appear to be specific to the angle and do not transfer into increased strength throughout the full range of motion.

Calisthenics is the oldest form of weight training. Using the body as resistance, it represents a safe, practical, and effective method of developing muscular strength and endurance. Because the resistance is low (body weight) and a high number of repetitions must be used to bring about fatigue, calisthenics is more effective for developing muscular endurance than strength. Calisthenics is also an ideal, safe strength- and endurance-training method for preadolescent children.

Professional athletes and fitness experts prefer isotonic movements with free weights for the development of muscular strength and endurance, muscle mass, and speed. Special equipment that allows either isotonic or isokinetic movement is excellent for rehabilitating from injury, focusing on specific body areas, and improving general body development. This equipment is relatively safe and can be used without a spotter or partner.

■ Home-Fitness Equipment

The home-fitness strength equipment boom has continued into the 21st century. Unfortunately, a multitude of approaches and claims make it difficult for consumers to make wise choices. It is also nearly impossible to rate each piece of strength-training equipment on the market today, let alone keep up with the new items appearing on a regular basis. One way to increase your chances of making a sound choice is to answer each of the following questions before consulting a certified strength and conditioning coach at your college or university:

1. What type of equipment is likely to best help you meet your training objectives? Do you favour isotonic workouts, isotonic and isokinetic methods combined, or machines that take full advantage of the negative phase of each exercise? If you have the space and work out with others, you may want to consider free weights and some special bench and squat racks.

2. How much do you want to spend? High-quality machines work much more smoothly, make the workout more enjoyable, and are much less likely to break down.

3. How much space do you have for your workout area? Depending on the area you are using, you may need to choose equipment that folds up or takes up limited space.

4. How safe is the equipment? Most home weight-training equipment can be safely used without a spotter or partner.

5. Does the item give you a complete strength-training workout? Some machines train only a few body areas, forcing exercisers to use free weights to supplement the machine.

6. How much weight or resistance is available for each exercise? If you can almost move the maximum resistance provided for a given exercise, you are certain to need additional weight in the near future as you progress. Some equipment items are not designed for additional weight, which forces you to add repetitions and possibly change your objectives. If you are primarily interested in adding muscle weight and strength, you need equipment that permits the adding of heavy weight.

7. Do you like using the equipment? Before purchasing any item, take the time to find a local fitness centre, high school, or university that will allow you to complete a workout or two on the equipment. A five-minute session in a store is not enough exposure to help you decide.

8. What do others who possess this equipment say about the item? Ask the salesperson for a few names of people who have purchased the item. Take the time to call and inquire. The information you get may keep you from impulsively purchasing an inferior item.

After you have thought through these questions, you are ready to meet with an expert and finalize your decision. One thing is certain: you will not experience the amazing results shown in TV commercials and infomercials unless you become a dedicated user over a period of years and combine your hard work with proper nutrition and aerobic exercise. (See Chapter 15 for a discussion of other home exercise equipment.)

Myth and Fact Sheet

Myth	Fact
1. Strength training will make you inflexible.	1. Strength training will actually improve your flexibility providing you go through the full range of motion on each exercise and stretch properly before and after each workout.
2. Strength training makes females unfeminine and masculine.	2. With only three to four strength-training sessions per week, it is impossible to acquire large, bulky muscles. A program using a moderate number of repetitions and weight will only improve your feminine appearance.
3. Strength training will convert your fat to muscle.	3. Fat (adipose) and muscle are separate tissue types. You cannot convert one to the other. When you burn more calories than you eat, fat cells shrink. Strength training causes muscle tissue to increase in size and helps your skin fit you better after weight loss.
4. Sit-ups are the best stomach-flattening exercise.	4. Although exercises such as the abdominal curl and crunch are helpful in flattening the stomach, they are not as effective as decreasing your caloric intake. Reduced calories will shrink the fat cells in your stomach area; the girth-control program described in this chapter will improve the muscular strength and endurance of your abdominal muscles. Both programs must be used to obtain a flat stomach.
5. If stomach exercises do not hurt, they will not work.	5. You can improve your abdominal strength and endurance without pain. In fact, it is good advice to back off when a burning sensation occurs to prevent muscle soreness and injury.
6. Without steroids, it is next to impossible to add muscle mass.	6. You can safely add 454–907 grams of muscle a month (up to 227 grams per week) without steroids through weight training and sound nutrition.
7. It's pointless to start a strength-training program because when you stop, your muscle will turn to fat.	7. As we indicated previously, fat cannot turn into muscle, nor can muscle change into fat. When you stop exercising, muscles will get smaller and fat cells will get larger.
8. Unlike men, women who engage in weight training progress very slowly.	8. The quality of muscle tissue and the ability to produce force is identical in men and women. When identical weight-training programs are used, women and men respond similarly.
9. Weight training burns very few calories and is of little help in losing weight.	9. In addition to the added muscle weight and increased calorie burn at rest, a weight-training workout expends a significant amount of calories. A one-hour session involving at least eight large-muscle exercises and three or more sets utilizes over 500 calories; just five workouts expends enough calories to lose 454 grams of fat.

Amount of Resistance (Weight) to Use

The weight with which you can perform a specific number of repetitions is called the RM (repetitions maximum). The 9-RM, then, is the amount of weight that would bring you to almost complete muscle failure on the ninth repetition—you could not perform even one additional repetition. After you decide on the range of repetitions for your training objective, your starting weight is the RM for the lower repetition (for example, with a six-to-nine cycle, your starting weight is 6-RM).

Number of Repetitions to Complete

The number of consecutive times you perform each exercise is called **repetitions**. A high number (10–20) with lighter weights favours the development of endurance, whereas a low number (3–5) with heavier weights tends to favour strength development.

Number of Sets to Complete

One group of repetitions for a particular exercise is a **set**. Depending on your training objectives and the method of progression you select, three to five sets are recommended. Sets should be performed consecutively for each exercise before moving on to another muscle group. To avoid excess muscle soreness and stiffness, beginners should start with one set and gradually work up to three over a period of 3–4 weeks.

Amount of Rest Between Sets

The time you take between sets is the **rest interval**. Muscle fibres will recover to within 50 percent of their capacity within 3–5 seconds and continue to near full recovery after about 2 minutes. In a program designed to increase strength only, the rest interval is less important and should approach 1 minute. For muscular endurance training, however, the rest interval should gradually decrease from 2 minutes to about 30 seconds over a 6-to-8-week period. Unless you slowly decrease the rest interval between repetitions or increase the number of repetitions, you will not improve muscular endurance.

Amount of Rest Between Workouts

For a total-body workout, you will receive the best results when you allow at least 48 hours of rest (alternate-day training) between workouts. With shorter rest periods, complete recovery is not taking place, and you are not receiving the full benefits of your workout. For split-body routines that emphasize the upper body one day and the lower body the next, it is possible to train for six consecutive days before taking a day of rest. If too much time (four or more days) elapses before the next workout, acquired strength and endurance gains begin to diminish.

Speed for Completing Exercises

For most training objectives, you should return the weight to the starting position (negative phase) twice as slowly as you completed the positive phase. For example, if it took you one second to bench-press the weight overhead, it should take two seconds to lower the weight. It is important to raise the weight slowly enough to eliminate the help of inertia in the positive phase and lower the weight under control to receive the full benefit of the negative phase. If you simply drop the weight in the negative phase of each exercise, your muscles are not being exercised during one-half of the workout and benefits are greatly reduced.

Application of the Principle of Specificity

To gain strength and endurance in a particular muscle, muscle group, or movement, you must specifically train the muscle or muscles in a similar movement. To improve sprinting speed by increasing your strength and endurance, for example, you must identify the muscles involved in sprinting and choose isotonic exercises that strengthen those muscles in a movement similar to the sprinting action.

Application of the Overload Principle

Strength gains occur either by muscle fibres producing a stronger contraction or by recruitment of a higher proportion of the available fibres for the contraction. The overload principle improves strength both ways, providing the demands on the muscle are systematically and progressively increased over time and the muscles are taxed beyond their accustomed levels. In other words, during each workout, your muscles must perform a higher volume of work than they did in the previous workout. This is achieved by increasing the amount of resistance (weight) on each exercise or the number of repetitions and/or sets.

Application of the Progressive Resistance Exercise (PRE) Principle

As training progresses and you grow stronger, you must continuously increase the amount of resistance (weight) if continued improvement is to occur. One way to apply the PRE principle is to choose your starting weight and the lower limit of repetitions for each exercise. If you are using three sets of 6–9 repetitions, for example, you would perform 6 repetitions for each exercise on your first workout. In the second, third, and fourth workouts, you would complete 7, 8, and 9 repetitions, respectively. Then you would add 2.3 kilograms of weight to each upper-body exercise and 4.5 kilograms to each lower-body exercise and return to three sets of 6 repetitions.

Numerous other methods of progression in weight training have been shown to be effective. The *rest-pause* method involves completion of a single repetition at near-maximal weight (1-RM) before resting one or two minutes, completing a second repetition, resting again, and so on until the muscle is fatigued and cannot perform one additional repetition. The *set system* involves use of multiple sets (3–10) of about five to six repetitions for each exercise.

The *burnout* method uses 75 percent of maximal weight for as many repetitions as possible. Without any rest interval, 4.5 kilograms are removed from the starting weight and another RM set is performed. The procedure is repeated until the muscle does not respond (burnout). Each designated muscle group is put through the same demanding process.

Supersets involve the use of a set of exercises for one group of muscles followed immediately by a set for their antagonist. For example, one set of arm curls (biceps) is followed by a set of bench presses (triceps). Each of the preceding methods has been effective in the development of muscular strength and endurance. To avoid boredom, add variation to your program and help overcome plateaus (periods when improvement is slow or nonexistent). It is good to alternate your program among these methods every three or four weeks.

■ Bodybuilding

Bodybuilders are generally more concerned with flex appeal (size, shape, definition, proportion) than they are with muscular strength. They use dumbbells, barbells, and resistance-designed machines to carve out and define individual muscles. Beauty of physique is much more important to them than feats of strength. Competitors perform posing routines and are judged on symmetry (body parts having been equally developed top and bottom, left and right), muscle definition, and poise. Female competitors complete their competition by engaging in a brief freestyle routine to music, a cross between sport and cabaret.

■ When to Expect Results

Just how fast you progress depends on your initial level of strength, your training habits, the intensity and length of your training program, and genetic factors that govern your potential for strength gains and the speed at which these gains occur. Strength gains of 8–50 percent have been reported. The fastest improvement occurs in individuals who have not engaged in weight training previously and whose programs involve large-muscle exercises, heavier weights, multiple sets, and more training sessions.

You should see significant strength gains after only 8–12 weeks of training. But be patient, because it will take approximately 12 months to change the general appearance of your body dramatically and to add 4.5–5.4 kilograms of muscle mass.

■ Signs of Overtraining

Those who notice a plateau or drop in performance over time may be experiencing the overtraining phenomenon. This is likely to occur when you train too aggressively, train too soon after being ill or injured, shorten the rest period between workouts, or simply fail to follow the guidelines presented in this chapter. The condition occurs because your body does not have adequate time to recuperate from one workout to another. Some of the signs of overtraining are extreme muscle soreness and stiffness following a workout, a gradual increase in soreness, loss of appetite, loss of weight, constipation or diarrhea, inability to complete a normal workout, and an unexplained drop in the amount of weight you can successfully lift in several exercises. If two or more of these symptoms develop, you should reduce the intensity, frequency, and duration of your workouts immediately. Short workouts with light weights two times per week for several weeks should give your body ample time to recover and allow you to resume your normal routine.

■ Maintenance of Strength and Endurance Gains

After you have acquired the level of muscular strength and endurance desired, one or two vigorous training sessions per week will maintain most of the improvement that has occurred.

*L*IFTING TECHNIQUES

■ Warm-Up and Cool-Down

To warm up properly, it is helpful to perform four or five minutes of walking and light jogging to raise body temperature and then to stretch for six to eight minutes (see Chapter 7). The first of three sets can be used as a light set with a high number of repetitions (15–20) and low weight (20-RM) for most workouts. You will need additional warm-up sets if you are going to execute maximum lifts. Stronger athletes also seem to need more warm-up sets. When warming up prior to maximum-lift

---

Repetitions The number of times a specific exercise is completed.

Set A group of repetitions for a particular exercise.

Rest interval The amount of time taken between sets.

BEHAVIOURAL CHANGE AND MOTIVATIONAL STRATEGIES

A number of things may interfere with your strength-training progress. Here are some common barriers (roadblocks) and strategies for overcoming them and moving toward your training goals.

Roadblock	Behavioural Change Strategy
You are aware of your need to engage in strength training but just cannot seem to stay interested enough to avoid skipping workouts.	The first month of any exercise program is the most difficult. Muscle soreness, discomfort, and a body that looks the same can discourage you at this stage. Try some of these techniques to overcome this critical period: 1. Set a realistic goal for each exercise, such as only a 4.5-kilogram gain in the amount of weight you can move for three weeks. 2. Take a tape measure and record the size of your upper arm, upper leg, and abdominal area. 3. Avoid remeasuring yourself until you have added 4.5 kilograms to most of the exercises in your program. You can be assured that you will meet this goal at your own pace and that, when you do, you will have acquired additional muscle mass. 4. Use a more realistic approach to determining your progress, such as merely feeling various muscle groups and pinching fat to assure yourself of a new firmness, more muscle, and less fat.
After three or four months of training, you seem to have levelled off or reached a plateau. Improvement is occurring so slowly that you are becoming discouraged and feel you have already improved as much as possible.	What you are experiencing happens to everyone. Initial gains in strength and endurance are always much greater than those you achieve months later. Consider some behavioural changes to help overcome this levelling-off: 1. Incorporate one fun day into your weekly schedule, preferably on the day you are most likely to skip. Use lighter weights, rest longer between sets and exercises, and enjoy yourself. 2. Find a partner or group of people at about your level to work out with, and encourage one another to put a strong effort in your remaining two workouts weekly. 3. Incorporate a *maximum lift day* into your workout routine once every four weeks to demonstrate how you are progressing in each exercise. Use this session to reestablish your 1-RM and record the results.
List other roadblocks you are experiencing that seem to be reducing the effectiveness of your strength-training program. 1. _____ 2. _____ 3. _____	Now list the behavioural change strategies that can help you overcome the roadblocks you listed. If you need to, refer back to Chapter 3 for behavioural change and motivational strategies. 1. _____ 2. _____ 3. _____

attempts, you should perform the first warm-up set with weights of 50–70 percent of the RM weight to be attempted, and the second set at 75–80 percent. If you are performing any of the Olympic lifts, as many as ten to twelve warm-up attempts may be needed before a maximum effort. A four-to-five-minute stretching period at the close of your workout will help prevent muscle soreness and aid in improving your range of motion.

Full Range of Motion

For each exercise, you should move through the full range of motion without locking out the joint. The arm curl, for example, should result in the weight being moved as close to the chest as possible on the positive phase before returning to the starting position, without locking the elbow joint. When you are lifting heavy arm or leg weights, you are much more likely to injure a joint that is fully extended at both the beginning and the ending phases of the exercise.

Proper Breathing

One recommended breathing procedure is to breathe out during the working or exertion phase of the exercise and inhale during the relaxation phase. If you are taking several breaths during the execution of one repetition, you are breathing too quickly and inhaling and exhaling at the wrong time. You should also avoid the tendency to hold your breath throughout the exertion phase. When you fail to exhale, the flow of blood to your heart is reduced, which, in turn, reduces blood flow to the brain and causes you to become dizzy and possibly to faint. Holding your breath is particularly dangerous when you are performing overhead exercises. For individuals with high blood pressure, proper breathing is essential during the completion of each repetition.

Sequence of Exercises

Exercises should be arranged to prevent fatigue from limiting your lifting ability. One approach is to exercise the large-muscle groups before exercising the smaller muscles. It is difficult to exhaust large-muscle groups when the smaller muscles that serve as connections between the resistance and the large-muscle groups have been prematurely fatigued. It is also important for the abdominal muscles, used in most exercises to stabilize the rib cage, to remain relatively unfatigued until the latter phases of the workout. A typical sequence that applies the concept of large to small is: (1) hips and lower back, (2) legs (quadriceps, hamstrings, calves), (3) torso (back, shoulders, chest), (4) arms (triceps, biceps, forearms), (5) abdominals, and (6) neck.

Form and Technique

It is important to carefully follow the specific form tips identified for each exercise in Figure 6.3. In addition, you can apply these general techniques to most exercises and equipment:

1. Assume the basic stance by placing your feet slightly wider than shoulder width apart with your feet parallel. The stronger leg is sometimes placed back in a heel–toe alignment.

2. Place your toes just under the bar in the starting phase of exercises in which the barbell is resting on the floor.

3. Keep your back erect (unless it contains the muscle group being exercised) with your head up and your eyes looking straight ahead.

4. Grasp the bar with your hands shoulder width apart using one of three grips:

   a. **Overhand** Grasp the bar until your thumbs wrap around and meet your index fingers. You may place your thumbs next to your index fingers without wrapping your hand around the bar if you prefer.

   b. **Underhand** Grasp the bar with your palms turned upward away from your body. Your fingers and thumbs are wrapped around the bar.

   c. **Mixed grip** Combine the overhand and underhand grip, with each hand assuming one of the grips.

5. Avoid leaning backward to assist a repetition.

6. Stress safety at all times, and use workout partners to spot and protect you when you are using heavy free weights. Specifically:

   a. Avoid attempting to lift more weight than you can safely handle.

   b. Secure collars and engage pins before attempting a lift.

   c. Avoid holding your breath during the lift.

   d. Return the barbell to the floor, rack, or starting position in a controlled manner.

   e. Bend your knees when moving heavy weight from one place to another for storage.

Hints for weight-training exercises are provided in Figure 6.3. These suggestions will help you prevent injury and improve the effectiveness of each exercise.

BARBELL AND DUMBBELL EXERCISES

Figure 6.3 shows specific exercises, describes the equipment needs, outlines the basic movement, gives helpful hints, and identifies the muscle groups involved. This information will help you choose exercises that train the important muscle groups in your sport or activity. Table 6.2 includes some of the many barbell and dumbbell exercises and their variations for a basic resistance program designed to improve your strength, muscular endurance, and muscle size.

Table 6.2 ✦ Basic and Alternative Weight-Training Programs: Programs for General Body Development

EXERCISES	REPETITIONS	STARTING WEIGHT (RM)(kg)	SPEED OF CONTRACTION
Basic Program			
Two-arm curl	6–10	3.6	Moderate
Military press	6–10	3.6	Moderate
Sit-ups (bent-knee)	25–50	13.6	Rapid
Bench press	6–10	3.6	Moderate
Squat	6–10	3.6	Rapid
Heel raise	15–25	9	Rapid
Dead lift (bent-knee)	6–10	3.6	Rapid
Alternative I			
Reverse curl	6–10	3.6	Moderate
Triceps press	6–10	3.6	Moderate
Sit-ups (bent-knee)	25–50	13.6	Rapid
Shoulder shrug	6–10	3.6	Moderate
Squat jump	15–25	9	Rapid
Knee flexor	6–10	3.6	Rapid
Knee extensor	6–10	3.6	Rapid
Pull-overs (bent-arm)	6–10	3.6	Moderate
Alternative II			
Wrist curl	6–10	3.6	Moderate
Side bender	6–10	3.6	Moderate
Lateral raise	6–10	3.6	Moderate
Straddle lift	6–10	3.6	Rapid
Supine leg lift	6–10	3.6	Rapid
Hip flexor	6–10	3.6	Rapid
Leg abductor	6–10	3.6	Rapid
Forward raise	6–10	3.6	Moderate

GIRTH CONTROL

Almost everyone wants a flat tummy. In fact, a flat stomach is strongly associated with fitness and wellness in our society. A large belly can make people appear much older than they really are. It also can be a sign of poor health—evidence of accumulating fat that may lead to hypertension, stroke, heart disease, adult-onset diabetes, and other ailments. Some fat around the midsection is not necessarily unhealthy. Practically everyone acquires at least a small spare tire (fat on both sides of the hips) and some abdominal fat. Becoming obsessed with this somewhat natural change is a mistake. In fact, as you reach the third and fourth decades of life, maintaining the flat stomach you had in your teens may be impossible.

Most people attempt to solve the girth-control problem by using unnatural and worthless devices such as girdles, corsets, weighted belts, rubberized workout suits, and special exercise equipment that promises a flat stomach with just minutes of use daily. Although it is not an easy task, you can bring back some of the lost youth in your abdominal area by completing the program described in Lab Activity 6.2: Obtaining a Flat, Healthy Stomach.

Figure 6.3 ✦ Barbell and Dumbbell Exercises

Bench press

Equipment: Barbell, bench rack, spotter

Movement: Using an overhand grip, slowly lower the bar to the chest, then press back to the starting position.

Hints: Bend knees at 90° and keep feet off the bench and the floor.

Muscle Groups: Pectoralis major, Triceps, Deltoid

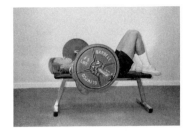 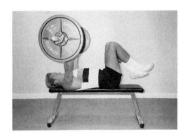

Incline bench press

Equipment: Incline bench, squat rack, spotter

Movement: Using an overhand grip, slowly raise and lower the bar to the chest (both feet flat on the floor).

Hints: Use a weight rack to support the weight above the bench. Avoid lifting the buttocks or arching the back while lifting.

Muscle Groups: Pectoralis major, Anterior deltoid, Triceps

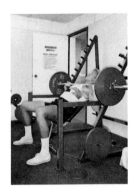 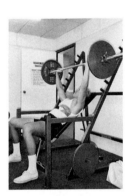

Power cleans

Equipment: Barbell

Movement: Using an overhand grip, pull the bar explosively to the highest point of your chest. Rotate hands under the bar and bend your knees. Straighten up to standing position. Bend the arms, legs, and hips to return the bar to the thighs, then slowly bend the knees and hips to lower to the floor.

Hints: Grasp the bar at shoulder width. Start with knees bent so hips are knee-level. Keep head up and back straight.

Muscle Groups: Trapezius, Erector spinae, Gluteals, Quadriceps

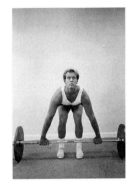 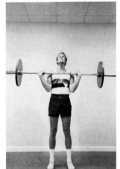 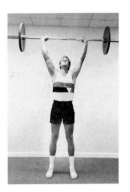

Dead lift

Equipment: Barbell

Movement: Using a mixed grip, bend knees so hips are close to knee level. Straighten knees and hips to standing position. Bend at knees and hips to return.

Hints: Keep the head up and back flat. Grasp bar at shoulder width.

Muscle Groups: Erector spinae, Gluteus, Quadriceps, Hamstrings

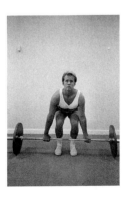 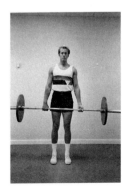

(continued)

Figure 6.3 ✦ Barbell and Dumbbell Exercises *(continued)*

Bent arm flys

Equipment: Dumbbells

Movement: Using an underhand grip, hold a dumbbell in each hand above the shoulders with the elbows slightly bent.

Hints: Keep elbows slightly bent at all times.

Muscle Groups: Pectoralis major

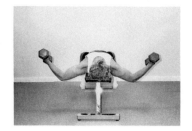 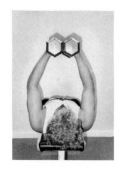

Barbell rowing

Equipment: Barbell

Movement: Using an overhand grip, hold the barbell directly below your shoulders. With elbows leading, pull the barbell to chest and hold momentarily. Then slowly return to the starting position.

Hints: Grasp bar slightly wider than shoulder width. Refrain from swinging or jerking the weights upward to the chest region.

Muscle Groups: Latissimus dorsi, Rhomboids, Trapezius

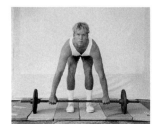 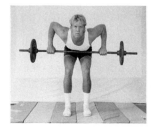

One dumbbell rowing

Equipment: Dumbbells

Movement: Using an underhand grip, kneel with one hand and one knee on exercise bench. Pull weight on support side upward to chest.

Hints: Hold dumbbell briefly at chest before returning.

Muscle Groups: Latissimus dorsi

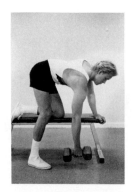 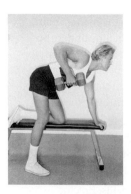

Shoulder shrug

Equipment: Barbell

Movement: Using an overhand grip, elevate both shoulders until they nearly touch the earlobes, then relax and return bar to the thighs.

Hints: Keep the extremities fully extended. Heavy weights (within limitations) will bring more rapid strength gains.

Muscle Groups: Trapezius

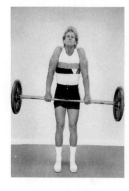

Figure 6.3 ✦ Barbell and Dumbbell Exercises *(continued)*

Military press

Equipment: Barbell

Movement: Using an overhand grip, slowly push bar overhead from chest until both arms are fully extended.

Hints: Keep neck and back erect, and knees extended and locked. Avoid jerky movements and leaning.

Muscle Groups: Deltoids, Triceps

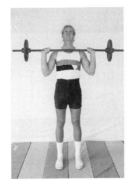 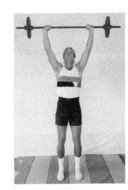

Bent-over lateral raise

Equipment: Dumbbells

Movement: Using an overhand grip, grasp dumbbell in each hand and draw arms to shoulder level. Slowly return to hanging position.

Hints: Keep knees and elbows slightly bent. Hold weights for 1–2 seconds before returning to hanging position.

Muscle Groups: Posterior deltoid, Latissimus dorsi, Rhomboids, Middle Trapezius

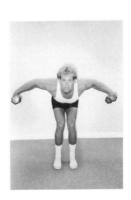

Two-arm curl

Equipment: Barbell

Movement: Using underhand grip, raise bar from thighs to chest level, and return.

Hints: Keep body erect and motionless throughout.

Muscle Groups: Elbow flexors

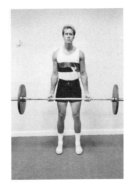 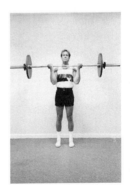

(continued)

Figure 6.3 ✦ Barbell and Dumbbell Exercises *(continued)*

Reverse curl

Equipment: Barbell

Movement: Using overhand grip, raise bar from thighs to chest level, and return.

Hints: Use less weight than in two-arm curl.

Muscle Groups: Upper arm flexors, Hand extensors, Finger extensors

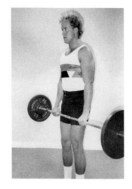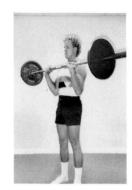

Seated dumbbell curl

Equipment: Dumbbells

Movement: Using an underhand grip, curl one or both dumbbells to the shoulder, then slowly return the weight to the sides of the body.

Hints: Keep the back straight throughout the movement.

Muscle Groups: Elbow flexors

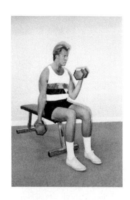

Close grip bench press

Equipment: Barbell, squat rack, spotter

Movement: Using a close overhand grip, slowly lower the barbell to the chest and press back to the starting position.

Hints: Grasp centre of bar (hands 5 to 10 centimetres apart). Bend knees at 90°; keep feet off the bench floor so as to avoid arching the back. Keep elbows in; extend arms fully.

Muscle Groups: Triceps, Anterior deltoid, Pectoralis major

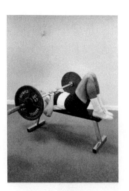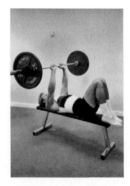

Standing or seated tricep

Equipment: Dumbbell

Movement: With both hands grasped around the inner side of one dumbbell overhead, lower the weight behind your head, then return.

Hints: Keep the elbows close together throughout the manoeuver.

Muscle Groups: Triceps

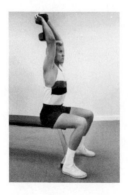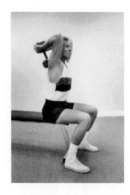

Figure 6.3 ✦ Barbell and Dumbbell Exercises *(continued)*

Barbell wrist curl

Equipment: Barbell

Movement: Using an underhand grip, let the bar hang down toward the floor and then curl toward you.

Hints: Grasp centre of bar (hands 5 to 10 centimetres apart). Keep forearms in steady contact with the bench while moving the weight.

Muscle Groups: Wrist flexors

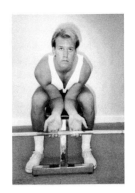 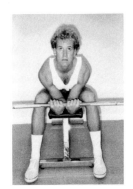

Reverse wrist curl

Equipment: Barbell

Movement: Using an overhand grip, and moving the wrists only, raise bar as high as possible, and return to the starting position.

Hints: Grasp barbell at shoulder width. Movement should only be at the wrist joint.

Muscle Groups: Forearm extensors

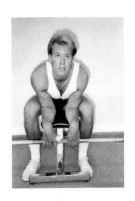 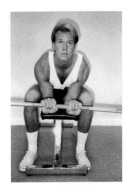

Front squat

Equipment: Barbell, squat rack, chair or bench, 5-to-8-centimetre board, spotters

Basic Movement: Using an overhand grip, flex legs to a 90° angle. Return to standing position.

Hints: Keep the heels up, and point the chin outward slightly. A chair or bench can be placed below the body (touch buttocks slightly to surface).

Muscle Groups: Quadriceps, Gluteals, Hamstrings

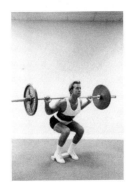 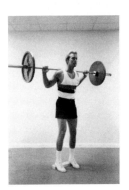

Lunge with dumbbells

Equipment: Dumbbells

Movement: Overhand grip; alternate stepping forward with each leg, bending the knee of the lead leg, and lowering your body until thigh of the front leg is level to the floor. Barely touch the knee of rear leg to the floor before returning to the starting position.

Hints: Keep your head up and upper body erect throughout the exercise. Avoid bending front knee more than 90°.

Muscle Groups: Quadriceps, Gluteals, Hamstrings

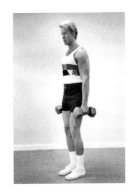 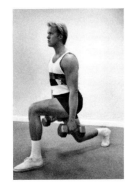

(continued)

Figure 6.3 ✦ Barbell and Dumbbell Exercises *(continued)*

Heel raise

Equipment: Barbell, squat rack, spotters, 5-to-8-centimetre board

Movement: Using an overhand grip, the body is raised upward to maximum height of the toes.

Hints: Alter the position of the toes from straight ahead to pointed in and out. Keep the body erect.

Muscle Groups: Gastrocnemius, Soleus

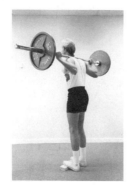 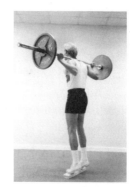

One dumbbell heel raise

Equipment: Dumbbell, 5-to-8-centimetre board

Movement: Using an overhand grip, shift entire body weight onto the leg next to the dumbbell, and raise the foot off the floor behind. Raise the heel of the support foot upward as high as possible and hold momentarily.

Hints: A wall is useful for balance, but avoid using free hand for assistance.

Muscle Groups: Gastrocnemius, Soleus

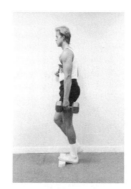 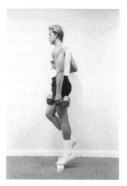

SUMMARY

The Importance of Strength and Endurance

Strength and endurance training provides health-related benefits for people of all ages. Such training burns calories, adds muscle mass, prevents the slowing of metabolism with age, and is an important aspect of controlling body weight and body fat throughout life. Over a period of 6–12 months of this training, your general physical appearance, body image, and self-concept will improve. Strength training also aids in the development of the skeletal system and in improving bone-mineral content. The added strength and endurance also increase energy and productivity on the job and in recreational activities and reduce the incidence of sports- and work-related injuries. And finally, strength and endurance training plays a major role in the rehabilitation of soft-tissue injuries such as muscle strains, tears, and contusions.

Factors Affecting Muscular Strength and Endurance

A muscle is composed of fibres and myofibrils bound together by layers of connective tissue. There are three general types of fibre tissue: slow-twitch, oxidative (aerobic); fast-twitch, glycolytic (anaerobic); and fast-twitch, oxidative, glycolytic (aerobic and anaerobic). Strength training predominantly affects the fast-twitch fibres while endurance training affects the slow-twitch fibres. Your strength and endurance potential is governed by genetics and the number, size, and distribution of your fast- and slow-twitch fibres. Everyone can increase muscle size, strength, and endurance with training.

Strength-Training Principles

Three basic training methods are commonly used to develop strength and endurance: isotonics, isokinetics, and isometrics. In an isotonic or isokinetic contraction, the muscle shortens during the positive phase as weight is brought toward the body and lengthens in the negative phase as the weight is returned to the starting position. No muscle shortening occurs when force is applied to an immovable object (isometric contraction). Isotonic and isokinetic workouts are more beneficial to sports performance than isometric workouts are.

Training variables can be altered to meet specific objectives. By manipulating the number of sets, repetitions, and rest intervals, and the speed of contraction, you can alter your programs to focus on strength, muscular endurance, general body development, muscle mass, speed and explosive power, or rehabilitation from injury.

Prior to purchasing home strength-training equipment, you should take the time to determine your training objectives, analyze your available space and funds, try out the equipment, and consult with a strength and conditioning coach.

Lifting Techniques

Sound lifting techniques with free weights or special equipment require careful warm-up and cool-down periods with stretching, the full range of motion on each repetition, proper breathing, use of a partner or spotter, and careful attention to ideal form in each exercise.

Barbell and Dumbbell Exercises

A variety of exercises can be chosen that focus on the major muscle groups of the body. One sound approach is first to identify the key muscles involved in the activity or those you want to train, and then to select specific weight-training exercises that activate these muscles, preferably in a similar movement.

Girth Control

To obtain a flat stomach, it is necessary to restrict your daily calories enough to cause fat cells in the abdominal area to shrink in size and to engage in a series of high-repetition abdominal exercises daily. You cannot change fatty tissue to muscle tissue, and muscle tissue will not change to fatty tissue when exercise ceases. Abdominal exercises alone will only improve the strength and endurance of your stomach muscles; little or no change will take place in the size of the stomach unless calories are also restricted.

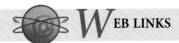

STUDY QUESTIONS

1. Exactly what is the difference between muscular strength and muscular endurance?

2. How is muscular endurance different from cardiorespiratory endurance?

3. List and explain three reasons that strength training should be incorporated into any fitness/wellness program.

4. What should you do/know before beginning a resistance training program?

5. What method(s) would you use to acquire stronger abdominal muscles?

6. If you know the origin and insertion of major muscle groups, you should be able to devise strength and endurance exercises for those groups. For each of the quadriceps, hamstrings, gastrocs, rectus femoris, biceps, triceps, deltoids, lats, describe proper strength/endurance training techniques.

WEB LINKS

Anatomy of Bones
www.meddean.luc.edu/lumen/MedEd/
GrossAnatomy/learnem/bones/main_bone.htm

Anatomy of Muscles
www.meddean.luc.edu/lumen/MedEd/
GrossAnatomy/dissector/mml/

Youth Strength Training Guidelines of the ACSM
www.acsm.org/pdf/YSTRNGTH.pdf

Strength Training for Women
www.newellness.com/physfitn/strntrng.htm

Body Building for Muscle Tone, Strength and Endurance
http://kirtland.cc.mi.us/~balbachl/weight.htm

Strength Training Guidelines from Health World Online (comprehensive site)
www.healthy.net/fitness/training/strength.htm

Lab Activity 6.1

Do You Need to Start a Strength-Training Program?

INSTRUCTIONS: *Answer each question below before reading the interpretation section to find out how badly you are in need of a strength-training program. Be sure to include your elaborations to the Yes/No answers; these elaborations will help you to better understand how you, personally, can benefit from a strength-training program.*

	Yes	No
1. Have you been on a diet within the past 6–12 months? Why? _____	_____	_____
2. Have you ever lost, then regained, 3.6–4.5 kilograms in the same year? What happened? _____ _____	_____	_____
3. Do you have difficulty controlling your body weight? How so? _____	_____	_____
4. Do you have excess, sagging skin on the back of your upper arms, thighs, back of your legs, stomach, or other body part? Where? _____	_____	_____
5. Are you interested in changing your appearance by adding muscle and reducing the size of fat deposits?	_____	_____
6. Would a firmer, more muscular body help your body image, how you feel about yourself, and how you think others feel about you? Why? _____	_____	_____
7. Would additional strength or muscular endurance improve your performance in any sports or recreational activities? Which ones and how? _____ _____	_____	_____
8. Would additional strength or muscular endurance help you perform better on the job and at home? Explain: _____ _____	_____	_____

(continued)

Lab Activity 6.1 *(continued)*
Do You Need to Start a Strength-Training Program?

	Yes	No
9. Are there any specific muscle groups in your body that you would prefer to strengthen? Which ones and why? _____	_____	_____
10. Have you sustained a soft-tissue injury within the past 12 months, such as an ankle sprain, a pulled muscle, or a contusion? What happened? _____	_____	_____

✦ Interpretation

If you answered yes to two or more of the questions, a strength and endurance program may be needed.

Questions 1–3 are concerned with body weight and fat. Strength and endurance training can help your skin fit better, help you focus on your body, help you shrink fat cells, and add muscle mass.

Questions 4–6 are concerned with body image and your interest in improving your appearance through strength and endurance training.

Questions 7–9 are concerned with the need for additional strength and endurance to aid performance on the job, at home, and in recreational activities.

Question 10 is concerned with the prevention of job-, home-, and sports-related injuries.

Lab Activity 6.2

Obtaining a Flat, Healthy Stomach

INSTRUCTIONS: *Take a moment to measure and record the size of your waist. Now apply the pinch test or use skinfold calipers one inch (2.5 centimetres) to the right of your bellybutton and on the left side of your hip to locate the excess fat. If you can pinch more than an inch in these areas, consider following the program described in this Lab Activity.*

A girth-control program is designed to flatten your stomach and improve the strength and endurance of your "abs" (abdominal muscles). It is based on two sound principles:

1. Consume fewer calories than you burn, and remain in a negative caloric balance daily for a few months. Keep in mind that fat or adipose tissue and muscle tissue are different tissue types; one cannot be transformed to the other no matter what you do. Reducing caloric intake to produce a fat loss of 454–907 grams per week (see Chapter 9) will shrink the size of your fat cells in the abdominal area. It is important to engage in an aerobic exercise program three to four times per week to help burn extra calories and to allow consumption of sufficient nutrients and calories to spare protein, thus reducing the amount of lean-muscle-tissue loss that occurs when you diet without exercise.

2. Supplement your dietary management with aerobic exercise (see Chapter 5) and the six abdominal exercises described in this Lab Activity. For each exercise, work toward 50 repetitions daily. Begin with the maximum number you can perform in one set and add 2–5 repetitions each day until you reach 50. Complete these exercises daily, and expect to train for three or four months before you notice significant results. Remember that these abdominal exercises only strengthen muscles that lie beneath the fat. Unless you reduce calories to shrink the fat cells, you will merely have firm abdominal muscles beneath the fat, with little reduction in the size of your stomach.

(continued)

LOWER ABDOMINALS

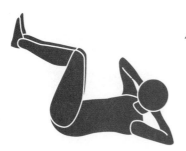 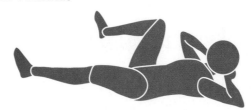

Reverse Curls

Lie on the floor with fingers locked behind your head. Knees are bent. Contract your lower abs to curl hips off the ground about 7–13 centimetres, raising knees to ceiling. Slowly return to the floor. Do not "whip" your legs. Let the abs do the work. Remember to press your lower back into floor throughout the exercise.

Knee Tucks

Lie on your back with hands supporting your head. Tuck one knee to your chest and extend the other straight several centimetres off the floor. Hold two counts and switch legs. Some hip flexor work is involved, but keeping the low back pressed to the floor will work the lower abs isometrically.

INTERNAL/ EXTERNAL OBLIQUES

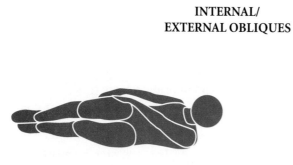 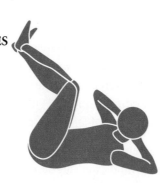

Oblique Twisters

Lie on your back, bend your knees, and point both knees to the left. Extend your arms over your right hip. Slowly curl shoulders and upper back off the floor to a half-upright position. Reverse the curl to return to the floor. Repeat with the opposite side.

Twisting Crunches

Lie on your back with knees bent, ankles crossed and fixed. Contract abs to lift shoulder and upper back off floor. Twist trunk, bringing left elbow to right knee. Repeat to opposite side.

UPPER ABDOMINALS

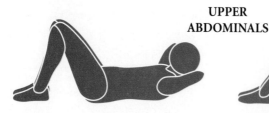

Crunches

Lie on your back with knees bent, feet flat on the floor. Hands support your head. Look at the ceiling and contract the abs to lift the shoulders and upper back off the floor. Lift one knee and bring it in toward your elbow. Press the low back to the floor, hold briefly, then return to floor.

Gravityfighters

Start with knees bent, feet flat, and body rounded to a position 45° off the floor. Arms are crossed over the chest, chin is tucked. The body is gradually lowered until the shoulder blades touch the floor. Reverse the movement to starting position.

7

Flexibility

JAMIL IS PROUD of the fact that he is muscular and athletic, but he is troubled by his lack of flexibility. In the past, he thought limited flexibility was a normal part of developing muscles and becoming strong. He now realizes that his inflexibility is interfering with his ability to enjoy recreational activities and competitive sports and to perform daily tasks such as picking up an object, tying his shoes, and even getting up out of a chair. Unfortunately, Jamil does not know what to do to improve his range of motion and correct the problem.

Flexibility is the range of motion around a joint. Of the five components of health-related physical fitness, it is the aspect most misunderstood and neglected by the exercising population, by athletes, and by health care professionals and practitioners. Like Jamil, few individuals understand the importance of developing and maintaining acceptable levels of joint flexibility, yet the health, injury, and performance consequences of doing so are quite evident.

In this chapter, we will provide solutions to all of Jamil's problems and examine the many aspects of joint flexibility, such as the factors affecting range of motion, its importance, assessment techniques, sound training principles, and choice of specific stretching exercises to help evaluate range of motion and devise a program that meets your specific health and fitness needs.

FACTORS AFFECTING FLEXIBILITY

Because flexibility is specific to each joint, having good hip flexibility is no guarantee you will be flexible in the shoulders, back, neck, or ankles. Depending on your stretching routine and choice of exercises, you may become highly flexible in some joints and remain inflexible in others. A number of factors combine to determine the range of motion around each joint.

Joint structure determines the limits of our range of motion (ROM) in all our joints and cannot be altered. *Ball-and-socket joints,* such as the hip and shoulder, allow the greatest ROM; *elliposoidal joints,* such as in the wrist, are among the least flexible, with an ROM of approximately 70–90 degrees. *Hinge joints,* such as the knee and elbow, have an ROM of approximately 130 degrees. Joints cannot be forced to extend movement beyond the limitations placed by their structure.

Age and gender advantages also clearly exist—the young are more flexible than older people, and females are more flexible than males. Older adults undergo a process called **fibrosis** that causes some muscle fibres to degenerate and be replaced with a less elastic fibrous connective tissue. Females may be more flexible than males because of anatomical differences and differences in the type and extent of activities they perform throughout life.

Muscle bulk, involving a large increase in muscle mass, can limit movement in a number of joints. Extremely large biceps and deltoids, for example, can make it difficult to stretch the triceps. A change in weight-training routine could reduce the amount of bulk; however, this is unadvisable for power athletes such as interior linemen in football, some positions in rugby, shot-putters, and discus and hammer throwers in track and field, and athletes in other sports in which muscle bulk, push weight, and power are important.

Connective tissue (tendons, ligaments, fascial sheaths) and even the skin may limit ROM. Changes in the **elasticity** (ability to return to the original form) and **plasticity** (inability to return to original form) of connective tissue occur with age and injury and may restrict ROM.

> **Fibrosis** A condition in which muscle fibres degenerate with age and are replaced by fibrous connective tissue.
>
> **Elasticity** The ability of connective tissue to return to its original form.
>
> **Plasticity** The inability of connective tissue to return to its original form.
>
> **Muscle extensibility** The ability of muscle tissue to stretch.

Improper weight-training techniques involving high-volume resistance training with limited ROM (as in bodybuilding) can restrict ROM in various joints. However, individuals who perform each weight-training exercise by going through the full ROM (see Chapter 6) for both the agonist and antagonist muscles (such as the biceps and triceps when performing barbell curls) not only do not reduce their flexibility but actually can increase their ROM. Exercises that overdevelop one muscle group while neglecting opposing groups produce the imbalance that restricts flexibility.

Improper stretching procedures also play a role in the decrease in ROM. Maximum benefits occur when each training session begins with a general aerobic warm-up period and 8–12 minutes of stretching, and concludes with another 4–5 minutes of stretching.

Activity levels also affect ROM throughout life. Active individuals are considerably more flexible than inactive ones. A sedentary lifestyle can lead to shortening of muscles and ligaments and restricted ROM. Poor posture, long periods of sitting or standing, or immobilization of a limb can have a similar effect.

Finally, excessive body fat can reduce ROM by increasing resistance to movement and creating premature contact between adjoining body surfaces.

Fortunately, everyone is capable of increasing ROM in particular joints. Regular stretching routines cause permanent lengthening of ligaments and tendons. Muscle tissue undergoes only temporary lengthening following a warm-up and stretching routine as **muscle extensibility** increases. Muscle temperature changes alone, attained through proper warm-up, can increase flexibility by 20 percent.

THE IMPORTANCE OF FLEXIBILITY

A regular stretching routine will help increase ROM, improve performance in some activities, help prevent soft-tissue injuries, aid muscle relaxation, and help you cool down at the end of a workout. It is a valuable part of a complete exercise program, and it provides some benefits to everyone.

Increased Range of Motion and Improved Performance

Because we have established the fact that ROM is joint-specific, a well-rounded flexibility program must devote attention to all the body's major joints: neck, shoulders, back, hips, knees, wrists, and ankles. You can increase your ROM in each of these major joints in six to eight weeks by following one of the recommended stretching techniques discussed in this chapter.

In sports such as gymnastics, diving, skiing, swimming, and hurdling and in other activities requiring a high level of flexibility, a stretching routine that focuses on the key joints can also help improve performance. Although there is little scientific evidence available, the association between flexibility and sports performance is almost universally accepted.

Injury Prevention

Regular stretching routines may help reduce the incidence of injury during exercise for athletes and others. Continuous exercise such as jogging, running, cycling, and aerobics tightens and shortens muscles, and tight muscles are more vulnerable to injury from the explosive movements common in sports. A brief aerobic warm-up period followed by stretching will not only increase range of motion but also provide some protection from common soft-tissue injuries such as strains, sprains, and tears. Some recent studies suggest that a longer warm-up period may actually be more beneficial than stretching for preventing injury (Shrier and Gossal, 2000). Regardless, it is clear that some combination of aerobic warm-up and stretching is essential for injury prevention. Striving to maintain a full, normal ROM in each joint with adequate strength, endurance, and power throughout the range will reduce your chances of experiencing an exercise-induced injury.

Lower-Back Pain The Back Association of Canada stresses the importance of flexibility for back fitness. Pain in the lower back occurs as frequently in our society as the common cold.

Eight out of ten Canadians will experience back pain at some point in their lives (Health Canada, 2000). Informal surveys of middle and high school athletes indicate that as many as 40 percent have experienced back problems severe enough to result in missed practice time. Although back pain affects all age groups, the elderly are the most vulnerable. The older you are, the more likely you are to have problems with your lower back. No one seems to be immune.

A brief description of your spinal column will help you understand why the back is so vulnerable to injury (see Figure 7.1). The human body has 24 vertebrae that extend from the base of the skull to the tail bone. The

Figure 7.1 ✦ The Vertebral Column and Muscle Support

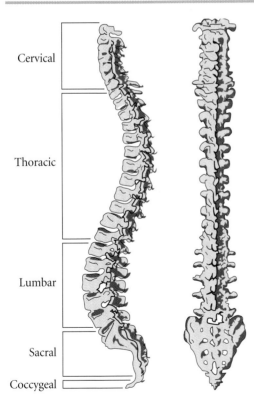

Cervical

Thoracic

Lumbar

Sacral

Coccygeal

The vertebrae that make up the spinal column are designed for support, strength, and flexibility.

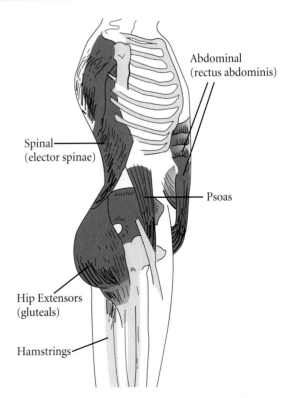

Abdominal (rectus abdominis)

Spinal (elector spinae)

Psoas

Hip Extensors (gluteals)

Hamstrings

Adequate strength and flexibility in the muscle groups of both the back and abdomen are essential for supporting the back and maintaining posture.

WELLNESS HEROES

David Sit

Flexibility is not only a physical property of the body; it can be part of lifestyle adaptation, as it was for David Sit at the University of Western Ontario. When David came to university, his lifestyle up to that point had always been rooted in physical activity. Whether playing tag during recess as a child or playing pick-up hockey with friends in high school, being active, having fun, and enjoying friendships were among the top priorities in David's life. The huge adjustments to university life, such as living away from home and the increased academic workload, resulted in his physical activity passion becoming relegated to a very low to nonexistent status. Poor decision-making and lack of time management skills resulted in scant time devoted to an active and healthy lifestyle.

While living in residence, he noticed that the majority of students faced the same adjustment problems and reoriented their priorities toward busy residence and academic life. Astutely, David observed lots of opportunities for leadership and academic development, but very little energy and very few programs seemed to be effective in promoting a more physically active and healthy lifestyle for students. Research confirmed that individuals form most of their health-related habits during the early adult years; thus, he reasoned that it is important to ensure that part of those habits be firmly established in healthy lifestyle behaviour patterns that are consistent over time and not buffeted by time or academic pressures. Particularly vulnerable were first-year students living in residence.

By third year, David came to realize that he had the tools and skills to create and implement a full-scale and university-wide health promotion program. Coincidentally, he was taking a course in health promotion and was the student president of his academic program in the bachelor of health sciences program. Drawing on his practical experience in rural health education, he founded the ATTAC Life Health Promotion Program (ATTAC was an acronym for Active Teams Towards Active Communities). ATTAC Life is a self-committing, peer-support program that is committed to promoting the importance of a well-balanced lifestyle. Some 200 students per year volunteer to become health promotion facilitators trained and responsible for motivating students in their "community" (residence, for example) to join them in physical activity programs each week. The basic idea is to provide opportunities for students to benefit from leadership, from social interaction, and from physical health improvements; even more, the ATTAC Life teams believe the various programs reduce stress levels, illness, class absenteeism, and improve self-esteem and overall confidence.

David's flexibility and initiative worked to develop a very successful program that benefits hundreds of students each year. Those who volunteer for program coordination roles are now receiving partial academic credit for work related to research and implementation of the program. And, the program has gone online to further increase the opportunity to attract students and share the program beyond one university ✦

Sources: Personal interview with David Sit; information from *Attac Life* Web site, January 2, 2003, accessed May 30, 2003 www.uwo.ca/hfs/attaclife/.

---

vertebrae form a double-*S*, reverse curve to ensure proper balance and weight bearing. If the vertebrae were placed directly on top of one another, the back would be only 5 percent as strong as it is, and one step would produce enough trauma and brain jolt to cause concussion. Shock absorbers, known as *discs*, are located between vertebrae. These capsules of gelatinous matter contain approximately 90 percent water in young people but only 70 percent in older individuals. With loss of water comes a loss of compressibility and increased vulnerability to injury, often referred to as *slipped, ruptured,* or *herniated* disc. Ruptured disc material may bulge through the rear portion of the outer ring and pressure nerves, thereby producing pain in the lower back that may radiate down into the legs and feet (**sciatica**).

Not all sufferers of lower-back pain have bone or disc disorders. In fact, the problem for most individuals involves muscles, tendons, or ligaments. No one cause can be isolated that triggers an episode of back pain. Some of the more common factors include physical injury, hard sneezing or coughing, improper lifting or bending, standing or sitting for long hours, sitting slumped in an overstuffed chair or automobile seat, tension, anxiety, depression, obesity, and disease (for example, arthritis and tumours). Some individuals simply have a genetically weak back involving one or more of the approximately 140 muscles that provide support to the back and control its movements. Typically, a muscle, ligament, or tendon strain or sprain causes nearby muscles to spasm to help support the back. An estimated seven out of ten back problems are due to the improper alignment of the spinal column and pelvic girdle caused by inflexible and weak muscles.

The exact cause of most lower-back pain, however, remains something of a mystery. Blaming back pain on pressure against a spinal nerve caused by one of the bulging spongy discs may be erroneous. Magnetic resonance imaging scans show that about one-third of young adults and practically all older adults who have no back pain have some bulging disks. A so-called normal back without some degree of bulging may be the exception. Other theories suggest that lower-back muscles spasm or that spinal nerve roots are compressed by arthritic spurs or bony overgrowth.

You can reduce your chances of developing lower-back pain by changing the way you stand, bend, lift objects, sit, rest, sleep, and exercise. Figure 7.2 summarizes the key factors for taking good care of your back. Study this figure carefully to make sure you are practising correct sitting, standing, and sleeping posture.

In the past, treatment for lower-back pain has involved a little bit of everything, from major surgery to traction, bed rest, and enzyme injections. Experts now feel that for most people who experience the sudden onset of lower-back pain, the best treatment may be no treatment at all. Like the common cold, chances are good that the condition will improve quickly. The use of a firm mattress, moderate application of heat and cold, and gentle massage until muscle spasms are eliminated or significantly reduced will prepare you for a series of daily exercises such as those shown in Figure 7.2 designed to strengthen the four key muscle groups supporting your back and the important abdominal muscles. Three other components may help your rehabilitation and prevention program: (1) exercising more, (2) decreasing your stomach fat by reducing your caloric intake, and (3) continuing to do lower-back exercises daily in addition to 30 minutes of aerobic activity three or four days per week after recovery. Only rarely is surgery needed to correct lower-back problems.

◄ The Cool-Down Phase

As we discussed in Chapter 4, the final 3–8 minutes of a workout should be a period of slowly diminishing intensity through the use of a slow jog or walk followed by a brief stretching period. By stretching at the end of your workout as the final phase of the cool-down, you are helping fatigued muscles return to their normal resting length and to a more relaxed state, while helping to prevent pulls, strains, and spasms.

THE ASSESSMENT OF FLEXIBILITY

Because range of motion is joint specific, no one test provides an accurate assessment of overall flexibility. Instead, each joint must be evaluated. This explains why so few physical fitness batteries employ a flexibility test. Only recently have test developers begun to include flexibility as part of health-related, physical fitness test batteries. Unfortunately, modern tests gen erally include only the **sit-and-reach test,** which measures only lower-back and hamstring (the large muscle group located on the back of the upper leg) flexibility. Although this test is quite valuable and accurate, primarily because it involves some of the muscle groups associated with lower-back pain, a more thorough test is also needed. In addition, the sit-and-reach test is not recommended for those with lower-back pain/flexibility problems.

A quick evaluation of your overall flexibility level, using a less objective approach, may be even more valuable in determining your needs and the effectiveness of your stretching program. You can do this by completing the seven subjective tests described in Lab Activity 7.1: Determining Your Total Body Flexibility at the end of the chapter. If you check Yes in any test, your flexibility is considered *good* in that joint. Strive to improve your flexibility in the areas where you checked No. Repeat this series of tests after you have followed a stretching routine for 6–8 weeks. You will discover how easy it is to increase your range of motion substantially.

FLEXIBILITY-TRAINING PRINCIPLES

◄ Who Should Stretch

Some individuals need to stretch more than others. People with lean body types and a high ROM may need very little stretching whereas stocky, more powerfully

---

Vertebrae The 24 bones of the spinal column, some of which are normally fused together (sacral and coccygeal vertebrae).

Sciatica Pain along the course of the great sciatic nerve (hip, thigh, leg, foot).

Sit-and-reach test A test designed to measure the flexibility of the lower-back and hamstring muscles.

Figure 7.2 ✦ Your Back and How to Care for It

Whatever the cause of lower back pain, part of its treatment is the correction of faulty posture. But good posture is not simply a matter of "standing tall." It refers to correct use of the body at all times. In fact, for the body to function in the best of health it must be so used that no strain is put upon muscles, joints, bones, and ligaments. To prevent lower back pain, avoiding strain must become a way of life, practised while lying, sitting, standing, walking, working, and exercising. When body position is correct, internal organs have enough room to function normally and blood circulates more freely.

With the help of this guide, you can begin to correct the positions and movements that bring on or aggravate backache. Particular attention should be paid to the positions recommended for resting, since it is possible to strain the muscles of the back and neck even while lying in bed. By learning to live with good posture, under all circumstances, you will gradually develop the proper carriage and stronger muscles needed to protect and support your hardworking back.

How to Stay on Your Feet Without Tiring Your Back

To prevent strain and pain in everyday activities, it is restful to change from one task to another before fatigue sets in. Homemakers can lie down between chores; others should check body position frequently, drawing in the abdomen, flattening the back, bending the knees slightly.

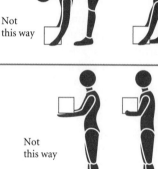
Not this way

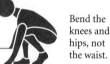
Bend the knees and hips, not the waist.

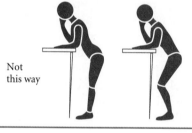
Not this way

Use of a footrest relieves swayback.

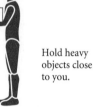
Not this way

Hold heavy objects close to you.

Not this way

Never bend over without bending the knees.

Check Your Carriage Here

In correct, fully erect posture, a line dropped from the ear will go through the tip of the shoulder, middle of hip, back of kneecaps, and front of anklebone.

Incorrect: Lower back is arched or hollow.

Incorrect: Upper back is stooped, lower back is arched, abdomen sags.

Incorrect: Note how, in strained position, pelvis tilts forward, chin is out, and ribs are down, crowding internal organs.

Correct: In correct position, chin is in, head up, back flattened, pelvis held straight.

To Find the Correct Standing Position

Stand one foot away from wall. Now sit against wall, bending knees slightly. Tighten abdominal and buttock muscles. This will tilt the pelvis back and flatten the lower spine. Holding this position, inch up the wall to standing position, by straightening the legs. Now walk around the room, maintaining the same posture. Place back against wall again to see if you have held it.

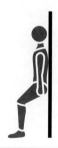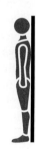

Figure 7.2 ✦ Your Back and How to Care for It *(continued)*

How to Sit Correctly

A back's best friend is a straight, hard chair. If you can't get the chair you prefer, learn to sit properly on whatever chair you get. *To correct sitting position from forward slump:* Throw head well back, then bend it forward to pull in the chin. This will straighten the back. Now tighten abdominal muscles to raise the chest. Check position frequently.

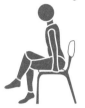
Relieve strain by sitting well forward, flatten back by tightening abdominal muscles, and cross knees.

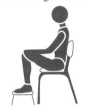
Use of footrest relieves swayback. Aim is to have knees higher than hips.

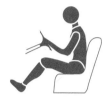
Correct way to sit while driving, close to pedals. Use seat belt or hard backrest, available commercially.

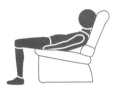
TV slump leads to "dowager's hump," strains neck and shoulders.

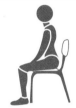
If chair is too high, swayback is increased.

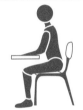
Keep neck and back in as straight a line as possible with the spine. Bend forward from the hips.

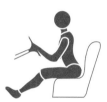
Driver's seat too far from pedals emphasizes curve in lower back.

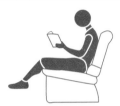
Strained reading position. Forward thrusting strains muscles of neck and head.

How to Put Your Back to Bed

For proper bed posture, a firm mattress is essential. Bedboards, sold commercially, or devised at home, may be used with soft mattresses. Bedboards, preferably, should be made of 1.9-centimetre plywood. Faulty sleeping positions intensify swayback and result not only in backache but also in numbness, tingling, and pain in arms and legs.

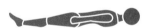
Incorrect: Lying flat on back makes swayback worse.

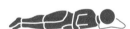
Correct: Lying on side with knees bent effectively flattens the back. Flat pillow may be used to support neck, especially when shoulders are broad.

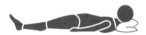
Incorrect: Use of high pillow strains neck, arms, shoulders.

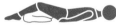
Correct: Sleeping on back is restful and correct when knees are properly supported.

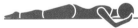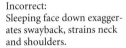
Incorrect: Sleeping face down exaggerates swayback, strains neck and shoulders.

Correct: Raise the foot of the mattress eight inches to discourage sleeping on the abdomen.

Incorrect: Bending one hip and knee does not relieve swayback.

Proper arrangement of pillows for resting or reading in bed.

When Doing Nothing, Do It Right

Rest is the first rule for the tired, painful back. The following positions relieve pain by taking all pressure and weight off the back and legs. Note pillows under knees to relieve strain on spine.

For complete relief and relaxing effect, these positions should be maintained from 5 to 25 minutes.

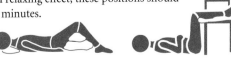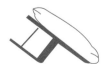
A straight-back chair used behind a pillow makes a serviceable backrest.

(continued)

Figure 7.2 ✦ Your Back and How to Care for It *(continued)*

Exercise—Without Getting Out of Bed

Exercises to be performed while lying in bed are aimed not so much at strengthening muscles as at teaching correct positioning. But muscles used correctly become stronger and in time are able to support the body with the least amount of effort.

Do all exercises in this position. Legs should not be straightened.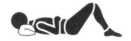

Bring knee to chest. Lower slowly but do not straighten leg. Relax.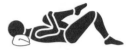

Exercise—Without Attracting Attention

Use these inconspicuous exercises whenever you have a spare moment during the day, both to relax tension and to improve the tone of important muscle groups.

1. Rotate shoulders forward and backward.
2. Turn head slowly side to side.
3. Watch an imaginary plane take off, just below the right shoulder. Stretch neck, follow it slowly as it moves up, around and down, disappearing below the other shoulder. Repeat, starting on left side.
4. Raise both shoulders to touch ears, drop them as far as possible.
5. At any pause in the day—waiting for an elevator to arrive, for a specific traffic light to change—pull in abdominal muscles, tighten, hold for the count of eight without breathing. Relax slowly. Increase the count gradually after the first week. Practise breathing normally with abdomen flat and contracted. Do this sitting, standing, and walking.

Bring both knees slowly up to chest. Tighten muscles of abdomen, press back flat against the floor. Hold knees to chest 20 seconds. Then lower slowly. Relax. Repeat five times. This exercise gently stretches the shortened muscles of the lower back, while strengthening abdominal muscles. Clasp knees, bring them up to chest at the same time coming to a sitting position. Rock back and forth.

Rules to Live By – From Now On

1. Never bend from the waist only; bend the hips and knees.
2. Never lift a heavy object higher than your waist.
3. Always turn and face the object you wish to lift.
4. Avoid carrying unbalanced loads; hold heavy objects close to your body.
5. Never carry anything heavier than you can manage with ease.
6. Never lift or move heavy furniture. Wait for someone to do it who knows the principles of leverage.
7. Avoid sudden movements, sudden "overloading" of muscles. Learn to move deliberately, swinging the legs from the hips.
8. Learn to keep the head in line with the spine when standing, sitting lying in bed.
9. Put soft chairs and deep couches on your "don't sit" list. During prolonged sitting, cross your legs to rest your back.
10. Your doctor is the only one who can determine when low back pain is due to faulty posture. He is the best judge of when you may do general exercises for physical fitness. When you do, omit any exercise which arches or over strains the lower back: backward or forward bends, touching the toes with the knees straight.
11. Wear shoes with moderate heels, all about the same height. Avoid changing from high to low heels.
12. Put a footrail under the desk and a footrest under the crib.
13. Diaper a baby sitting next to him or her on the bed.
14. Don't stoop and stretch to hang the wash; raise the clothesbasket and lower the wash-line.
15. Beg or buy a rocking chair. Rocking rests the back by changing the muscle groups used.
16. Train yourself vigorously to use your abdominal muscles to flatten your lower abdomen. In time, this muscle contraction will become habitual, making you the envied possessor of a youthful body profile!
17. Don't strain to open windows or doors.
18. For good posture, concentrate on strengthening "nature's corset" – the abdominal and buttock muscles. The pelvic roll exercise is especially recommended to correct the postural relation between the pelvis and the spine.

MYTH AND FACT SHEET

Myth	Fact
1. Stretching exercises are an excellent warm-up activity.	1. Stretching exercises are only one part of a sound routine to warm up the body. To prevent injury and muscle soreness, avoid stretching cold muscles. Begin with a general warm-up routine that involves large-muscle groups, such as walking or jogging, for at least 5 minutes or until sweating is evident; then follow with 5–10 minutes of stretching to complete the warm-up phase.
2. Stretching is only needed before vigorous activity.	2. It is important to stretch before any workout. Stretching is also an excellent cool-down activity at the end of a workout, particularly after strength training.
3. Using your body's weight to bounce into the stretch helps increase flexibility.	3. Ballistic stretching (bouncing) actually causes the muscle to shorten by stimulating a muscle spindle (an end organ in a muscle sensitive to stretching). The technique is unsound and may result in joint injury.
4. It is important to become as flexible as possible.	4. Joint laxity (looseness around a joint) and too much flexibility may decrease joint stability. Yoga-type exercises are often unsound and may lead to injuries associated with overstretching.
5. Strength training decreases flexibility.	5. Acquiring muscle mass does not automatically decrease joint movement. When weight-training exercises are performed correctly through the full range of motion, flexibility is improved.
6. Lost flexibility is an inevitable part of aging.	6. Inactivity causes much more loss than aging. Now that more of the greying population remains active, some previous findings are being reconsidered.

built athletes with limited motion need 5–10 minutes of flexibility exercise before making any radical moves such as bending over to touch the toes or explosive jumping or sprinting. Almost every healthy individual of any age or level of fitness can benefit from a regular stretching routine. Routines can be gentle, easy, relaxing, and safe or extremely vigorous. Daily stretching will help maintain flexibility throughout life and help prevent joint stiffness.

When to Stretch

Stretching exercises are used as part of a warm-up routine to prepare the body for vigorous activity, during the cool-down phase of a workout to help muscles return to a normal relaxed state, as a way to improve ROM in key joints, and as an aid to rehabilitation after injury.

Warm-Up and Cool-Down Flexibility (stretching) exercises are often too closely associated with warm-up. Consequently, most individuals make the mistake of stretching cold muscles before beginning a workout rather than first warming the body up with some large-muscle activity such as walking or jogging for 5–8 minutes or until perspiration is evident. At this point, body temperature has been elevated 2–4 degrees, and muscles can be safely stretched.

Keep in mind that you warm up to stretch; you do not stretch to warm up. Table 7.1 provides a suggested order for stretching for those who engage in jogging, walking, cycling, swimming, racquet and team sports, and strength training. Most organized aerobics classes follow a similar routine that involves a slow, gentle warm-up to cause sweating, followed by careful stretching, vigorous aerobics, and a cool-down period. Joggers and runners may choose to cover the first 0.8 kilometres or so

Table 7.1 ✦ Suggested Order for a Typical Exercise Session

Program	Workout order	Explanation
4.8-Kilometre Jog (or Run, Cycle, or Swim)		
Slow jog (0.8 km)	1	This will elevate body temperature, produce some sweating, and warm the muscles around the joints for stretching.
Stretch (8–12 min)	2	Muscles can now be safely stretched.
Fast jog (3.2 km)	3	The pace can now be increased to elevate the heart rate above the target level for the aerobic portion of the workout.
Cool-down jog (slow 0.8 km)	4	This final portion of the run can be used to help the body slowly return to the pre-exercise state.
Cool-down stretch (4–5 min)	5	This concentrated, slow, stretching session will help prevent muscle soreness and improve range of motion.
Racquet Sports (or Team Sports or Strength Training)		
Slow, deliberate strokes or movement	1	Movements specific to the sport are used to elevate body temperature and produce sweating.
Stretch (5 min)	2	Muscles can now be safely stretched using sport-specific flexibility exercises.
Actual play or workout	3	Muscles are now prepared for vigorous, explosive movement.
Cool-down (5 min)	4	This final portion of the workout should involve a return to slow, deliberate stroking or movements.
Cool-down stretch (4–5 min)	5	This concentrated, slow, stretching session will help prevent muscle soreness and improve range of motion.

at a very slow pace, then do stretching exercises before completing the run, as opposed to the more common routine of stretching cold muscles prior to the jog or run. Ideally, the majority of a stretching routine should follow the jog, run, cycle, swim, or strength-training or aerobics session and take place at the end of a workout during the cool-down phase. Stretching at the end of your workout when muscle-tissue temperature is high may effectively improve range of motion and reduce the incidence of muscle soreness the following day.

Stretching to Improve Range of Motion If your main purpose is to improve body flexibility, you can safely stretch anytime you desire—early in the morning, at work, after sitting or standing for long periods of time, when you feel stiff, after an exercise session, or while you are engaged in passive activities such as watching television or listening to music. Remember, you must first elevate body temperature and produce some sweating by engaging in large-muscle-group activity before you stretch.

Rehabilitation from Injury When you are recovering from soft-tissue injuries, focus attention on the reduction of pain and swelling, a return to normal strength, and achievement of a full, unrestricted range of motion. Unless regular stretching begins as soon as pain and swelling have been eliminated, some loss of flexibility in the injured joint is almost certain.

◼ What Stretching Technique to Use

You can choose one of several different techniques that have been shown to increase joint flexibility effectively (see Figure 7.3). Each method has its advantages and disadvantages.

Figure 7.3 ✦ A Comparison of Different Stretching Techniques

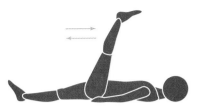

Ballistic Stretching

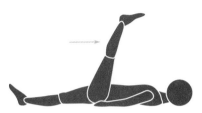

Static Stretching

PNF Stretching (Contract–Relax)

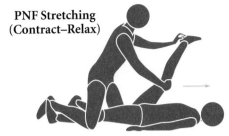

Concentric contraction of the hip flexors during contract–relax PNF stretching.

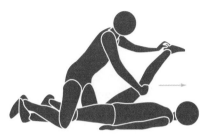

Increased ROM in the hamstrings during the passive stretch of contract–relax PNF stretching.

PNF Stretching (Hold–Relax)

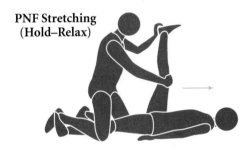

Easy stretch of hamstrings during hold–relax PNF stretching.

PNF Stretching (Reversal–Hold–Relax)

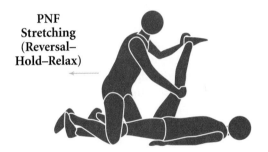

Isometric action of the hamstrings during slow–reversal–hold–relax PNF stretching.

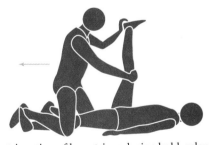

Isometric action of hamstrings during hold–relax PNF stretching.

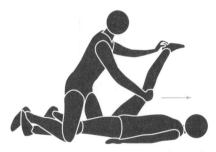

Concentric contraction of the quadriceps during slow–reversal–hold–relax PNF stretching.

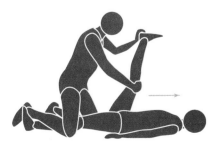

Increased ROM in the hamstrings during the passive stretch of hold–relax PNF stretching.

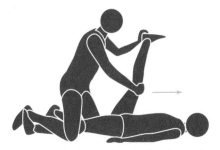

Increased ROM in the hamstrings during the passive stretch of slow–reversal–hold–relax PNF stretching.

Ballistic Stretching The technique of **ballistic stretching** employs bouncing or bobbing at the extreme ROM or point of discomfort. When they stretch the hamstring muscles, for example, individuals bounce vigorously three or four times as they reach for their toes in an attempt to aid the stretch forcefully. This method has several disadvantages. A muscle that is stretched too far and too fast in this manner may actually contract and create an opposing force, causing soft-tissue injury. An injury may also occur if the force generated by the jerking motions becomes greater than the extensibility of the tissues. Ballistic stretching is also likely to result in muscle soreness the following day.

Dynamic stretching is similar to ballistic stretching in that it involves movement; however, these movements are specific to a sport or movement pattern. Athletes, for example, choose exercises that mimic the movement patterns in their sport, such as the hurdler's stretch for track, back-scratch stretch for tennis and volleyball, specific kicking movements for soccer and football, and so on. The so-called bouncing movement at the end of the stretch must be controlled and unforceful to prevent injury.

Static Stretching While performing each exercise, you can concentrate on three unique phases of **static stretching**: (1) easy stretching, in which you move slowly into the stretch and apply only a steady, light pressure; (2) developmental stretching, in which you increase the intensity of the pressure and continue in a "stretch-by-feel" phase; and (3) drastic stretching, in which you increase the pressure further and hold for 10–30 seconds to the point of some discomfort. In phase 3, if pain occurs, simply release the pressure and return to phase 2 for the remainder of the hold. For each exercise, move slowly from the starting position into the stretch, staying relaxed and breathing normally throughout and continuing until a stretching of the muscle is felt. From the easy stretch, move to the developmental stretch by increasing the intensity for 10–15 seconds without bouncing. Move to the drastic stretch for the final 10 seconds of the 30-second stretch, decreasing the intensity and returning to the developmental stretch if you feel pain.

Proprioceptive Neuromuscular Facilitation (PNF) Stretching Proprioceptive neuromuscular facilitation (PNF) stretching is a two-person technique that combines alternating contraction and relaxation of the agonist and antagonist muscles. The interaction of the agonist and antagonist muscles results in decreased resistance and increased ROM when stretching a particular muscle. Both PNF and static stretching techniques will increase your ROM. Some studies have indicated that PNF techniques produce greater improvements. The main difference in the two techniques is that static stretching requires relaxation of the agonist muscle (the muscle being stretched) while PNF utilizes relaxation and isometric or concentric contraction of the agonist and relaxation of the antagonist muscle (the muscle not being stretched). The main disadvantage of PNF stretching is the need for an experienced partner and for supervision to eliminate "horseplay" and avoid injury due to overstretching.

Three unique types of PNF are used. In the *hold–relax* technique, your partner performs an easy stretch of your right hamstring (see Figure 7.3). With the command "push," you exert a 3-to-4-second isometric contraction of your hamstring (your partner does not allow your leg to move), followed by a 10-second easy stretch on the command "relax" (your partner pushes backward on your right leg). Complete three to five repetitions without lowering your leg before repeating the exercise on your other leg.

The *contraction–relax* technique (see Figure 7.3) begins in the same starting position with your partner providing an easy 4-to-6-second stretch before giving the signal "back" for you to contract your hip flexors for 4–6 seconds as your partner continues to push your leg forward. On the command "relax," your partner provides another easy stretch against your hamstring for 10 seconds. You then lower your leg to the starting position. Complete three to five repetitions with each leg.

The *reversal–hold–relax* technique (see Figure 7.3) begins in the same starting position, with your partner performing an easy stretch until you experience slight discomfort. Your partner now tells you to "push" against the hand for 6–10 seconds (isometric action of the hamstring against an immovable object—the hand). Near the end of the 10-second period, your partner gives the command "back" to signal you to contract your quadriceps and hip flexors in an attempt to pull your leg back and lift the heel of your right foot off the hand. Your partner simultaneously pushes against your straight leg. At this point, with your quadriceps contracted, your hamstrings are relaxed and the ROM of the stretch is increased. Continue to contract your muscles until your partner says "relax," at which time a 10-second easy push is applied. Complete two to three repetitions before moving to your other leg.

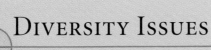

DIVERSITY ISSUES

Flexibility: Improving the Lives of People of All Ages

An infant or young child has an amazing degree of flexibility. These youngsters may place their feet behind their heads or nibble on their toes—acts most adults can only admire, for, as we age, our degree of flexibility diminishes until even toe-touching becomes difficult.

Like most components of fitness, loss of flexibility occurs more rapidly and to a much higher degree among the sedentary population. Individuals of all ages, but especially the elderly, who engage in regular stretching routines can maintain a fairly high level of joint flexibility throughout life. In fact, flexibility is one of the easiest fitness components to improve. Even sedentary, inflexible individuals can greatly improve joint movement after only a few weeks of regular stretching.

Common ailments among the elderly, such as joint stiffness, pain, and inflexibility, can be improved through regular exercise and stretching. In fact, stretching can improve mobility, make daily chores easier, and increase self-efficiency. Flexibility begins to decrease dramatically in sedentary university-age men and women. Even minor injuries to the joints produce scar tissue and begin to reduce flexibility. As midlife approaches, joint stiffness becomes common, often to the point of limiting recreational pursuits and daily chores. This dramatic loss of flexibility over the aging process is primarily due to inactivity and failure to maintain an active program of stretching.

One dramatic example of the importance of maintaining adequate flexibility throughout life is lower-back pain—one of the most prevalent health complaints in Canada. By middle age, approximately one in two individuals suffers from this ailment and experiences pain, discomfort, and decreased work and recreational efficiency. In most cases, lower-back pain is caused by poor lower-back flexibility and inadequate abdominal-muscle tone. Simply engaging in a 5-to-10-minute stretching routine three times weekly in young adulthood can maintain or improve flexibility levels and help prevent lower-back and other joint-related health problems in later years. ✦

◗ How Much Intensity to Use

Proper stretching should take the form of slow, relaxed, controlled, and relatively pain-free movement. It is important to disregard the "no pain, no gain" mentality when you stretch because improvement occurs without undue pain. Joint pressure should produce only mild discomfort. Too much pain or discomfort is a sign you are overloading soft tissue and are at risk of injury. After experiencing mild discomfort with each stretch, relax the muscles being stretched before the next repetition. You will learn to judge each exercise by the *stretch-and-feel method*, easing off the push if pain becomes intense or increases as the phase progresses.

◗ How Long to Stretch

Depending on the stretching technique you choose, the length of your workout will be determined by the number of repetitions (ballistic stretching) and/or the length of time each repetition is held in the stretched position (static and PNF stretching). The amount of time the position is held should progress from 10 seconds at first to 30 seconds after two or three months of regular stretching. A 30-to-60-second stretch appears to only slightly increase the benefits and may be impractical.

Ballistic stretching Flexibility exercises employing bouncing and jerking movements at the extreme range of motion or point of discomfort.

Static stretching Flexibility exercises in which a position is held steady for a designated period of time at the extreme range of motion.

Proprioceptive neuromuscular facilitation (PNF) stretching A two-person stretching technique involving the application of steady pressure by a partner at the extreme range of motion for a particular exercise and steady resistance to the pressure.

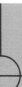

BEHAVIOURAL CHANGE AND MOTIVATIONAL STRATEGIES

A number of things may interfere with your flexibility-training progress. Here are some of these barriers (roadblocks) and strategies for overcoming them to keep you moving toward your training goals.

Roadblock	Behavioural Change Strategy
You are aware of your need to engage in flexibility training but just can't seem to stay interested long enough to avoid skipping workouts.	The first month of any exercise program is the most difficult. If you are beginning a new exercise program, it is normal to feel overloaded and anxious to complete the workout. At this point, you feel that 5–10 minutes of stretching takes valuable time and you are unable to see its benefits. Try some of the following techniques to get past this critical period: 1. Arrive at the exercise site early with plenty of time to enjoy your workout. 2. After you walk or jog a few minutes, take 5–10 minutes to relax, wind down, and enjoy stretching the major joints. 3. Make a mental note of how far beyond your toes you can reach, how difficult it is to reach behind your back and touch both hands, or how far forward you are able to move when stretching your calf muscles. Having these mental notes will help make you aware of improvement in future workouts. 4. Force yourself to stretch carefully prior to every workout until it becomes habit and you discover the benefits of stretching.
At the end of a workout, your calves feel tight and are sometimes sore.	A feeling of tightness or even some mild soreness should only occur after your first three or four workouts. If it continues, examine every phase of your program. Are you properly warmed up prior to beginning your stretching session? Are you using static or PNF stretching exercises rather than ballistic movements? Are you stretching for 3–5 minutes at the end of your workout? Are you performing the correct exercises? Are you stretching both the calf muscles and the Achilles tendon? You should find the answer to the problem in one or more of these questions.
List other roadblocks you are experiencing that seem to be limiting the effectiveness of your flexibility-training program. 1. _____ 2. _____ 3. _____	Now list the behavioural change strategies that can help you overcome these roadblocks. If you need to, refer back to Chapter 3 for behavioural change and motivational strategies. 1. _____ 2. _____ 3. _____

If your main purpose for stretching is to prepare your body for vigorous exercise and to maintain the existing ROM in the major joints, 5–12 minutes is sufficient time. For athletes and other individuals striving to increase their ROM, 10–30 minutes of careful stretching may be necessary. Several different stretching exercises may be performed for each joint.

How Flexible to Become

Just how much flexibility someone needs depends on the individual. The gymnast, ballet dancer, and hurdler must be more flexible than a person who merely wants to maintain a high enough level to reap the health benefits, perform daily activities, and engage in regular exercise.

According to professionals in Canada's health-related industries, there is an increasing number of injury cases associated with excessive stretching and attempts to acquire high levels of flexibility compared to injury cases associated with failure to stretch. This may be partially due to a renewed interest in stretching and the popularity of various forms of yoga and aerobics that tend to overemphasize flexibility or use questionable stretching exercises (Baker, 1999).

How Often to Stretch

Those who are just beginning a flexibility-training program should do their routine three to four times a week. After several months, two or three workouts a week will maintain the flexibility you have acquired. As we pointed out previously, stretching should also be a part of the regular warm-up routine prior to participation in aerobics, sports, or other forms of exercise.

*F*LEXIBILITY EXERCISES

It is important to choose at least one stretching exercise for each of the major muscle groups and to apply exercises equally to both sides of the body. Although there are hundreds of different stretches in use, many are

unsafe and should be avoided. This section identifies the proper way to stretch and some of the more commonly used exercises that have been shown to be potentially harmful along with safe alternatives.

What Exercises to Use

It is important to focus on a stretching routine that will increase the range of motion in particular joints of your choice. Stretching routines are also available that are designed for a specific sport or activity. After you warm up properly and are perspiring, complete each exercise slowly, beginning with a 10-second hold and adding 2–3 seconds to your hold time each workout until you can comfortably maintain the position at your extreme ROM for 30 seconds. You can begin with the neck and progress downward to the shoulders and chest, trunk and lower back, groin and hips, abdomen, and upper and lower legs.

What Exercises to Avoid

As we pointed out previously, stretching can be harmful when the routine is too vigorous or too lengthy or when bouncing at the extreme ROM is used. The wrong choice of exercises also imposes serious risk of injury to joints. In fact, many popular stretching exercises used in the past are considered potentially harmful. Unfortunately, most people acquire their stretching knowledge by watching others. This informal, copycat approach has spawned a series of popular but dangerous exercises capable of damaging the knees, neck, spinal column, ankles, and lower back. Figure 7.4 identifies nine of the most popular "Hit List" stretching exercises that should be avoided and offers a safe substitute that will effectively stretch the same muscle group.

Figure 7.4 ✦ Dangerous Popular Stretching Exercises and Suggested Replacements

OLD METHOD		NEW METHOD	

Neck roll (circling)

Danger: Drawing the head backward could damage the discs in the neck area, and may even precipitate arthritis.

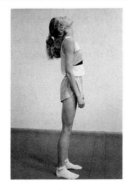

Forward neck roll

Description: Bend forward at the waist with the hands on the knees. Gently roll the head.

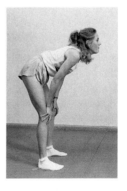

(continued)

Figure 7.4 ✦ Dangerous Popular Stretching Exercises and Suggested Replacements (*continued*)

OLD METHOD	NEW METHOD

Quadricep stretch

Danger: If the ankle is pulled too hard, muscle, ligament, and cartilage damage may occur.

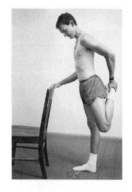

Opposite leg pull

Description: Grasp one ankle with your opposite hand. Instead of pulling, attempt to straighten the leg.

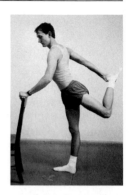

Hurdler's stretch

Danger: Hip, knee, and ankle are subjected to abnormal stress.

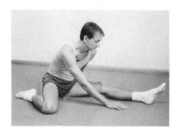

Everted hurdler's stretch

Description: Bend the leg at the knee and slide the foot next to the other foot. Pull yourself forward slowly by using a towel, or by grasping the toe.

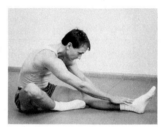

Deep knee bend (or any exercise that bends the knee beyond a right angle)

Danger: Excessive stress is placed on ligament, tendon, and cartilage tissue.

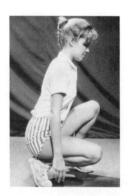

Single knee lunge

Description: Place one leg in front of your body and extend the other behind. Bend forward at the trunk as you bend the lead leg to right angles.

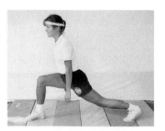

Yoga plow

Danger: This exercise could overstretch muscles and ligaments, injure spinal discs, or cause fainting.

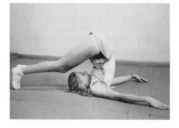

Extended one-leg stretch

Description: Lead leg extended and slightly bent at the knee. With your foot on the floor, draw the knee of the other leg toward your chest. Bend forward at the trunk as far as possible.

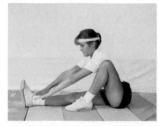

Figure 7.4 ✦ Dangerous Popular Stretching Exercises and Suggested Replacements *(continued)*

OLD METHOD	NEW METHOD

Straight-leg sit-up

Danger: Produces back strain and sciatic nerve elongation. It also moves the hip flexor muscles and does not flatten the abdomen.

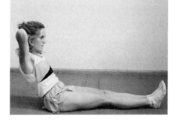

Bent-knee sit-up

Description: Cross both hands on your chest, with the knees slightly bent. Raise the upper body slightly to about 25° on each repetition.

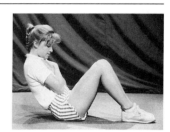

Double leg raise

Danger: Stretches the sciatic nerve beyond its normal limits, and places too much stress on ligaments, muscles, and discs.

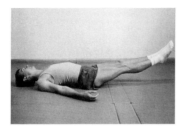

Knee-to-chest stretch

Description: Clasp both hands behind the neck. Draw the knee toward the chest, and hold that position of maximum stretch for 15–30 seconds.

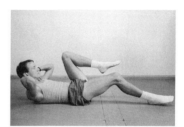

SUMMARY

■ Factors Affecting Flexibility

A number of factors combine to place some limitation on the degree of flexibility you attain. After age, sex, heredity, and injury, your choice of lifestyle has the greatest influence on ROM in your joints. By engaging in a regular aerobic exercise program, stretching before and after your workout, and maintaining normal body weight and fat, you can remain relatively flexible throughout your life.

■ The Importance of Flexibility

Regular involvement in stretching exercises two to three times a week will increase joint flexibility, help improve performance in sports, aid in the prevention of soft-tissue injuries, help you prevent and recover from lower-back problems, and assist your muscles in returning to a relaxed state following a workout. Stretching can provide some benefit to almost everyone and make daily chores at home and at work easier and safer.

■ The Assessment of Flexibility

To properly evaluate your body's flexibility, one test should be used for each of the major joints. Although the sit-and-reach test is one of the most common and accurate, it only measures hamstring and lower-back flexibility. Tests are also needed to measure ROM in the neck, elbows, wrists, groin, trunk, hips, and shoulders.

■ Flexibility-Training Principles

Two to three sessions a week in addition to the stretching routine you normally perform before an aerobic workout will improve your flexibility. You should stretch for about five minutes before every workout but only after your body temperature has been elevated, as indicated by the presence of perspiration following some large-muscle activity such as jogging. It is important to avoid stretching cold muscles. A more concentrated 10-minute session should be used during the cool-down phase of a workout.

All three of the most common methods of stretching (ballistic, static, and PNF) have been shown to be equally effective in improving joint ROM. Ballistic and PNF methods are more likely to result in injury and muscle soreness than static stretching is.

Stretching should produce only mild discomfort. Pain is an indication of risk of injury from overextending soft tissue. Stretching for too long a period of time in an attempt to obtain an extremely high degree of flexibility may also result in injury. Extreme flexibility is unimportant for most individuals, and yoga-style contortions should be avoided.

Effective stretching involves warming up, stretching before and after exercise, stretching slowly and gently, holding the stretch for 10–30 seconds, and relaxing the body parts other than the muscle group you are stretching.

▪ Flexibility Exercises

A sound program requires at least one exercise for each major joint and emphasis on both sides of the body. Exercises can be chosen that focus on the particular joints you identify as inflexible or important to your personal life, job, sport, or activity. Although not everyone who uses so-called banned stretching exercises will suffer an injury, it is wise to avoid those known to have the potential to damage a joint.

STUDY QUESTIONS

1. Describe the basic structure of the back bones.

2. What are the most common causes of back pain?

3. Describe three daily activities that can contribute to lower-back problems. For each activity, describe the proper method to perform those activities in a safer way.

4. What is the basic difference between stretching and warm-up? How do you cool down?

5. How does PNF stretching work? That is, what is the theory behind PNF stretching?

6. Describe some of the more effective exercises or exercise methods one might use to become more flexible.

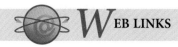# WEB LINKS

How to Stretch
www.enteract.com/~bradapp/docs/rec/ stretching/http://www.sport-fitness-advisor.com/ flexibilitytraining.html www.mckinley.uiuc.edu/health-info/fitness/ exercise/imprflex.html www.savvyknowledge.com/fitness_software/ stretching_and_flexibility.htm www.mckinley.uiuc.edu/health-info/ fitness/back/stretch.html

Types of Stretching
www.bath.ac.uk/~masrjb/Stretch/stretching_4.html

Lower Back Pain Explanation/Analysis
http://familydoctor.org/flowcharts/531.html www.methodisthealth.com/rehab/lowback.htm

The Alexander Technique for Lower Back Care
www.idellepacker.net/backcare.html

The College of Family Physicians of Canada/Le Collège des médecins de famille du Canada
www.cfpc.ca/programs/education/pated/low_back.asp

REFERENCES

J. Baker, "Yoga's Harder Than You Think," *The Gazette* (Montreal), February 1999. Available at **http.stretchingtips. com/press.html**. Accessed March 13, 2003.

Henderson, Bob, *Stretching*, Bolinos, CA: Shelter Publications, Inc., 1984, 2000 ed.

"Preventing Sports Injury." Sept 23, 2002. Information from the *Capital Health* Web site. **www.cha.ab.ca**. Accessed March 5, 2003.

Shrier, Ian, and Kav Gossal. "Myths and Truths of Stretching." *The Physician and Sportsmedicine* 28, 8 (2000).

Lab Activity 7.1

Determining Your Total Body Flexibility

INSTRUCTIONS: *You can test aspects of your flexibility subjectively alone or with a partner. The only equipment needed is a straight-backed chair and a ruler. Score each test by checking Yes or No, depending on whether you can meet the standard cited.*

   Warm up properly before testing your flexibility. Walk, jog, or participate in a low-to-moderate-level aerobic activity for 5–10 minutes or until you perspire. Now complete your warm-up by gently stretching out your body as shown in Figure 7.4.

		Yes	No
1. Neck Lower your chin to sandwich your flattened hand against your chest.		____	____
2. Elbow and wrist Hold your arms out straight with palms up and little fingers higher than your thumbs.	Right arm/wrist	____	____
	Left arm/wrist	____	____
3. Groin While standing on one leg, raise the other leg to the side as high as possible. You should be able to achieve a 45-degree angle between the two legs.	Right leg	____	____
	Left leg	____	____
While you are sitting on the floor, put the soles of your feet together and draw your heels as close to your body as possible. Try to touch your knees to the floor or to press your upright fists to the floor using your knees.		____	____
4. Trunk While sitting in a straight chair with your feet wrapped around the front legs, twist your body 90 degrees without allowing your hips to move.	Right twist	____	____
	Left twist	____	____
5. Hip While standing, hold a yardstick or broom handle with your hands shoulder-width apart. Without losing your grasp, bend down and step over the stick (with both feet, one at a time) and then back again.		____	____
6. Shoulder In a standing position, attempt to clasp your hands behind your back by reaching over the shoulder with one arm and upward from behind with the other. Repeat, reversing the arm positions.	Right arm top	____	____
	Left arm top	____	____

8

Nutrition

During Rita's freshman year, cafeteria food became unappealing. She had gained 4 kilograms, had low energy, and was aware she was eating too much fat. She also was sick a number of times and wondered whether any of these illnesses were related to her poor eating habits. To be honest, Rita had to admit, she simply didn't know enough about proper nutrition. Even if she discontinued the university meal plan, she would not know what to do.

This chapter focuses on Rita's concerns and presents an overview of sound nutrition to help her (and others like her) make appropriate choices in the cafeteria or prepare a nutritional program. Discussion is provided on the basic food components, the energy or macro nutrients (carbohydrates, fats, proteins), the nonenergy or micro nutrients (vitamins, minerals, water), food density, dietary guidelines for good health and high energy, food labelling, nutrition–disease relationships, nutrition and aging, and special needs of the active person.

KINDS OF NUTRIENTS

Six categories of nutrients—carbohydrates, fats, proteins (the energy or macro nutrients), vitamins, minerals, and water (the nonenergy or micro nutrients)—satisfy the basic body needs:

- Energy for muscle contraction
- Conduction of nerve impulses
- Growth
- Formation of new tissue and tissue repair
- Chemical regulation of metabolic functions
- Reproduction

The body's use of these nutrients for conversion into tissue, production of energy for muscle contraction, and maintenance of chemical machinery is called **metabolism**.

THE ENERGY NUTRIENTS (MACRO NUTRIENTS)

Carbohydrates and fat provide the body with its two main sources of energy. All food has energy potential, measured in calories. When you see the term *calorie* on a food label or in terms of the number of calories the body needs or burns, it refers to kilocalories (kcal). One kilocalorie is the amount of heat required to raise the temperature of 1 kilogram of water 1 degree Celsius. Because the term *kilocalorie* is generally reserved for laboratories and technical journals, the term **calorie** will be used now throughout this chapter. The energy in one peanut, for example, can add 1 degree of heat to 9 litres of water. Only carbohydrates, fats, and protein contain calories; vitamins, minerals, and water do not.

Just how much energy do these nutrients provide? Carbohydrates and protein contain 4 calories per gram, fat contains 9 calories per gram, and alcohol contains 7 calories per gram.

Recall that basal metabolism (BMR) is the minimum energy the body needs to support the ongoing activities of the cells when the body is at rest, or work that goes on continuously without awareness. This represents the largest (60 percent or more) portion of your daily caloric expenditure and amounts to about 1200–1400 calories daily for an individual whose total energy expenditure is 2000 calories. BMR is increased by factors such as drugs (caffeine and other stimulants), fever, growth (higher in children and pregnant women), height and weight, ingestion of a meal (the **thermic effect of food**), sex (males possess more lean muscle tissue), mus-

cle mass, stress, and the thyroid hormone. BMR is decreased by age and reduced caloric intake (fasting, starvation, low-calorie diets).

Your metabolic rate or metabolism refers to the energy expended to maintain all physical and chemical changes occurring in the body. This includes basal metabolism, exercise metabolism (the **thermic effect of exercise**), and calories expended following ingestion of food. It is estimated that your total daily caloric expenditure breaks down as follows:

- Basal metabolism: 60–65 percent
- Thermic effect of exercise: 25–30 percent
- Thermic effect of food: 5–10 percent

You can determine your daily total caloric needs by completing Lab Activity 8.1: Estimating Caloric Expenditure at the end of this chapter.

◼ Carbohydrates

Carbohydrates are organic components of various elements that provide a continuous supply of energy in the form of glucose (sugar) to trillions of body cells. **Simple carbohydrates (monosaccharides and disaccharides)** come concentrated—such as refined sugar, which is made from cane or beet sugar, molasses, and honey—and natural—such as the sugars in some fruits, vegetables, and grains. **Complex carbohydrates (polysaccharides)** are chains of sugar molecules found in fruits, vegetables, and grains. Carbohydrates are broken down into six simple carbon-sugar molecules to permit absorption into the bloodstream. After food is eaten, the blood-sugar level is elevated, and there is an increase in the amount of glucose transported to the cells. Excess sugar is converted to glycogen and stored for future use in the liver and muscles. Once maximum storage capacity is reached, excess sugars are converted to body fat and stored in **adipose tissue**.

Simple Versus Complex Carbohydrates Simple carbohydrates (sugars) are consumed in four forms: sucrose, glucose, fructose, and lactose. Annual intake of refined sugar, maple sugar, and honey in Canada is approximately 40 kilograms per person. Consumed in these large quantities, sugar contributes directly to dental cavities, excessive weight, and body fat and indirectly to such degenerative diseases as diabetes and heart disease. As you can see from Table 8.1, it is not unusual for a person to consume the equivalent of 50 teaspoons (247 mL) of sugar per day.

Sugar intake should be managed from infancy. Infants seem to be born with a preference for sweet foods, and it is not until early adulthood that the desire for sugar slowly decreases. You can reduce your own sugar intake by reading the labels for sweeteners and sugars in

Table 8.1 ✦ Sugar Content of Common Foods and Drinks

Food/Drink	Size	Approximate Content (mL)
Beverages:	341 mL	
Pop		25–45
Sweet cider		21.25
Jams and jellies, candies	15 mL	20–30
Milk chocolate	43 mL	12.5
Fudge	28 mL	22.5
Hard candy	114 mL	100
Marshmallow	1	7.5
Fruits and canned juices:		
Dried raisins, prunes, apricots, dates	3–5	20
Fruit juice	227 mL	12.5–17.5
Breads:		
White	1 slice	1.25
Hamburger/ hot dog bun	1	15
Dairy products:		
Ice cream cone	Single dip	15
Sherbet	One scoop	45
Desserts:		
Pie (fruit, custard cream)	1 slice	20–65
Pudding	114 mL	15–25

complex carbohydrates are the body's chief source of fuel. Sugar, on the other hand, provides empty calories and very little long-term energy.

Complex carbohydrates should make up at least 45 percent of your total daily calories. Simple carbohydrates should be reduced from 24 percent to 10 percent of total calories.

Fibre As the indigestible portion of complex carbohydrates, dietary or **insoluble fibre** is a nonnutritive substance that cannot be broken down by the enzymes in the human body. Six of the seven types of fibre are carbohydrates. Only lignin, found in fruit and vegetable skins and the woody portions of plants, is a noncarbohydrate.

In 2002, the Food and Nutrition Board, overseen by the Standing Committee on the Scientific Evaluation of Dietary Reference Intakes, recommended that Canadian and American men and women should consume 38 and 25 grams of fibre a day, respectively.

Table 8.2 provides an overview of key information on fibre, including water-soluble and -insoluble

Metabolism The sum of energy expended in carrying on the normal body processes: converting nutrients into tissue, fuelling muscle contraction, and maintaining the body's chemical machinery.

Calorie A "large" calorie, equal to 1000 "small" calories; 1 calorie is the amount of heat required to raise the temperature of 1 kilogram of water 1 degree Celsius.

Thermic effect of food The increase in the basal metabolic rate following the ingestion of a meal; lasts 1–4 hours.

Thermic effect of exercise The increase in metabolism brought about by activity or muscular movement during the day.

Simple carbohydrates (monosaccharides and disaccharides) Sugars; chains of sugar molecules (one or two) found in concentrated sugar and the sugar that occurs naturally in food.

Complex carbohydrates (polysaccharides) Starch and fibre; chains of sugar molecules (three or more) found in fruits, vegetables, and grains.

Adipose tissue Fatty tissue; fat cells.

Nutrition density Foods that are high in nutrients and low in calories.

Insoluble fibre The undigestible portion of food after it is exposed to the body's enzymes.

products you are considering (the terms *sucrose, glucose, dextrose, fructose, corn syrup, corn sweetener, natural sweetener,* and *invert sugar* all mean that the product contains sugar), substituting water and unsweetened fruit juices for sodas and punches, buying fruit canned in its own unsweetened juice, cutting back on desserts, purchasing cereals low in sugar, reducing the amount of sugar called for in recipes, and avoiding sweet snacks. If you never again consumed concentrated sugars, it would have absolutely no effect on sound nutrition.

Complex carbohydrates are your major source of vitamins (except vitamin B_{12}) and minerals, an important long-term energy source and the only source of fibre. Complex carbohydrates burn efficiently, leave no toxic waste in the body, and do not tax the liver or raise blood-fat levels. Fruits, vegetables, and grains also have high **nutrition density,** providing a high percentage of our needed daily nutrients in a low number of calories. In the past 75 years, our intake of complex carbohydrates has declined by about 30 percent while sugar intake has increased by a similar amount. Unlike sugars,

Table 8.2 ✦ All About Fibre

CHARACTERISTIC	DESCRIPTION
Water-insoluble	Cellulose, forming the cell walls of many plants, is the most abundant insoluble fibre. Cellulose and lignin (from the woody portion of plants, parts of fruit and vegetable skins, and whole grains) cannot be broken down, digested, or made to provide calories for the body.
Water-soluble	Fibre types such as pectin, gums, and mucilages dissolve or swell when placed in water. Dried beans and peas (7 grams per 100 mL), oat bran, and the flesh of fruits and vegetables are excellent sources of water-soluble fibre.
Dietary fibre	Undigested residue after the action of the body's enzymes; much more concentrated than crude fibre (1 gram of crude fibre = 2–3 grams of dietary fibre). Dietary fibre (water-insoluble) is reported on most labels that list fibre content.
Daily needs	25–38 grams. It is important to increase your daily intake slowly if you are unaccustomed to adequate fibre to avoid frequent bowel movements and diarrhea. Add several grams daily over a period of a few weeks to give your system a chance to adjust.
Nutritional advantages of consuming adequate fibre	*Water-insoluble* fibre increases transit time (digestion and elimination of food) and decreases the amount of time the bacteria in the food has to act on intestinal walls. It helps prevent colon and rectal cancer and *diverticulosis* (outpouchings in the wall of the large intestine), provides bulk to the stools, helps eliminate constipation, helps maintain normal bowel movement, and helps to control and maintain normal body weight and fat. *Water-soluble* fibre is associated with lower cardiovascular disease, lower blood cholesterol, and lower blood pressure. It also may improve blood-sugar tolerance by delaying glucose absorption and help prevent obesity by prolonging eating time and replacing calories from fat.
Dangers of excess fibre	Excess fibre binds to some trace minerals and causes excretion prior to the absorption of these minerals. Excessive fibre intake causes poor absorption of nutrients, interferes with the absorption of some drugs, reduces the ability to digest and absorb food by speeding up digestive time, and causes irritation of the intestinal wall. The high phosphorous content of high-fibre foods may create special problems for some individuals, such as those with kidney problems.
Food sources	Complex carbohydrates (fruits, vegetables, grains) are the sole source of fibre. Both water-insoluble and water-soluble fibre are contained in some food sources, such as in the skin of fruits and vegetables (insoluble) and in the flesh of fruits and vegetables (soluble). Raw fruits and vegetables are a major source of insoluble fibre such as in dried beans and peas (7 grams per 100 mL). Oat bran and grains are a major source of soluble fibre.
	Many hot and cold cereals (unprocessed bran, 100 percent bran, shredded wheat, oatmeal) contain 2–5 grams of fibre per serving. Legumes provide about 8 grams per portion (114 mL of garbanzo beans, kidney beans, or baked beans). Fruits provide about 2 grams per serving (1 small apple, banana, orange; 2 small plums, 1 medium peach, 114 mL strawberries, 10 large cherries). Vegetables also provide about 2 grams per serving (broccoli, brussels sprouts, 2 stalks of celery, small cob of corn, lettuce, green beans, small potato, tomato), and 1 gram of fibre is provided by 10 peanuts, 57 mL walnuts, 12.5 mL of peanut butter, and 1 pickle. Additional foods with fibre are breads (whole wheat, whole grain), crackers, and flours (wheat germ, wild rice, cornmeal, buckwheat, millet, rice, raisin, popcorn). Cooking does not significantly reduce the fibre content of foods.

Sources: Jerry Greenberg and George B. Dintiman, *Exploring Health: Expanding the Boundaries of Wellness* (Englewood Cliffs, NJ: Prentice-Hall, 1992); Food and Nutrition Board and Institute of Medicine. Dietary Reference Intakes for Energy, Carbohydrate, Fiber, Fat, Fatty Acids, Cholesterol, Protein and Amino Acids (Washington Macronutrients National Academy Press, 2002).

Figure 8.1 ✦ Controlling Blood-Glucose Levels

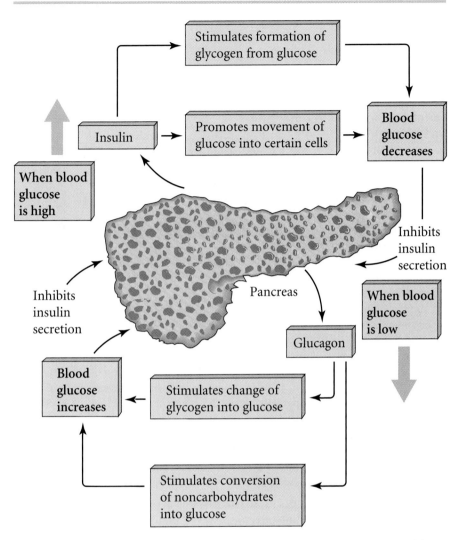

Source: From David C. Nieman, Diane E. Butterworth, and Catherine N. Nieman, *Nutrition*, rev. 1st ed., © 1992 Wm. C. Brown Communications, Inc., Dubuque, IA. All rights reserved. Reprinted by permission of The McGraw-Hill Companies.

varieties, recommended daily intake, nutritional advantages of adequate amounts, dangers of excess intake, and the food sources for both types. Complete Lab Activity 8.2: Estimating Your Daily Fibre Intake at the end of this chapter to discover whether your diet contains enough fibre.

Blood-Glucose Control Blood-glucose levels are carefully regulated by the pancreas. When blood-sugar levels are too high, the pancreas releases a hormone called **insulin**, which promotes the movement of glucose into certain cells, dropping blood-sugar levels. When levels are too low, the pancreas secretes a hormone called **glucagon**, which stimulates the conversion of stored liver glycogen into glucose and the conversion of non-

carbohydrates into glucose to raise the blood-sugar level (see Figure 8.1). The pancreas of individuals who

Insulin A natural hormone produced in the pancreas gland that aids in the digestion of sugars and other carbohydrates; secreted when blood sugar is too high.

Glucagon A natural hormone secreted by the pancreas that stimulates the metabolism of sugar; secreted when blood sugar is too low, a condition that causes the release of liver glycogen and its transformation into glucose.

have **Type I** (insulin-dependent) **diabetes mellitus** fails to produce insulin, so it must be injected to control blood-glucose levels. The pancreas of most individuals who have adult-onset, **Type II** (non-insulin-dependent) **diabetes mellitus** produces insulin; glucose uptake at the cellular level, however, does not occur normally, and blood-sugar levels remain high. For most of us, the pancreas does its job and, in conjunction with proper diet, maintains blood glucose at normal levels regardless of what we eat and how much we exercise.

Although the use of the term is controversial, foods with a high **glycemic index**, such as those containing high amounts of concentrated sugars (maple syrup, table sugar, honey, molasses, bagels, raisins, white potatoes, sweet corn, corn flakes), cause a rapid rise in blood-glucose levels if they are not consumed with adequate amounts of protein or foods with a low glycemic index (apples, cherries, chick peas, lentils, dates, figs, peaches, plums, green beans, kidney/navy beans, red lentils, skim milk). A rapid increase in blood-glucose levels can lead to both fatigue and hunger. (See Chapter 9 for more information on the control of hunger and appetite and the role of changes in blood-glucose levels.)

Alcohol In 2001, Canadians drank an average of just over 83 litres of alcohol. Over 80 percent of this was beer, 11 percent wine, and over 7 percent spirits. Close to 80 percent of Canadians aged 18 and over consume alcohol. Just over half claim to consume five or more drinks at a single occasion, and 12 percent report drinking daily. For light drinkers (one or two beers, small glasses of wine, or average-size cocktails) who are well nourished and in good health, the occasional consumption of alcohol will have little effect on nutrition except for the additional 250–300 calories. Any amount of alcohol, however, affects metabolism. With larger amounts, your nutritional status becomes compromised, and a number of problems occur. These include: protein deficiency; failure of intestinal cells to absorb thiamin, folate, and vitamin B_{12}; excretion of increased quantities of magnesium, calcium, potassium, and zinc by the kidneys; dislodgement of vitamin B_6, creating a deficiency that lowers the production of red blood cells; reduced capacity of the liver to activate vitamin D; and many other changes. Although proper nutrition is important for those who consume alcohol, it does not prevent changes in the excretion, absorption, and utilization of numerous nutrients.

Fats

Fat is a critical nutrient that provides a tremendous source of energy to the human body. Fat also stores and transports vitamins A, D, E, and K; carries linoleic acid

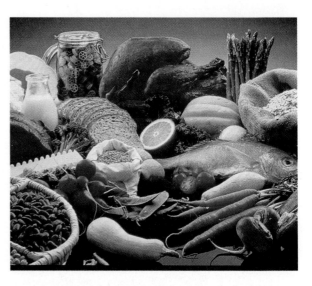

To maintain sound nutrition, choose lower-fat foods whenever possible.

(an essential fatty acid); increases the flavour and palatability of foods; provides sustained relief from hunger; and helps to keep protein from being used as energy. The fatty tissue in our bodies supports organs, cushions them from injury, and aids in the prevention of heat loss. Fat is in most body tissue, with bone marrow containing 96 percent, liver 2.5 percent, and blood 0.5 percent. Unfortunately, too much body fat and high blood-fat levels can shorten life and increase vulnerability to numerous chronic and degenerative diseases, such as cardiorespiratory disease and cancer.

The Fat in Food The fat in food is classified as **saturated, polyunsaturated**, and **monounsaturated. Cholesterol** is used in the synthesis of sex hormones, vitamin D, and bile salts. It is also associated with artery clogging and heart disease (see Chapter 13). Cholesterol is a **nonessential nutrient**. Blood levels depend on the cholesterol consumed by people and that produced by their livers (see Table 8.3). The intake of saturated fat stimulates the liver to produce more cholesterol.

According to Health Canada's Office of Nutrition Policy and Promotion (2002), Canadians appear to consume, on average, a higher percentage of fat than recommended. Current levels are estimated at approximately 38 percent of total energy, which is well above the recommended level of 30 percent. There has, however, been a trend toward lower proportions of energy derived from fat since the 1974 Family Food Expenditure Survey, which found that the average proportion of energy contributed by fat was over 43.5 percent. The proportion of fat from vegetable sources is increasing in relation to total fat intake, whereas animal sources of fat have been declining in popularity. Although the average

Table 8.3 ✦ A Few High-Cholesterol Foods

FOOD	AMOUNT	CHOLESTEROL (mg)
Liver, beef	85 g	372
Kidney, beef	85 g	315
Eggs (whole or yolk only)	1 large	252
Sponge cake	½ of cake	162
Shrimp, canned	85 g	128
Frankfurter	2 (113 g)	112
Lemon meringue pie	⅙ of 9-inch pie	98
Crab, canned	85 g	85
Veal (lean)	85 g	84
Beef (lean)	85 g	77
Chicken, dark (no skin)	85 g	77
Pork, lean	85 g	75
Butter	15 mL	35

Source: "Keeping Cholesterol at Bay," off *Aim This Way* Web page, accessed April 27, 1999 **http://aimthisway.com/aimthisway/keepcholatba.html**.

level of saturated fats is falling, it is currently estimated at 13 percent of total energy intake, which exceeds the recommended level of 10 percent. The average amount of cholesterol in foods purchased is estimated at 442 milligrams per day per person in contrast to the recommended maximum of 300 milligrams per day. Total and saturated fat levels in the Canadian diet need to be significantly reduced to meet the recommendation for no more than 30 percent of energy from total fat and no more than 10 percent energy from saturated fat.

The five kinds of foods containing the highest percentage of their calories in fat are hamburgers and meatloaf (63 percent); hot dogs, ham, and luncheon meats (58 percent); whole milk (54 percent); doughnuts, cakes, and cookies (54 percent); and beefsteak and roasts (50 percent). Another major source of saturated fat in our diet is the food eaten in fast-food restaurants. Most hamburgers, hot dogs, and chicken and fish sandwiches served by major fast-food chains in Canada contain more than 50 percent fat and are very high in calories. Even McDonald's McLean Deluxe Sandwich (taken off the menu due to poor sales) contained 320 calories and 10 grams of fat (90 calories) for a total of 28 percent fat. Other popular sandwiches and their percent of calories from fat include McDonald's Filet-O-Fish (440 calories, 53 percent fat), Burger King's Broiler Chicken Sandwich (379 calories, 42 percent fat), Burger King's Double Whopper with Cheese (935 calories, 59 percent fat), Wendy's Grilled Chicken Sandwich (340 calories, 34 percent fat), Wendy's Big

Classic (570 calories, 52 percent fat), Kentucky Fried Chicken's Lite 'n Crispy Drumsticks (242 calories, 52 percent fat), and Kentucky Fried Chicken's Chicken Sandwich (482 calories, 50 percent fat).

Trans Fatty Acids For decades, people have used margarine rather than butter to reduce their consumption of unhealthy saturated fat. Although both products contain the same number of calories, margarine contains much less saturated fat. Research now suggests that a type of fat found in margarine may increase cholesterol levels as much as butter does. **Trans fatty acids** are formed during processing when manufacturers add hydrogen to highly unsaturated vegetable oil to ensure consistency and to prevent rancidity. During the process of hydrogenation, the oil creates a new chemical configuration, known as trans fatty acids. This chemical forms in all oils that are hydrogenated, such as margarine, shorten-

Diabetes mellitus A disease caused by insufficient production of insulin by the endocrine portion of the pancreas; **Type I** (insulin-dependent) or **Type II** (non-insulin-dependent).

Glycemic index An index expressing the effects of various foods on the rate and amount of increase in blood-glucose levels.

Saturated fat Fat that contains glycerol and saturated fatty acids; found in large quantities in animal products (such as meat, milk, butter, and cheese) and in small quantities in vegetable products, with the exception of coconut oil, a highly saturated vegetable source. High intake is associated with elevated blood-cholesterol levels.

Polyunsaturated fat Fat containing two or more double bonds between carbons; found in large quantities in vegetable oils, nuts, fish, and margarines.

Monounsaturated fat Fat containing one double bond between carbons; found in foods such as avocados, cashews, and peanut and olive oils.

Cholesterol One of the sterols, or fatlike chemical substances, manufactured in the body and consumed from foods of animal origins only; high intake is associated with elevated blood-cholesterol levels and heart disease.

Nonessential nutrient Nutrients the body can manufacture in sufficient quantities without there being any of that substance in the diet.

Trans fatty acid A fatty acid that is created when hydrogen is added to an unsaturated fat.

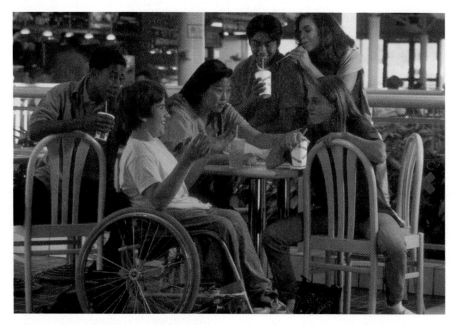

Malls are convenient to shoppers but generally offer foods high in calories, fat, and salt.

ing, baked goods, commercial frying fats, and fats used by some fast-food outlets to cook french fries. In fact, any product that lists partially hydrogenated vegetable oil among its ingredients contains trans fatty acids.

Research now suggests that high levels of trans fatty acids not only may raise levels of "bad" cholesterol (LDL) almost as much as saturated fats but also may lower levels of the "good" cholesterol (HDL). One study went a step further and indicated that women whose diets are high in trans fatty acids were more likely to suffer heart disease than women who ate little margarine and other foods high in trans fatty acids. In January 2003, Health Canada indicated that to make a claim about a food's associated reduction in the risk of heart disease, that food must be low in or completely free of both saturated fat and trans fatty acids.

However, some questions still remain, and much more research is needed on the effects of trans fatty acids before firm conclusions can be drawn. Because trans fatty acids account for only 2–8 percent of total calories compared to 12–14 percent for saturated fat, which research shows clearly to elevate blood-cholesterol levels, individuals should continue to strive to reduce daily saturated fat intake to less than 10 percent of their total calories and total fat to less than 30 percent of their total calories.

In the meantime, the Food and Consumer Products Manufacturers of Canada encourage the public to read the nutrient content claims on food labels and replace saturated and trans fatty unsaturated fats with unhydrogenated monosaturated and polyunsat-urated fat. It is wise to take notice of and reduce your intake of products that have the words "partially hydrogenated" in their list of ingredients. Soft, tub margarine is also a wiser choice than stick margarine; the harder the margarine, the more hydrogenation was involved.

◼ Protein

Protein, from the Greek word *proteios*, or *primary*, is critical to all living things. In the human body, it is used to: repair, rebuild, and replace cells; aid in growth; balance fluid, salt, and acid–base; and provide needed energy when carbohydrates and fats are insufficient or unavailable. Protein is produced in the body through building blocks called **amino acids**. Some of these are produced in the body; others are derived only from food sources. **Nonessential amino acids** can be manufactured by the body if not obtained from the diet. **Essential amino acids**, 8–10 of which must be present in the body in the proper amount and proportion to the nonessential acids for normal protein metabolism to proceed, cannot be manufactured by the body and must be acquired through diet. All 22 amino acids must be present simultaneously (within several hours) in order for the body to synthesize them into proteins that will be used for optimal maintenance of body growth and function.

Sources of Protein Humans obtain protein from both animal and plant foods. In general, animal protein is superior to plant protein because it contains all the essential amino acids in the proper proportions. If one essential amino acid is missing or present in the incorrect proportion, protein construction may be blocked.

Eggs are the complete protein by which all other protein is judged. Milk, cheese, other dairy products, meat, fish, and poultry compare favourably with eggs as excellent sources of protein. Although eggs contain about 213 milligrams of cholesterol and 5 grams of fat (60 percent), they are a low-calorie (75 calories) source of protein, vitamin A, riboflavin, vitamin B_{12}, iron, zinc, phosphorus, calcium, potassium, and other nutrients. It is still advisable to consume no more than two to three eggs per week, and never more than one per day, to eliminate or substitute other food products in recipes calling for eggs as an ingredient, and to purchase small eggs rather than medium, large, or extra large. The Canadian Working Group on the Prevention and Control of Cardiovascular Disease has advised the adult population to decrease their average blood cholesterol from the current 5.3 mmol/L (millimoles per litre) to 4.9 mmol/L. This goal will be difficult to accomplish if the population starts off each day with sausages and a couple of eggs rather than cold or hot cereal.

Protein containing all essential amino acids is termed a **complete**, or high-quality, **protein**; protein from most vegetable sources is low in some amino acids and will not support growth and development when used as the only source of protein. This sort of protein is called **incomplete**, or low-quality, **protein**. Terms such as **low** and **high biological value** are also used to describe the quality of protein.

Approximately 54 grams of protein are recommended daily for university-age males, and 46–48 grams for females. To determine your specific protein needs, multiply your body weight in kilograms by 0.8 grams. A woman, for example, who weighs 60 kilograms needs 48 grams ($60 \times 0.8 = 48$) of protein daily. Larger individuals, pregnant and lactating women, adolescents, and those who are ill may need slightly more. Physically active individuals generally do not require additional protein unless the weather is hot and profuse sweating that produces additional nitrogen loss occurs. Those living in extremely hot climates may also need slightly more protein. Canadians consume 15 percent of their total energy intake as protein, which is at the upper end of recommended levels. Approximately 12–15 percent of the total daily calories in your diet should come from protein.

It is not difficult for most people to obtain their recommended daily intakes of protein. Meat contains about 7 grams per ounce; milk has 8 grams per glass; and protein is plentiful in eggs and dairy products and present in small quantities in vegetables and grains. Two glasses of milk, 1 ounce of cheese, and 3 ounces of beef, chicken, or fish provide all the protein the average person needs per day.

Vegetarian Diets Believing that vegetables are healthier than meats, that it is morally wrong to consume meat, or that meat is contaminated with growth-enhancing drugs, more and more people in Canada are resorting to some form of vegetarianism.

There are three basic kinds of vegetarian: the **vegan**, the **lactovegetarian**, and the **ovolactovegetarian**. All vegetarians must plan their diets carefully because it is more difficult for them to consume adequate protein, iron, and vitamin B_{12} than it is for people who are not vegetarians. Because dairy products and eggs are excellent protein sources, lacto- and ovolactovegetarians have much less difficulty than strict vegans do. Vegans must use complementary protein combinations of vegetables and grains to include proper amounts of protein in their diets. Traditional complementary protein diets include combinations of soybeans or tofu with rice (China and Indochina), peas with wheat (the Middle East), beans with corn (Central and South America), and rice with beans, black-eyed peas, or tofu

Amino acids The basic component of most proteins.

Nonessential amino acids Amino acids that can be manufactured by the body if they cannot be acquired from food sources.

Essential amino acids Amino acids that cannot be manufactured by the body and therefore must be acquired from food sources.

Complete protein A food source that contains all essential amino acids in the correct proportions.

Incomplete protein A food source that does not contain all essential amino acids or contains several in incorrect proportions.

Low biological value A protein source such as corn and wheat that does not contain all essential amino acids or contains some in low proportions.

High biological value A protein source such as meat that contains all eight essential amino acids in the correct proportions.

Vegan A strict vegetarian who consumes only fruits, vegetables, and grains.

Lactovegetarian An individual who eats fruits, vegetables, grains, and dairy products but avoids eggs and meat products.

Ovolactovegetarian An individual who eats fruits, vegetables, grains, dairy products, and eggs but avoids meat products.

(the United States and the Caribbean). Other protein combinations readily available to Canadian vegans include peanut butter and whole-grain bread, whole-wheat bread, black beans, and black-bean and rice soup. These combinations of complete proteins are excellent substitutes for meat, egg, and dairy proteins.

Because fruits, vegetables, and grains contain no cholesterol, little saturated fat, and a lot of fibre, vegans tend to avoid heart disease for a decade longer than meat eaters do. Vegetarians may also be able to avoid certain kinds of digestive-system cancers; however, vegans are especially prone to dangerous deficiencies in iron, calcium, and vitamin B_{12} (available only in animal products). In order to combat serious nutrient shortages, vegans should follow certain daily dietary recommendations and include in their diets:

- 454 mL of legumes daily for proper levels of calcium and iron
- 227 mL of dark greens daily to meet iron requirements (for women)
- At least 1 gram of fat daily for proper absorption of vitamins
- A supplement of fortified plant foods (like soy or nut milks or a multiple vitamin and mineral) to obtain vitamin B_{12}

The Energy Systems Practically all the energy your muscles use is formed by the chemical reactions of two unique pathways of energy formation: the **glycolysis** and the **citric acid cycle.**

The majority of energy formed by glycolysis is derived from glucose, and because it is anaerobic, it can be produced quickly. The glucose used to fuel glycolysis comes from blood glucose, glycogen (the stored form of glucose), glycerol (a small fraction of stored fat molecules), and several amino acids. Most university-age people have approximately 1400 calories of stored glycogen in the muscles and 300 stored in the liver (liver glycogen can be used to supply glucose to muscles). Short, intense anaerobic exercises such as sprinting, weight training, pull-ups, diving, and push-ups are fuelled by the glycolysis energy cycle.

The citric acid cycle uses three different types of fuel: glucose fragments produced by glycolysis, fatty acids, and

Glycolysis energy cycle The anaerobic energy pathway fuelled primarily by glucose.

Citric acid energy cycle The aerobic energy pathway fuelled primarily by fat, small quantities of glucose fragments, and certain amino acids.

certain amino acids. Fatty acids drawn from the body's fat stores are by far the largest supplier of energy in this aerobic cycle. Only in the aerobic cycle, in which oxygen is present, can fat be burned as fuel. Activities such as walking, jogging, running, lap swimming, aerobic dance, cycling, basketball, and soccer are fuelled by fat in the citric acid cycle. These aerobic activities are ideal for weight and fat loss. Fat cannot be burned in the anaerobic cycle because oxygen is not present.

Nutritional Habits of University Students Personal lifestyle choices, including dietary habits, are often established in early adulthood (Troyer et al., 1990). Consequently, the nutritional practices of university students are important issues because these practices are likely to continue into their adult years, either contributing to or detracting from their health (Haberman and Luffey, 1998). Unfortunately, as a group, university students are not consuming a well-balanced diet; although protein intake seems sufficient, a review of the literature revealed that this group eats too much fat and not enough complex carbohydrates.

While most researchers agree that university students consume appropriate servings of protein (Brevard and Ricketts, 1996; Glore et al., 1993; Quinn and Jenkins, 1991), the findings are less desirable when it comes to fat and complex carbohydrate consumption.

Between 34 percent and 40 percent of university students' daily calories come from fat (Lowry et al., 2000; Troyer et al., 1990; Quinn and Jenkins, 1991) compared to the ideal of no more than 30 percent. In a study of Canadian university students in Nova Scotia, it was found that in addition to not meeting the standards set forth in *Canada's Food Guide to Healthy Eating*, more than 75 percent of students ate fried food at least once per week, and 42 percent consumed fried food three or more times each week. Not surprisingly, more than 35 percent of these respondents revealed that they had gained at least 10 pounds in the previous year, during which they lived in a university residence (Makrides et al., 1998).

In addition to overconsuming fat, university students underconsume complex carbohydrates (Brevard and Ricketts, 1996; Quinn and Jenkins, 1991) and fibre (Glore et al., 1993). In particular, students do not consume adequate servings of fruits and vegetables each day (Makrides et al., Haberman and Lufey, 1998; Lowry et al., 2000; Dinger and Waigandt, 1997).

University is a time for learning, socializing, and balancing a variety of academic and personal stressors. With a healthy diet and moderate exercise, students can better achieve their goals and have the energy for a well-balanced life.

MYTH AND FACT SHEET

Myth	Fact
1. Organically grown foods are superior.	1. Organic farmers avoid pesticides, use natural soil enhancers such as compost instead of fertilizers, and rotate crops more frequently. The resulting claim is that their food products are more nutritious and have fewer health hazards. Nutrition scientists disagree. Research indicates that pesticide levels are similar in organically and conventionally grown foods, soil nutrients from natural fertilizers (manure) are the same as chemical fertilizers, nutritional differences do not exist, and conventionally grown products look and taste better—and cost less.
2. You should attempt to eliminate all fat in your diet.	2. Because fat is a nutrient found in many foods, it would be impossible to completely cut it from your diet. Dietary fat also performs some important functions for the body such as aiding satiety by slowing the rate of stomach emptying and cueing you to stop eating, providing some essential nutrients that are soluble in fat and found mainly in these fat-containing foods (essential fatty acids and the fat-soluble vitamins A, D, E, and K), and lending flavour and aroma to food. Once fat is formed in the body, it performs many other functions, such as providing a concentrated source of stored energy, a major component of cell membranes, nourishment for skin and hair, insulation from temperature extremes, and a cushion for vital organs to protect them from shock. You should restrict dietary fat to less than 30 percent of your total calories, but you should not attempt to avoid it entirely.
3. You should consume margarine instead of butter to stay healthier.	3. Until recently, margarine was considered a much wiser selection than butter. Although both are 100 percent fat and contain the same amount of calories, margarine contains little or no saturated fat, which increases blood cholesterol levels in the human body. The so-called trans fatty acids formed in margarine when hydrogen is added to a highly unsaturated vegetable oil have been shown in some studies to raise our bad cholesterol (LDL) levels and lower our good cholesterol (HDL) levels. Until further evidence is available, you should continue to reduce your consumption of all types of fat, choose tub or soft margarine over hard-stick margarine, use margarine sparingly, and try to avoid products that list the words "partially hydrogenated" or "hydrogenated" in their ingredients.
4. Consuming a chocolate bar or nondiet pop before exercise gives you extra energy.	4. If you eat large amounts of sugar at one time, such as an entire chocolate bar, the blood releases too much insulin, starting a series of complex chemical reactions. As a result, too much glucose is removed from the blood and stored in the fat cells and liver. This process can leave you with less energy than you would have had without eating the chocolate bar or drinking the pop. Sugar also draws fluid from other body parts into the gastrointestinal tract and may contribute to dehydration, distention of the stomach, cramps, nausea, and diarrhea. To avoid these problems, dilute concentrated fruit juices with twice the recommended water, add an equal volume of water to commercial drinks, and eat only small quantities of sugar. Sugar is absorbed faster than the muscles can use it; thus, frequent small amounts are preferable to single doses. Your blood-glucose level will reach a peak about half an hour after consumption and then rapidly decline. Eating large quantities of sugar causes more rapid decline and greater shortage of glucose for energy.

THE NONENERGY NUTRIENTS (MICRO NUTRIENTS): VITAMINS, MINERALS, AND WATER

■ Vitamins

Vitamins are essential in helping chemical reactions take place in the body and are required in very small amounts. Water-soluble vitamins (vitamin C and the B-complex vitamins) need to be consumed in the proper amounts over a 5-to-8-day period because they are easily dissolved in water, not stored for long periods of time, and eliminated in the urine (see Table 8.4). Fat-soluble vitamins (vitamins A, D, E, and K) are stored in large amounts in fatty tissues and the liver and are absorbed through the intestinal tract as needed (see Table 8.5). Although Tables 8.4 and 8.5 represent up-to-date information, it is important to note that a group of Canadian and American scientists are currently compiling a new comprehensive set of nutrient reference values for healthy populations. These dietary reference intakes (DRIs) will soon replace our current recommended nutrient intakes (RNIs), and *Canada's Food Guide to Healthy Eating* is being reviewed to make sure that it will accommodate the new DRIs.

Regardless of the claims, vitamin C does not cure or prevent the common cold. Large supplements of other vitamins and minerals are being examined for their disease-fighting potential and their ability to assist in medical treatment. It is important to realize three important things about taking vitamin supplements. First, the best way to obtain adequate vitamins and minerals is from food, not from supplements. Food has the added benefit of containing fibre and water and many other chemicals. Second, the vast majority of people in Canada get all the vitamins and minerals they need from their diets and do not need supplements. Third, vitamin and mineral toxicity problems are found predominantly in those who take supplements (especially fat-soluble supplements).

■ Minerals

Minerals are present in all living cells. They serve as key components of various hormones, enzymes, and other substances that aid in regulating chemical reactions within cells. Mineral elements play a part in the body's metabolic

> **MFP factor** A factor in meat, fish, and poultry that enhances the absorption of nonheme iron present in the same foods and other foods eaten at the same time.

processes, and deficiencies can result in serious disorders. *Macrominerals*, such as sodium, potassium, calcium, phosphorus, magnesium, sulfur, and chlorides, are needed by the body in large amounts (more than 5 grams). *Trace minerals* are needed in small amounts (less than 5 grams). A minimum of 14 trace minerals must be ingested for optimum health. Iron, iodine, copper, fluoride, and zinc are the ones most important for body function. The body is composed of about 31 minerals, 24 of which are considered essential for sustaining life (see Tables 8.6 and 8.7).

Iron Iron is one of the body's most essential minerals. Approximately 85 percent of our daily iron intake is used to produce new hemoglobin (the pigment of the red blood cells that transports oxygen); the remaining 15 percent is used for the production of new tissue or held in storage. Iron needs also vary according to age and sex. Table 8.8 summarizes these variables. Iron deficiency results in loss of strength and endurance, rapid fatigue during exercise, shortening of the attention span, loss of visual perception, impaired learning, and numerous other physical disorders. Although the importance of sufficient dietary iron is common knowledge, many women may not get enough iron in their diet. In Canada, iron intake has been reduced by the removal of iron-containing soils from the food supply and the diminished use of iron cooking utensils. Whereas animals can ingest iron from muddy water and soil, humans must rely solely on food.

Iron deficiency anemia, a major health problem in Canada, is common in low birth weight infants, infants fed with whole cow's milk, disadvantaged children, women of childbearing age, pregnant women, and low-income people. People must also be aware, however, that too much iron can be dangerous. Iron toxicity is rare, but a condition called *iron overload* occurs when the body is overwhelmed with too much iron given from blood transfusions or when too much iron is absorbed because of hereditary defects, heavy supplementation, and alcohol abuse (which increases absorption). Iron overload can cause tissue and liver damage. Rapid ingestion of large amounts of iron can also cause sudden death. Iron overdose is the second most common cause of accidental poisoning in small children. High blood-iron levels may also be related to heart disease in men.

Iron is more easily absorbed from meat, fish, and poultry (heme iron) than it is from vegetables (nonheme iron). Twice the volume of vegetable iron is absorbed when vegetables and meats are consumed during the same meal. Vitamin C also promotes iron absorption and can triple the amount of nonheme iron absorbed from foods eaten at the same meal. The **MFP factor** also enhances the absorption of nonheme iron from other foods eaten with meat, fish, and poultry.

Table 8.4 ✦ Summary of Information on Water-Soluble Vitamins

NAME	RNI FOR ADULTS	SOURCES	STABILITY	COMMENTS
Thiamine	0.4 mg per 1000 kcal	Pork, liver, organ meats, legumes, whole-grain and enriched cereals and breads, wheat germ, potatoes. Synthesized in intestinal tract.	Unstable in presence of heat, alkali, or oxygen. Heat-stable in acid solution.	As part of cocarboxylase, aids in removal of CO_2 from alpha-keto acids during oxidation of carbohydrates. Essential for growth, normal appetite, digestion, and healthy nerves.
Riboflavin	0.5 mg per 1000 kcal	Milk and dairy foods, organ meats, green leafy vegetables, enriched cereals and breads, eggs.	Stable to heat, oxygen, and acid. Unstable to light (especially ultraviolet) or alkali.	Essential for growth. Plays enzymatic role in tissue respiration and acts as a transporter of hydrogen ions. Coenzyme forms FMN and FAD.
Niacin (nicotinic acid and nicotinamide)	7.2 NE per 1000 kcal	Fish, liver, meat, poultry, many grains, eggs, peanuts, milk, legumes, enriched grains. Synthesized by intestinal bacteria.	Stable to heat, light oxidation, acid, and alkali.	As part of enzyme system, aids in transfer of hydrogen and acts in metabolism of carbohydrates and amino acids. Involved in glycolysis, fat synthesis, and tissue respiration.
Vitamin B_6 (pyridoxine, pyridoxal, and pyridoxamine)	15 µg per gram protein	Pork, glandular meats, cereal bran and germ, milk, egg yolk, oatmeal, and legumes. Synthesized by intestinal bacteria.	Stable to heat, light, and oxidation.	As a coenzyme, aids in the synthesis and breakdown of amino acids and in the synthesis of unsaturated fatty acids from essential fatty acids. Essential for conversion of tryptophan to niacin. Essential for normal growth.
Folate	M: 200 µg F: 180 µg	Green leafy vegetables, organ meats (liver), lean beef, wheat, eggs, fish, dry beans, lentils, cowpeas, asparagus, broccoli, collards, yeast. Synthesized in intestinal tract.	Stable to sunlight when in solution; unstable to heat in acid media.	Appears essential for biosynthesis of nucleic acids. Essential for normal maturation of red blood cells. Functions as a coenzyme: tetrahydrofolic acid.
Vitamin B_{12}	1 µg	Liver, kidney, milk and dairy foods, meat, eggs. Vegans require supplement.	Slowly destroyed by acid, alkali, light, and oxidation.	Involved in the metabolism of single-carbon fragments. Essential for biosynthesis of nucleic acids and nucleoproteins. Role in metabolism of nervous tissue. Involved with folate metabolism. Related to growth.
Pantothenic acid	Level not yet determined but 4–7 mg believed safe and adequate.	Present in all plant and animal foods. Eggs, kidney, liver, salmon, and yeast are best sources. Possibly synthesized by intestinal bacteria.	Unstable to acid, alkali, heat, and certain salts.	As part of coenzyme A, functions in the synthesis and breakdown of many vital body compounds. Essential in the intermediary metabolism of carbohydrate, fat, and protein.
Biotin	Not known but 30–100 µg believed safe and adequate.	Liver, mushrooms, peanuts, yeast, milk, meat, egg yolk, most vegetables, banana, grapefruit, tomato, watermelon, and strawberries. Synthesized in intestinal tract.	Stable.	Essential component of enzymes. Involved in synthesis and breakdown of fatty acids and amino acids through aiding the addition and removal of CO_2 to or from active compounds, and the removal of NH_2 from amino acids.
Vitamin C (ascorbic acid)	30–40 mg	Acerola (West Indian cherry-like fruit), citrus fruit, tomato, melon, peppers, greens, raw cabbage, guava, strawberries, pineapple, potato.	Unstable to heat, alkali, and oxidation, except in acids. Destroyed by storage.	Maintains intracellular cement substance with preservation of capillary integrity. Cosubstrate in hydroxylations requiring molecular oxygen. Important in immune responses, wound healing, and allergic reactions. Increases absorption of nonheme iron.

Note: RNI=recommended nutrient intake; mg=milligrams; NE=niacin equivalents; µg=micrograms.

Sources: Kathleen L. Mahan and Marian Arlin, *Food Nutrition and Diet Therapy* (Philadelphia: W. B. Saunders Company, 1992), pp. 105–106. Used by permission. Health and Welfare Canada, *Nutrition Recommendations: The Report of the Scientific Review Committee* (Ottawa: Canadian Government Publishing Centre, 1990), Tables 5 and 6, pp. 25, 27. Adapted and reproduced with the permission of the Minister of Public Works and Government Services Canada, 2003. *Health Canada assumes no responsibility for any errors or omissions which may have occurred in the adaptation of its material.*

Table 8.5 ✦ Summary of Information on Fat-Soluble Vitamins

NAME	RNI FOR ADULTS[a]	SOURCES	STABILITY	COMMENTS
Vitamin A (retinol; α-, β-, γ-carotene)	M: 1000 RE F: 800 RE	Liver, kidney, milk fat, fortified margarine, egg yolk, yellow and dark green leafy vegetables, apricots, cantaloupe, peaches.	Stable to light, heat, and usual cooking methods. Destroyed by oxidation, drying, very high temperature, ultraviolet light.	Essential for normal growth, development, and maintenance of epithelial tissue. Essential to the integrity of night vision. Helps provide for normal bone development and influences normal tooth formation. Toxic in large quantities.
Vitamin D (calciferol)	M: 5 μg F: 2.5–5 μg	Vitamin D milk, irradiated foods, some in milk fat, liver, egg yolk, salmon, tuna, sardines. Sunlight converts 7-dehydrocholesterol to cholecalciferol.	Stable to heat and oxidation.	Really a prohormone. Essential for normal growth and development; important for formation of normal bones and teeth. Influences absorption and metabolism of phosphorus and calcium. Toxic in large quantities.
Vitamin E	M: 7–10 mg F: 6–7 mg	Wheat germ, vegetable oils, green leafy vegetables, milk fat, egg yolk, nuts.	Stable to heat and acids. Destroyed by rancid fats, alkali, oxygen, lead, iron salts, and ultraviolet irradiation.	Is a strong antioxidant. May help prevent oxidation of unsaturated fatty acids and vitamin A in intestinal tract and body tissues. Protects red blood cells from hemolysis. Role in reproduction (in animals). Role in epithelial tissue maintenance and prostaglandin synthesis.
Vitamin K (phylloquinone and menaquinone)	M: 80 μg F: 65 μg	Liver, soybean oil, other vegetable oils, green leafy vegetables, wheat bran. Synthesized in intestinal tract.	Resistant to heat, oxygen, and moisture. Destroyed by alkali and ultraviolet light.	Aids in production of prothrombin, a compound required for normal clotting of blood. Toxic in large quantities.

[a]M=male; F=female; RE=retinol equivalents

Note: One retinol equivalent corresponds to the biological activity of 1 microgram of retinol, 6 micrograms of beta-carotene, or 12 micrograms of other carotenes.

Sources: Kathleen L. Mahan and Marian Arlin, *Food Nutrition and Diet Therapy* (Philadelphia: W. B. Saunders Company, 1992), p. 105. Used by permission. Health and Welfare Canada, *Nutrition Recommendations: The Report of the Scientific Review Committee* (Ottawa: Canadian Government Publishing Centre, 1990), Tables 5 and 6, pp. 25, 27.

Table 8.6 ✦ Micronutrients Essential at Levels of 100 mg/day or More

MINERAL	LOCATION IN BODY AND SOME BIOLOGIC FUNCTIONS	RNI[a] OR ESADDI[b] FOR ADULTS	FOOD SOURCES	COMMENTS ON LIKELIHOOD OF A DEFICIENCY
Calcium	99% in bones and teeth. Ionic calcium in body fluids essential for ion transport across cell membranes. Calcium is also bound to protein, citrate, or inorganic acids.	800 mg; 1200 mg for women 19–24 years	Milk and milk products, sardines, clams, oysters, kale, turnip greens, mustard greens, tofu.	Dietary surveys indicate that many diets do not meet recommended dietary allowances for calcium. Since bone serves as a homeostatic mechanism to maintain calcium level in blood, many essential functions are maintained, regardless of diet. Long-term dietary deficiency is probably one of the factors responsible for development of osteoporosis in later life.
Phosphorus	About 80% in inorganic portion of bones and teeth. Phosphorus is a component of every cell and of highly important metabolites, including DNA, RNA, ATP (high-energy compound), and phospholipids. Important to pH regulation.	M: 1000 mg F: 850 mg 1200 mg for women 19–24 years	Cheese, egg yolk, milk, meat, fish, poultry, whole-grain cereals, legumes, nuts.	Dietary inadequacy not likely to occur if protein and calcium intake are adequate.
Magnesium	About 50% in bone. Remaining 50% is almost entirely inside body cells with only about 1% in extracellular fluid. Ionic magnesium functions as an activator of many enzymes and thus influences almost all processes.	M: 240–250 mg F: 200–210 mg	Whole-grain cereals, tofu, nuts, meat, milk, green vegetables, legumes, chocolate.	Dietary inadequacy considered unlikely, but conditioned deficiency is often seen in clinical medicine, associated with surgery, alcoholism, malabsorption, loss of body fluids, certain hormonal and renal diseases.
Sodium	30 to 45% in bone. Major cation of extracellular fluid and only a small amount is inside cell. Regulates body fluid osmolarity, pH, and body fluid volume.	500–3000 mg	Common table salt, seafoods, animal foods, milk, eggs. Abundant in most foods except fruit.	Dietary inadequacy probably never occurs, although low blood sodium requires treatment in certain clinical disorders. Sodium restriction necessary practice in certain cardiovascular disorders.
Chloride	Major anion of extracellular fluid, functioning in combination with sodium. Serves as a buffer, enzyme activator; component of gastric hydrochloric acid. Mostly present in extracellular fluid; less than 15% inside cells.	750–3000 mg	Common table salt, seafoods, milk, meat, eggs.	In most cases dietary intake has little significance except in the presence of vomiting, diarrhea, or profuse sweating, when a deficiency may develop.
Potassium	Major cation of intracellular fluid, with only small amounts in extracellular fluid. Functions in regulating pH and osmolarity, and cell membrane transfer. Ion is necessary for carbohydrate and protein metabolism.	2000 mg	Fruits, milk, meat, cereals, vegetables, legumes.	Dietary inadequacy unlikely, but conditioned deficiency may be found in kidney disease, diabetic acidosis, excessive vomiting, diarrhea, or sweating. Potassium excess may be a problem in renal failure and severe acidosis.
Sulfur	Most dietary sulfur is present in sulfur-containing amino acids needed for synthesis of essential metabolites. Functions in oxidation-reduction reactions. Also functions in thiamin and biotin, and as inorganic sulfur.	Need for sulfur is satisfied by essential sulfur-containing amino acids.	Protein foods such as meat, fish, poultry, eggs, milk, cheese, legumes, nuts.	Dietary intake is chiefly from sulfur-containing amino acids and adequacy is related to protein intake.

[a]RNI = recommended nutrient intake. [b]ESADDI = estimated safe and adequate daily dietary intake.
Sources: Kathleen L. Mahan and Marian Arlin, *Food Nutrition and Diet Therapy* (Philadelphia: W. B. Saunders Company, 1992), p. 137. Used by permission. Health and Welfare Canada, *Nutrition Recommendations: The Report of the Scientific Review Committee* (Ottawa: Canadian Government Publishing Centre, 1990), Tables 5 and 6, pp. 25, 27.

Table 8.7 ✦ Micronutrients Essential at Levels of a Few mg/day

MINERAL	LOCATION IN BODY AND SOME BIOLOGIC FUNCTIONS	RNIᵃ OR ESADDIᵇ FOR ADULTS	FOOD SOURCES	COMMENTS ON LIKELIHOOD OF A DEFICIENCY
Iron	About 70% is in hemoglobin; about 26% stored in liver, spleen and bone. Iron is a component of hemoglobin and myoglobin, important in oxygen transfer; also present in serum transferrin and certain enzymes. Almost none in ionic form.	M: 9 mg F: 8–13 mg	Liver, meat, egg yolk, legumes, whole or enriched grains, dark green vegetables, dark molasses, shrimp, oysters.	Iron-deficiency anemia occurs in women in reproductive years and in infants and preschool children. May be associated in some cases with unusual blood loss, parasites, and malabsorption. Anemia is last effect of deficient state.
Zinc	Present in most tissues, with higher amounts in liver, voluntary muscle, and bone. Constituent of many enzymes and insulin; of importance in nucleic acid metabolism.	M: 12 mg F: 9 mg	Oysters, shellfish, herring, liver, legumes, milk, wheat bran.	Extent of dietary inadequacy in this country not known. Conditioned deficiency may be seen in systemic childhood illnesses and in patients who are nutritionally depleted or have been subjected to severe stress, such as surgery.
Copper	Found in all body tissues; larger amounts in liver, brain, heart, and kidney. Constituent of enzymes and of ceruloplasmin and erythrocuprein in blood. May be integral part of DNA or RNA molecule.	1.5–3 mg	Liver, shellfish, whole grains, cherries, legumes, kidney, poultry, oysters, chocolate, nuts.	No evidence that specific deficiencies of copper occur in the human. Menkes' disease is genetic disorder resulting in copper deficiency.
Iodine	Constituent of thyroxine and related compounds synthesized by thyroid gland. Thyroxine functions in control of reactions involving cellular energy.	160 μg	Iodized table salt, seafoods, water and vegetables in nongoitrous regions.	Iodization of table salt is recommended especially in areas where food is low in iodine.
Manganese	Highest concentration is in bone; also relatively high concentrations in pituitary, liver, pancreas, and gastrointestinal tissue. Constituent of essential enzyme systems; rich in mitochondria of liver cells.	2.5–5.0 mg	Beet greens, blueberries, whole grains, nuts, legumes, fruit, tea.	Unlikely that deficiency occurs in humans.
Fluoride	Present in bone and teeth. In optimal amounts in water and diet, reduces dental caries and may minimize bone loss.	1.5–4.0 mg	Drinking water (1 ppm), tea, coffee, rice, soybeans, spinach, gelatin, onions, lettuce.	In areas where fluoride content of water is low, fluoridation of water (1 ppm) has been found beneficial in reducing incidence of dental caries.
Molybdenum	Constituent of an essential enzyme xanthine oxidase and of flavoproteins.	75–250 μg	Legumes, cereal grains, dark green leafy vegetables, organs.	No information.
Cobalt	Constituent of cyanocobalamin (vitamin B_{12}), occurring bound to protein in foods of animal origin. Essential to normal function of all cells, particularly cells of bone marrow, nervous system, and gastrointestinal system.	2.0 μg of vitamin B_{12}	Liver, kidney, oysters, clams, poultry, milk.	Primary dietary inadequacy is rare except when no animal products are consumed. Deficiency may be found in such conditions as lack of gastric intrinsic factor, gastrectomy, and malabsorption syndromes.
Selenium	Associated with fat metabolism, vitamin E, and antioxidant functions.	M: 70 μg F: 55 μg	Grains, onions, meats, milk, vegetables variable—depends on selenium content of soil.	Keshan disease is a selenium-deficient state. Deficiency has occurred in patients receiving long-term total parenteral nutrition without selenium.
Chromium	Associated with glucose metabolism.	0.05–0.2 mg	Corn oil, clams, whole-grain cereals, meats, drinking water variable.	Deficiency found in severe malnutrition, may be factor in diabetes in the elderly and cardiovascular disease.
Tin Nickel Vanadium Silicon	} Now known to be essential but no RNIs established.			

ᵃRNI = recommended nutrient intake. ᵇESADDI = estimated safe and adequate daily dietary intake.

Sources: Kathleen L. Mahan and Marian Arlin, *Food Nutrition and Diet Therapy* (Philadelphia: W. B. Saunders Company, 1992), pp. 137–138. Used by permission. Health and Welfare Canada, *Nutrition Recommendations: The Report of the Scientific Review Committee* (Ottawa: Canadian Government Publishing Centre, 1990), Tables 5 and 6, pp. 25, 27.

Table 8.8 ✦ Dietary Reference Intakes (DRIs) for Iron (mg/d)

AGE	RECOMMENDED DIETARY ALLOWANCE (RDA)		ESTIMATED AVERAGE REQUIREMENT (EAR)		TOLERABLE UPPER INTAKE LEVEL(UL)
	MALES	FEMALES	MALES	FEMALES	ALL
7–12 months	11	11	6.9	6.9	40
1–3 years	7	7	3.0	3.0	40
4–8 years	10	10	4.1	4.1	40
9–13 years	8	8	5.9	5.7	40
14–18 years	11	15	7.7	7.9	45
19–30 years	8	18	6.0	8.1	45
31–50 years	8	18	6.0	8.1	45
51–70 years	8	8	6.0	5.0	45
70 years	8	8	6.0	5.0	45
18 years, pregnant	–	27	–	23.0	45
19–50 years, pregnant	–	27	–	22.0	45

Note: RDAs for vegetarians (those who do not include meat, fish or poultry in their diet) are 1.8 times greater than for individuals consuming a mixed diet.

Source: Institute of Medicine, Dietary Reference Intakes for Vitamin A, Vitamin K, Arsenic, Boron, Chromium, Copper, Iodine, Iron, Manganese, Molybdenum, Nickel, Silicon, Vanadium, and Zinc (prepublication copy). National Academy Pr. Washington, 2001. Reprinted with permission from (Dietary Reference Intakes) © (2002) by the National Academy of Sciences. Courtesy of the National Academies Press, Washington, D.C.

Supplementation Some people take large doses of vitamins and minerals in the belief that these are necessary to correct dietary deficiencies or to prevent or cure a variety of ills. More commonly, the multiple-vitamin/mineral pill is taken as an *insurance policy* against improper nutrition. Unfortunately, consuming too many vitamins and minerals, especially fat-soluble vitamins, which the body stores for long periods of time, can be toxic. The **megavitamin** approach may result in **hypervitaminosis**. The body also has an adequate reserve storage system for key vitamins and minerals to prevent health problems (see Table 8.9). This reserve capacity helps prevent deficiencies when you fail to eat right for a few days or weeks, but it should not be relied on for long periods of time.

With very few exceptions, individuals who experience toxicity problems from overdose of a specific vitamin or mineral are involved in heavy supplementation. It is extremely difficult to produce toxic reactions from food intake alone. Table 8.10 can help you decide whether you should consider use of supplementation.

▪ Water

The most critical food component is water. Though it has no nutritional value, water is necessary for energy production, temperature control, and elimination. Although water is present in all foods, experts recommend a minimum of 6–8 glasses of it daily, and 12–15 glasses when you are trying to change your body composition. For a more detailed discussion of daily water needs, see the section "Special Needs of the Active Individual" later in this chapter.

*F*OOD DENSITY

You can easily determine whether a food item or meal is nutritionally dense by examining the caloric and nutrient content. A high-density food or meal is one that provides a high percentage of key vitamins and minerals you need daily for a small percentage of your daily caloric intake. A good cold cereal with skim milk, for example, provides about 190 calories and 20–30 percent

Megavitamin intake Consuming 10–100 times the RNI for a particular vitamin.

Hypervitaminosis The toxic side-effects that result from the consumption of excess vitamins.

Table 8.9 ✦ Extent of Body Reserves of Nutrients and Nutrient/Health Consequences of Depletion

NUTRIENT	APPROXIMATE TIME TO DEPLETE	POTENTIAL HEALTH IMPLICATIONS
Amino acids	3–4 hours	Although you awake each morning with your amino acids depleted, no health consequences occur.
Calcium	2500 days	The majority of the body's calcium storage is in the skeletal system; drawing on this storage supply for long periods of time will adversely affect the bones.
Carbohydrates	12–15 hours	Short-term depletion causes no problems because the body can switch to protein and fat for energy. Long-term use of protein for energy can cause serious health problems.
Fat	25–50 days	Adipose tissue provides approximately 100 000–150 000 kcal of energy and is the body's greatest reserve source of fuel.
Iron	125 days (women) 750 days (men)	Women possess a smaller reserve capacity due to monthly loss of iron in blood during menstruation.
Sodium	2–3 days	After prolonged sweating without food intake, muscle cramps, heat exhaustion and heat stroke may occur.
Vitamin C	60–120 days	Most excess intake of this water-soluble vitamin is excreted in urine.
Vitamin A	90–360 days	Excess intake of this fat-soluble vitamin is stored in the fat cells.
Water	4–5 days	Death.

Table 8.10 ✦ People for Whom Vitamin and Mineral Supplements May Be Beneficial

- Women with heavy menstrual bleeding (extra iron)
- Women taking oral contraceptives (may need extra vitamin B_6)
- Pregnant women (extra iron, folic acid and calcium)
- Malnourished individuals, including dieters, elderly people with a low caloric intake, chronic alcoholics and those with other chemical dependencies
- Strict vegetarians (many need extra iron, zinc, calcium and vitamin B_{12})
- Newborn infants (may be deficient in vitamin E and vitamin K)
- Individuals with chronic disorders, such as patients with osteoporosis (may need extra vitamin D, calcium, magnesium and trace minerals)
- Hospitalized patients. Patients in hospitals and institutionalized people may become deficient in one or more vitamins.
- People who smoke (extra vitamin C)

Source: Robert A. Ronzio, *The Encyclopedia of Nutrition and Good Health* (New York: Facts On File, Inc., 1997), p. 442. © 1997 by Robert A. Ronzio. Reproduced with the permission of facts on file.

of practically all vitamins, minerals, carbohydrates, and protein for the day. Because the cold-cereal breakfast contains only 190 calories and about 8 percent of a 120-pound woman's daily energy needs, the meal is said to be nutritionally dense. Fruits, vegetables, and grains are examples of foods that are dense for a given nutrient or group of nutrients. Potato or corn chips and cake are examples of low-density foods that supply a high percentage of your daily calories and a low percentage of key nutrients.

Cold or hot cereal is an excellent way to start the day. Read the labels and choose cereals that contain no sugar, fat, or sodium and at least 2 grams of protein and 3 grams of fibre.

DIETARY GUIDELINES FOR GOOD HEALTH

Describing a practical plan for healthy eating is not as difficult as it may sound. Complicated tables and elaborate analysis are impractical for most people. Although some initial recordkeeping may be needed, a good system should allow some quick, daily spot checking without time-consuming analysis. A basic understanding of *Canada's Food Guide to Healthy Eating* and how to use food labels provides such a method.

■ *Canada's Food Guide to Healthy Eating*

Canada's Food Guide to Healthy Eating (see Figure 8.2) is intended to encourage an overall pattern of healthy eating—that is, of the average of what is eaten over time. Choices may be balanced over a day, or even over several days, and provided healthy eating is incorporated into a person's lifestyle, the other or "sometimes" foods such as those plentiful during religious and other celebrations can be balanced by lower-fat choices over the next few days. The *Guide* is designed to meet the needs of different people in various stages of life and includes ranges in both the number and the size of servings, which makes it flexible and easy to tailor to individual needs.

Most people will meet their nutritional needs by choosing a number of servings that falls somewhere between the lower and upper ends of the range. People with lower energy needs, such as older women, will choose the lower number of servings for each group; people with higher energy needs, such as athletes or male adolescents, will choose the higher number of servings for each group.

■ Food Labelling

Food labels are the most effective and important means of communicating information between food consumers and food merchants. The purpose of food labelling is threefold: first, to provide basic product information, including the list of ingredients, life dates, country of origin, and manufacturer information; second, to provide health/safety and nutrition information, including instructions for safe storage and handling, and the macro-nutrient and micro-nutrient profiles; and third, to promote the product. Product promotions come in the form of claims such as "low fat," "cholesterol-free," and "Product of Canada."

Figure 8.2 ✦ Canada's Food Guide to Healthy Eating

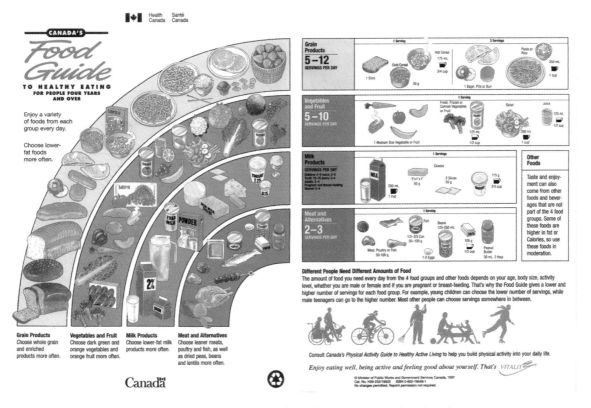

Source: Courtesy of Health Canada, Ministry of Public Works and Government Services, Canada

In Canada, three federal departments are responsible for the development and enforcement of food labelling requirements: Health Canada, Industry Canada, and the Canadian Food Inspection Agency. Health Canada is responsible for administering health and safety standards and developing food label policies related to health and nutrition under the *Food and Drug Act*. Industry Canada is responsible for administering the *Consumer Packaging and Labelling Act* respecting basic food label information, net quantity, metrication, and bilingual labelling. The Canadian Food Inspection Agency is responsible for administering food labelling policies related to misrepresentation and fraud with respect to food labelling, packaging and advertising, and the general agrifood and fish labelling provisions respecting grade, quality, and composition. These three agencies work together to ensure that Canada's strict food labelling standards are upheld.

As of January 1, 2003, amendments to Canada's Food and Drug Act made it mandatory for most prepackaged foods to bear a "Nutrition Facts" table on the label. (Single-ingredient foods such as fresh fruit and vegetables and raw, unground meat and poultry are exempt.) The Nutrition Facts table will usually appear in a standard format such as that in Figure 8.3, although at the time of printing the format had not yet been finalized. Each food label must now list, based on a serving of the food as offered for sale or that will reasonably be consumed by one person in a single eating occasion, the food energy in calories and the amounts of 13 key nutrients found in the food. These nutrients are fat, saturated and trans fats, cholesterol, sodium, carbohydrate, fibre, sugars, protein, vitamins A and C, calcium, and iron. In addition, the label must display the percentage of the recommended daily intake (% Daily Values) of these nutrients provided by this food. As a reference standard

Figure 8.3 ✦ The Nutrition Label

Serving Size

Is your serving the same size as the one on the label? If you eat double the serving size listed, you need to double the nutrient and calorie values. If you eat one-half the serving size shown here, cut the nutrient and calorie values in half.

Calories

Are you overweight? Cut back a little on calories! Look here to see how a serving of the food adds to your daily total. A 5'4", 138-lb. active woman needs about 2200 calories each day. A 5'10", 174-lb. active man needs about 2900. How about you?

Total Carbohydrate

When you cut down on fat, you can eat more carbohydrates. Carbohydrates are in foods like bread, potatoes, fruits and vegetables. Choose these often! They give you more nutrients than *sugars* like soda pop and candy.

Dietary Fibre

Grandmother called it "roughage," but her advice to eat more is still up-to-date! That goes for both soluble and insoluble kinds of dietary fibre. Fruits, vegetables, whole-grain foods, beans and peas are all good sources and can help reduce the risk of heart disease and cancer.

Protein

Most Canadians get more protein than they need. Where there is animal protein, there is also fat and cholesterol. Eat small servings of lean meat, fish and poultry. Use skim or low-fat milk, yogurt, and cheese. Try vegetable proteins like beans, grains and cereals.

Vitamins & Minerals

Your goal here is 100% of each for the day. Don't count on one food to do it all. Let a combination of foods add up to a winning score.

Nutrition Information Nutritionelle
Per 114-gram serving (1/2 cup)
4 servings per container

Energy/Energie	90 cal
	378 kJ
Protein/Proteines	3 g
Fat/Matières grasses	4 g
Polyunsaturates/polyinsaturés	1 g
Monounsaturates/monoinsaturés	1.5 g
Saturates/saturés	1.5 g
Cholesterol	0 mg
Carbohydrate/Glucides	13 g
Sugars/sucres	3 g
Starch/amidon	5 g
Dietary fibre/fibres alimentaires	5 g
Sodium	2,400 mg
Potassium	1,700 mg

Percentage of Recommended Daily Intake
Pourcentage de l'apport quotidien recommandé

Vitamin A/vitamine A	70%
Vitamin D/vitamine D	65%
Niacin/niacine	25%
Calcium	6%
Iron/fer	5%
Zinc	5%

More nutrients may be listed on some labels.

Total Fat

Aim low: Most people need to cut back on fat! Too much fat may contribute to heart disease and cancer. Try to limit your *calories from fat*. For a healthy heart, choose foods with a big difference between the total number of calories and the number of calories from fat.

Saturated Fat

A new kind of fat? No — saturated fat is part of the total fat in food. It is listed separately because it's the key player in raising blood cholesterol and your risk of heart disease. Eat less!

Cholesterol

Too much cholesterol — a second cousin to fat — can lead to heart disease. Challenge yourself to eat less than 300 mg each day.

Sodium

You call it "salt," the label calls it "sodium." Either way, it may add up to high blood pressure in some people. So, keep your sodium intake low — 2400 to 3000 mg or less each day.*

*The AHA recommends no more than 3000 mg sodium per day for healthy adults

Daily Value

Feel like you're drowning in numbers? Let the Daily Value be your guide. Daily Values are listed for people who eat 2000 or 2500 calories each day. If you eat more, your personal daily value may be higher than what's listed on the label. If you eat less, your personal daily value may be lower.

For fat, saturated fat, cholesterol and sodium choose foods with a low % *Daily Value*. For total carbohydrate, dietary fiber, vitamins and minerals, your daily value goal is to reach 100% of each.

g = grams (About 28 g = 1 ounce)
mg = milligrams (1000 mg = 1 g)

Key Words: *Fat Free:* Less than 0.5 g of fat per serving; ***Low Fat:*** 3 g of fat or less per serving and no more than 15% fat on a dry basis; ***Fat-Reduced:*** At least 25% less fat than original product; ***Light or Lite:*** The package must indicate to what this refers, given that these claims can refer to anything about the product including taste, texture, colour, or fat content.

Sources: Food and Drug Administration, American Heart Association, 1993. Canadian Food Inspection Agency, "Guide to Food Labelling and Advertising," *1997 Health Canada Fact Sheet: New Definition of "Fat-Free" Foods* (1997). Health Canada, Health Protection Branch, Food Program, June 1997.

for food labelling purposes only, RDIs are intended to give the consumer an idea or rough estimate of the macro-nutrient contribution the food will make to their daily diet and serves as a uniform standard to help the public more readily compare the nutrient value of foods. Because people are of different sizes and have different nutritional requirements, RDIs are not intended to indicate the actual needs of any given individual.

As in past years, the Act regulates nutrition claims that labels may display, such as "light," "low-fat," etc. For the first time in Canada, however, the new legislation permits certain diet-related health claims, such as "A healthy diet rich in a variety of vegetables and fruit may help reduce the risk of some types of cancer." Foods making such health claims must adhere to strict standards laid out in the legislation.

Together with *Canada's Food Guide to Healthy Eating*, food labels provide the tools needed to make appealing food choices that are also nutritionally sound. However, these tools are of little value unless people take the time to read them, to understand how to use them, and then actually to use them.

◼ Dietitians of Canada

Dietitians of Canada (DC) is a national organization that represents dietitians across Canada committed to the health and well-being of Canadians through food and nutrition. It provides professional development and support to over 5000 registered dietitians. Through courses, resources, and networks, dietitians are kept up to date on key issues and develop the skills needed for meeting the current needs and nutritional interests of the public.

According to DC's report, "Speaking of Food and Eating: A Consumer Perspective" (Dietitians of Canada, 1998), consumer interest in nutrition is high. Eighty-nine percent of Canadians say nutrition and health are important when they are choosing what to eat. Information on nutrition in the marketplace is abundant, but consumers are tired of getting conflicting messages. They are looking for clear, practical, reliable information. Personal consultations with dietitians can provide this type of advice.

In Canada, dietitians are employed in health settings such as hospitals, public health departments, outpatient clinics, doctors' offices, and home care and community health centres. They also work in business settings such as the food industry, food services, commodity marketing boards, and fitness centres. Many dietitians also work in private practice, research, and media.

To find out more about Dietitians of Canada, have your nutrition questions answered, or find a dietitian in your area, visit the DC Web site (see Web links at the end of this chapter).

N UTRITION–DISEASE RELATIONSHIPS

Scientific evidence associating diet with numerous diseases has increased in the past decade. Although cause-and-effect relationships are still rather uncommon, dietary risk factors have been identified for a number of diseases and disorders (see Table 8.11), and the consumption of various nutrients has been associated with the prevention of some diseases.

High-fat diets have been linked to cardiorespiratory disease and cancer; high sodium and alcohol intake to a small percentage of the hypertense population; and high calorie intake and obesity to high blood pressure, diabetes, cardiorespiratory disease, and cancer. On the other hand, diets high in complex carbohydrates (fruits, vegetables, and grains) that contain vitamin A, beta-carotene, and dietary fibre have been tied to the prevention of cancer (colon, stomach, and so on), diverticulitis, and constipation; and low-fat diets to the prevention of cardiorespiratory disease and certain types of cancer.

Osteoporosis is a serious nutrition-related disorder that affects a large number of women after menopause. The Osteoporosis Society of Canada advocates the prevention of osteoporosis by means of: adequate intake of calcium, vitamin D, and fluoride; weight-bearing exercise; a reduction in bone toxins produced by cigarettes and alcohol; and hormone therapy. The idea is to reach menopause with as much bone mass as possible through a drug-free lifestyle, sound nutrition, and regular aerobic exercise. Although hormone-replacement therapy is effective in treating osteoporosis, many women choose to avoid or abandon such therapy due to the side-effects (weight gain, depression, menstrual bleeding and cramps, a slightly higher risk of breast cancer).

Consumers must resist the temptation, however, to consume very large amounts of any nutrient identified as having the potential for disease prevention or treatment until supportive evidence is found. In early 1996, National Cancer Institute researchers shut down a $42-million vitamin study of 18 000 smokers almost two years early, because too many of those being given high doses of beta-carotene supplements were dying. The government declared that beta-carotene supplements do not protect people against cancer or heart disease and might increase smokers' risk of deadly tumours. Another study of 22 000 individuals receiving megadoses (10 times the average recommended daily intake) of beta-carotene for 12 years found no evidence of either harm or benefit from beta-carotene supplementation. A study of 34 000 postmenopausal women produced similar results, indicating that those who ate foods rich in vitamin E, especially nuts and seeds, had

Table 8.11 ✦ Nutrition Risk Factors Associated with the Development of Diseases and Disorders

DISEASE OR DISORDER	NUTRITION RISK FACTORS
Heart disease and atherosclerosis ("hardening of the arteries")	Diets high in animal fat and cholesterol; obesity
Cancer[a]	Diets high in fat and low in vitamin A, beta-carotene, dietary fibre, and certain types of vegetables
Diabetes (in adults)	Obesity
Cirrhosis of the liver	Excessive alcohol consumption, malnutrition
Infertility	Underweight, obesity, zinc deficiency (in men)
Health problems of pregnant women and newborns	Maternal underweight, obesity, malnutrition, and excessive use of vitamin and mineral supplements or alcohol
Growth retardation in children	Diets low in calories, protein, iron, zinc
Tooth decay	Frequent consumption of sweets, diets low in fluoride
Iron-deficiency anemia	Diets low in iron
Constipation	Diets low in fibre and fluids
Obesity	Excessive calorie intake
Underweight	Deficient calorie intake
Hypertension	Diets high in sodium, excessive alcohol consumption, obesity
Osteoporosis	Diets low in calcium and vitamin D

[a]The development of most types of cancer, notably excluding leukemia, have been associated with nutrition risk factors.
Source: Judith E. Brown, *The Science of Human Nutrition.* © 1990 by Harcourt Brace & Company. Reproduced by permission of the publisher.

less than one-half the risk of death from heart disease as women who ate minimal amounts. No benefit was found among women who took vitamin E pills (*U.S. News & World Report*, 1996).

Evidence suggests that supplementation in many areas does not adequately replace the complex mix of chemicals and high-fibre, low-fat content of foods such as fruits, vegetables, and grains. The fact that phytochemicals and antioxidants found in many foods may help prevent disease does not necessarily mean that heavy intake through supplementation will produce similar effects. Once again, you should strive for moderation, variation, and balance in all aspects of your diet.

NUTRITION AND AGING

Scientists have been searching for decades for ways to slow the aging process. Evidence from the study of

rodents and rhesus monkeys indicates that those who want to live longer and healthier lives should stop eating before they are full and reduce their caloric intake. Dietary restriction has been shown to both increase an animal's fitness and slow the aging process. According to Richard Weindruch of the University of Wisconsin in Madison, this is the only intervention that slows down the rate of aging in warm-blooded animals. For example, female mice on a maximally calorie-restricted diet lived to an age of 45 months, nearly 20 months longer than mice who consumed as much as they wanted. Calorie-restricted mice and rats also maintained better cardiovascular fitness, improved glucose utilization, and stronger immune responses—processes that falter with aging. The incidence of cancer was also reduced. Experts feel that calorie restriction is the most effective inhibitor of carcinogenesis known in rodents and rhesus monkeys.

Just how much were calories restricted? The mice received well-balanced meals with 65 percent fewer calories than their unrestricted counterparts. Some began at an early age and others after they reached sexual maturity. Early restriction caused stunted bone growth and delayed sexual maturation.

To date, there have been no long-term studies involving humans to suggest such a drastic reduction in calories. Reducing daily caloric intake to 800 for an individual who needs 2000 calories would make it quite difficult to obtain proper nutrition and energy levels. Previous studies reduced the calories of mice and rats by only 30–40 percent, which would be much more realistic for humans. In any case, until more evidence is available, simply follow the guidelines in this chapter, avoid overnutrition and overfatness, and exercise five or more times weekly (*The Journal of NIH Research*, 1995; ACSM, 2000).

SPECIAL NEEDS OF THE ACTIVE INDIVIDUAL

Active individuals who follow the nutritional plan already presented in this chapter have a few special nutritional needs. There are several other areas of concern for those who exercise three to seven times a week:

- Eating enough calories for energy and body repair in order to benefit fully from the conditioning program
- Eating a sufficient amount of carbohydrates and fats to spare the body from burning protein
- Drinking sufficient fluids to prevent dehydration, heat-related illness, and early fatigue
- Replacing electrolytes (potassium, sodium, chloride) lost in perspiration
- Considering the use of iron supplements (for women)

■ Eating Enough Calories

If you are neither losing nor gaining weight, you are taking in the correct number of calories daily to maintain your present weight and fat level. That is, your energy intake and output are in balance. An individual will experience a reduction in weight and often fat level when the energy taken in is less than the energy put out. When this occurs, the individual is in negative energy balance. The opposite is also true: the positive energy balance of an individual consuming more calories than are being used often results in an elevated fat level and body weight.

You can estimate the number of calories you need from Table 8.12. Multiply your body weight by the calories recommended per kilogram for your activity level. This is only an estimate of your needs. Your body has an infallible computer that accurately registers your caloric intake daily; the output is body-weight changes. Refer to Lab Activity 8.1 for a more accurate indication of your energy expenditure.

Your source of calories is also an important factor in providing sufficient energy for exercise. The percentage of calories from carbohydrates (55%), fats (30%), and protein (15%), is sufficient for most exercising individuals. Increasing your complex carbohydrate (fruits, vegetables, grains) intake from 48 percent to 60 percent of total calories will increase your energy level. Total fat intake should be decreased by 10–12 percent.

■ Protein Sparing

Eating sufficient fruits, vegetables, and grains is extremely critical for the exercising individual. When the body does not have adequate carbohydrates available for energy, it will convert dietary protein and lean protein mass (muscle) to glucose to supply the nervous system.

Table 8.12 ✦ Approximate Number of Calories Needed Daily per .454 kg of Body Weight

AGE RANGES	7–10	11–14	15–22	23–35	36–50	51–75
Males						
Very active	21–22	23–24	25–27	23–24	21–22	19–20
Moderately active	16–17	18–19	20–23	18–19	16–17	11–15
Sedentary	11–12	13–14	15–18	13–14	11–12	10–11
Females						
Very active	21–22	22–23	20–21	20–21	18–19	17–18
Moderately active	16–17	18–19	16–18	16–17	14–15	12–13
Sedentary	11–12	13–14	11–12	11–12	9–10	8–9

Sedentary=no physical activity beyond attending classes and desk work.

Moderately active=involved in a regular exercise program at least 3 times weekly.

Very active=involved in a regular aerobic exercise program 4–6 times weekly, expending more than 2500 calories per week during physical activity.

When this occurs, loss of lean muscle tissue takes place throughout the body, including major organs such as the heart. Failing to spare protein for long periods of time may jeopardize health. A sufficient amount of complex carbohydrates in your diet will spare protein, provide a high level of energy, and protect your health.

Carbohydrate Loading or Supercompensation

The body has an adequate supply of energy available in the form of glucose and glycogen for performing regular exercise or competing in a sport. Glucose (sugar in the blood available for energy) and glycogen (the chief storage form of carbohydrate) are available in the blood, muscles, and liver and provide sufficient energy for most anaerobic workouts.

Individuals who compete in marathons, triathlons, and other endurance contests lasting several hours need additional energy and can benefit from a technique called **carbohydrate loading**, or **supercompensation**. New evidence indicates that the depletion stage may be unnecessary. By merely increasing carbohydrate intake

3–4 days before an important exercise activity or competition, you will more than double your liver and muscle glycogen stores. Such an increase provides approximately 3060 calories of energy—enough for practically any endurance event. Two large, high-carbohydrate meals (300 grams, 1200 calories per meal) are recommended daily for 3–4 days.

Replacing Fluids (Water)

Water needs depend on the individual and on factors such as body weight, activity patterns, sweat loss, loss through expired air and urine, and amount of liquid consumed through other foods and drinks (see Figure 8.4).

The active individual needs a minimum of 8–10 glasses (2 quarts or more) of water daily—much more in hot, humid weather. It is not unusual to lose 1–2 litres of water per hour when exercising in extremely hot, humid weather. Drinking too much water generally poses no problem; water is rarely toxic, and the kidneys merely excrete it efficiently. The kidneys are also capable of conserving water when the body is deprived by excreting more highly concentrated urine. If the colour

Figure 8.4 ✦ Water Intake and Loss

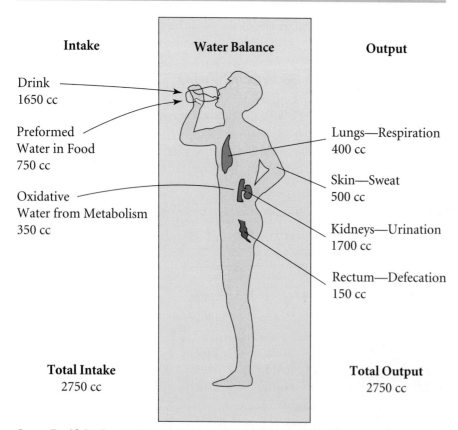

Intake — Water Balance — Output

Drink
1650 cc

Preformed
Water in Food
750 cc

Oxidative
Water from Metabolism
350 cc

Lungs—Respiration
400 cc

Skin—Sweat
500 cc

Kidneys—Urination
1700 cc

Rectum—Defecation
150 cc

Total Intake
2750 cc

Total Output
2750 cc

Source: David C. Nieman, Diane E. Butterworth, and Catherine N. Nieman, *Nutrition*, rev. 1st ed., © 1992 Wm. C. Brown Communications, Inc., Dubuque, IA. All rights reserved. Reprinted by permission of The McGraw-Hill Companies.

of your urine is darker than a manila folder, you need to consume additional water (not fluid from other drinks). It bears stating again that the body needs plain water for heat regulation and proper functioning of systems.

If you exercise in hot, humid weather, thirst sensations will underestimate your needs. By the time you are thirsty, a water deficit has been created that cannot be undone for several hours. Forced drinking (hydrating), even when no thirst sensation exists, will minimize water deficit, keep body temperature 1 or 2 degrees lower in hot weather, result in more efficient performance, and delay fatigue. The most beneficial approach is to force down an extra 16–32 ounces of water within 15 minutes before you begin to exercise. Earlier consumption may fill the bladder and make you uncomfortable during the activity.

Water will not interfere with your performance; drink it freely before, during, and after your workout. It is the single most important substance in preventing heat-related illnesses and in restoring the body to normal following exercise in hot, humid weather. For the quickest absorption of fluid, drink plain water chilled to about 4.4° C (40° F). (For additional discussion on water and its role in preventing heat exhaustion, muscle cramps, and heat stroke, see Chapter 12.)

◼ Maintaining Electrolyte Balance

Electrolytes lost through sweat and water vapour from the lungs must be replaced. It is the proper balance of each electrolyte that prevents dehydration, cramping, heat exhaustion, and heat stroke. Too much salt without adequate water, for example, actually draws fluid from the cells, precipitates nausea, and increases urination and potassium loss. A salt supplement is therefore rarely needed in spite of the weather or intensity and duration of exercise. The salt that occurs naturally in food, salt in processed food, and that used from the salt shaker will provide sufficient sodium even for active individuals.

Potassium is critical to maintaining regular heartbeat, and it also plays a role in carbohydrate and protein metabolism. Profuse sweating over several days can deplete potassium stores by as much as 3 milligrams per day. The average diet provides only 1.5–2.5 milligrams daily. If you sweat profusely and exercise almost daily, you may need five to eight servings of potassium-rich foods each day. Excellent sources of potassium include orange juice, skim milk, bananas, dried fruits, and potatoes. A potassium supplement is not recommended because too much potassium is just as dangerous as too little.

Ionic chloride is part of hydrochloric acid and serves to maintain the strong acidity of the stomach. Loss of too much chloride upsets the acid–base balance of the body. Adding chlorine to public water provides this valuable element and makes water safe for human consumption.

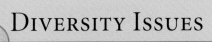

DIVERSITY ISSUES

Factors Affecting Our Food Choices

Culture has a tremendous influence on our food choices. Many eating habits arise from traditions, values, norms, and belief systems of the cultures in which we live. With the exception of a small percentage of those in Canada who occasionally sample chocolate-covered grasshoppers or other such delicacies, for example, the consumption of insects is viewed as repulsive. In many countries and cultures, however, the insect world offers a new protein source, new tastes, and new dishes such as locust dumplings (northern Africa), red-ant chutney (India), and fried caterpillars (South Africa). Most people can take a more conservative approach and sample almost any type of food in Canada by travelling only a few kilometres because ethnic cuisine is common in Canadian culture.

Religion also dictates a number of dietary practices in various cultures. Buddhism preaches vegetarianism and the consumption of all plant foods except for the five pungent foods that are considered unclean: garlic, leeks, scallions, chives, and onions. Hinduism prohibits the consumption of beef, and most Hindus are vegetarians. Islamic food laws do not allow "unclean" foods such as swine, animals killed without the blood fully drained from their bodies, meat-eating animals with fangs (lions, wolves), birds with sharp claws, and land animals without ears. Dietary laws of Judaism prohibit the eating of swine, carrion eaters, and shellfish and require foods to be "kosher" (prepared according to certain methods).

As you can see, many factors influence people's eating habits. The important thing is for all of us to understand, respect, and learn from these individual differences in dietary practices rooted in strong cultural heritages. ✦

Carbohydrate loading (supercompensation) An attempt to reduce carbohydrate intake to near zero for 2–3 days (depletion stage) before resorting to a high-carbohydrate diet for 3–4 days (loading phase) to raise glycogen stores in skeletal muscles and the liver to increase energy levels on the day of competition.

BEHAVIOURAL CHANGE AND MOTIVATIONAL STRATEGIES

People in the 2000s are more educated about nutrition than previous generations have been. Unfortunately, knowledge about proper nutrition does not readily translate into sound eating behaviour. Busy schedules, lack of money, fad diet and nutrition information, easy access to fast-food restaurants, youthful feelings of indestructibility, culture and religion, and many other factors help explain why, in spite of this knowledge, the typical diet of people in Canada is too high in saturated fat, cholesterol, total fat, calories, sodium, and sugar and too low in complex carbohydrates (fruits, vegetables, grains) and water. These problems are very much related to present and future health, behaviour, mood, and energy level. With only minimum effort, some of these problems can be corrected.

Roadblock	Behavioural Change Strategy
Some people simply do not seem to like water and therefore consume less than three of the recommended six to eight glasses daily. Most liquid consumed is coffee, tea, or high-calorie (132 cal per 300 mL serving) pop, juices, milk, beer, and other alcoholic drinks. Avoiding water allows more room for calories and salt, sugar, and fat.	You can change your liquid consumption patterns slowly and reacquire your taste for water. For a 7-day period, try: 1. Placing your favourite glass in the bathroom and drinking one full glass of water immediately on rising in the morning and just before bedtime. You are now already drinking more water than most people do. 2. Not passing by a water fountain, even if you are not thirsty. Take at least five swallows (about 85 mL). 3. Placing a cold pitcher of water in the front of your refrigerator so it is the first thing you see. 4. Drinking at least one glass of water with each meal.
So much of what we eat is processed food, which is typically high in sodium. There seems to be no way of avoiding the problem.	Although high sodium intake may not be as much of a health hazard as originally suspected, it is a good idea to cut back. About one-third of the salt you consume comes from processed food, another third comes from table salt, and one-third occurs naturally in food. There are a number of things you can do: 1. Restrict your visits to fast-food restaurants to no more than once a month. 2. Avoid or use very little table salt, substituting herbs and spices such as lemon and orange. Use a salt substitute that does not contain sodium or potassium. Plan on taking several weeks to become adjusted to not adding table salt to your food. 3. Read food labels and purchase products with no or low salt. 4. Avoid luncheon meats, smoked meats, hot dogs, sausages, and high-salt cheeses.
Although you are aware of the association between high total fat, high saturated fat, high cholesterol diets, and heart disease, it is simply too difficult to avoid high fat in the diet.	It does seem that way, particularly if you eat on the run and do not have time to plan meals. There are some specific things you can do that are certain to reduce the percentage of calories you consume from fat daily: 1. Take the time to glance at the label of every product you purchase. If it does not say it has zero grams of fat, do not buy it. 2. If you eat ice cream, purchase one of the brands that use artificial fat; the taste is excellent and the product is nearly fat- and cholesterol-free. 3. Pack a lunch every day consisting of fruit, vegetables, and a low-calorie sandwich. This will keep you from skipping a meal or running to a fast-food restaurant during the day. 4. Reduce your intake of invisible fat by reducing your consumption of chocolate, eggs, red meat, poultry skin, and dairy products. 5. Cut the skin off the raw poultry before cooking, avoid frying, and choose cooking methods that do not require the use of oils.

Roadblock	Behavioural Change Strategy
	6. Use paper towels to soak up the fat when you cook hamburger and other meats.
List some roadblocks that interfere with your following sound nutritional practices.	Now list behavioural change strategies that can help you overcome the roadblocks you just listed. If you need to, refer back to Chapter 3 for behavioural change and motivational strategies.
1. _____	1. _____
2. _____	2. _____
3. _____	3. _____

Water alone will not restore electrolyte balance. One alternative is to use commercially prepared, concentrated electrolyte drinks, provided you alter their contents. Some of these drinks contain too much sugar and should be diluted with twice the normal amount of water to increase absorption time and prevent a rapid drop in blood-glucose level shortly after consumption.

Although useful before and after exercise, the addition of electrolytes to water is of minimal value during a workout. Research suggests that electrolyte replacement is also secondary in importance to water replacement during rehydration after exercise. Fruit juices have the same pitfalls as commercial electrolyte drinks, and the concentrated varieties should be diluted with at least twice the amount of water suggested on the container.

▌Replacing Iron

Iron deficiency can lead to loss of strength and endurance, early fatigue during exercise, shortening of attention span, loss of visual perception, and impaired learning. Adolescent girls are more apt to be iron-deficient than women are at any other age. Female athletes of all ages should discuss with their physician the need for an iron supplement during menstruation.

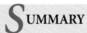

S UMMARY

▌Basic Food Components

Six categories of nutrients satisfy the basic body needs: the energy nutrients (carbohydrates, fats, proteins) and the nonenergy nutrients (vitamins, minerals, water).

Carbohydrates and fats provide the main sources of energy (calories) to perform work. Simple carbohydrates found in concentrated sugar provide empty calories to the diet and very little nutrition in terms of key vitamins and minerals. Complex carbohydrates (fruits, vegetables, grains) are our only source of fibre and a major supplier of long-term energy. Complex carbohydrates are nutritionally dense foods, providing low calories and a high percentage of our daily needs in vitamins and minerals. Both water-insoluble (dietary) and water-soluble fibres provide important health benefits.

Dietary fat is a critical nutrient and a source of high energy for the human body. Fat is classified as saturated, polyunsaturated, or monounsaturated. Cholesterol, a type of fat, is found in animal sources and also manu-factured by the human liver. Trans fatty acids are formed when low-saturated-fat vegetable oils are hydrogenated to make them more solid at room temperature. These fatty acids, present in margarine and all foods with the phrase "partially hydrogenated" or "hydrogenated" on their labels, have been shown to raise the "bad" LDL cholesterol and lower the "good" HDL cholesterol as well as contribute to the incidence of heart disease.

Protein can be obtained from both animal and plant foods. In the human body, protein is used for: the repair, rebuilding, and replacement of cells; growth; fluid, salt, and acid–base balance; and energy in the absence of sufficient dietary carbohydrates and fat. Protein from meat, eggs, and dairy products is termed *complete* because it contains all the essential amino acids in the correct proportion. The correct combinations of various vegetables and grains also compose complete protein sources. With proper planning, vegetarians can easily obtain sufficient protein in their diets without consuming meat, eggs, or dairy products.

Vitamins help chemical reactions take place in the body and are needed in only small amounts. A balanced diet provides the necessary vitamins and minerals needed daily for most people.

Minerals are present in all living cells and serve as components of hormones, enzymes, and other substances aiding chemical reactions in cells. Macrominerals are needed in large amounts, whereas 14 trace minerals are required in small quantities for optimum health. Your daily mineral needs can also be obtained through a balanced diet.

Although it has no nutritional value, water is necessary for all energy production, temperature control, and elimination. You should consume a minimum of six to eight glasses of water daily, exclusive of all other beverages.

Food Density

A food is said to be nutritionally dense if it contains a low percentage of the daily caloric needs and a high percentage of key nutrients such as protein, vitamins, and minerals. Complex carbohydrates are the most nutritionally dense foods; foods high in sugar and fat are the least dense.

Dietary Guidelines for Good Health

You can be assured of sound nutrition by planning your diet around *Canada's Food Guide to Healthy Eating*. The recommended servings from each of four key food groups and the limited use of the fifth group ("other foods") will provide you with excellent nutrition. *Canada's Food Guide* coupled with food labels offers a less complicated approach to sound nutrition for the layperson than complicated tables and calculations.

Dietary recommendations have also been made in terms of percentage of total calories to guide your intake of carbohydrates, protein, fat, and alcohol.

Nutrition and Disease

The evidence associating nutritional practices with various diseases and disorders and linking sound nutrition to the prevention of some of these diseases continues to mount. Diets that are high in complex carbohydrates and low in fat, cholesterol, sodium, and calories offer the greatest benefits.

Nutrition and Aging

Laboratory studies with rhesus monkeys and rodents have uncovered a favourable effect of undernutrition on the aging process. Laboratory animals whose caloric intake was reduced by 30–60 percent but that were given a balanced diet extended their lives by nearly 50 percent, maintained their fitness levels and function of their immune systems, and showed a remarkable resistance to cancer.

Special Needs of the Active Individual

Physically active individuals who follow the nutritional guidelines presented in this chapter have only a few special needs. Sufficient calories must be consumed to support activity levels and to prevent weight and muscle loss; adequate carbohydrates and fat must be consumed to prevent the loss of lean muscle mass; water intake should be increased dramatically; electrolyte balance must be maintained; and care must be taken to obtain sufficient dietary iron.

STUDY QUESTIONS

1. Collect a week's worth of empty food containers (with nutrition labels). From these containers, create a breakfast, lunch, and dinner that meet both *Canada's Food Guide* recommendations and the caloric intake recommendations for macro nutrients (note: add fresh fruits and vegetables to the list as you see fit).

2. What are the special nutritional needs of an active individual?

3. What are the six types of nutrients, and into which categories do they fall?

4. Differentiate among the different types of vegetarian diets.

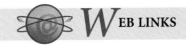

WEB LINKS

Dietitians of Canada
www.dietitians.ca

Danone Institute of Canada
www.danoneinstitute-can.com

Health Canada's Food & Nutrition Page
www.hc-sc.gc.ca/english/lifestyles/food_nutr.html

Canada's Food Guide to Healthy Eating
www.hc-sc.gc.ca/hppb/nutrition/pube/foodguid/index.html

Food Labels and the Food Guide
www.hc-sc.gc.ca/hppb/nutrition/labels/index.html

The Office of Nutrition Policy and Promotion
www.hc-sc.gc.ca/hppb/nutrition/index.html

REFERENCES

American College of Sports Medicine. *ACSM's Guidelines for Exercise Testing and Prescription, 6th Edition.* Philadelphia: Lippincott, Williams & Wilkins, 2000.

Brevard, P.B., and C.D. Ricketts. "Residence of College Students Affects Dietary Intake, Physical Activity, and Serum Lipid Levels." *Journal of the American Dietetic Association* 96 (1996): 35–38.

Dietitians of Canada. "Speaking of Food and Eating: A Consumer Perspective." Canadian Foundation for Dietetic Research and Kraft Canada Inc., 1998.

Dinger, M.K., and A. Waigandt. "Dietary Intake and Physical Activity Behaviors of Male and Female College Students." *American Journal of Health Promotion*, 11, 5 (1997): 360–362.

Food and Drug Act: Regulations Amending the Food and Drug Regulations (Nutrition Labelling, Nutrient Content Claims and Health Claims), Canada Gazette, December 11, 2002. Available at **http://canadagazette.gc.ca/partII/2003/20030101/html/sor11-e.html**. Accessed March 13, 2003.

Gibson, R. for the National Institute of Nutrition. (2001). Iron Concerns in Canada. **www.nin.ca**

Glore, S.R., C. Walker, and A. Chandler. "Dietary Habits of First-Year Medical Students as Determined by Computer Software Analysis of Three-Day Food Records." *Journal of American College Nutrition* 12 (1993): 517–520.

Haberman, S., and D. Luffey. "Weighing In College Students' Diet and Exercise Behaviors." *Journal of American College Health* 46 (1998): 189–191.

Health Canada. Office of Nutrition Policy and Promotion. (2002). **www.hc-sc.gc.ca**

"Health Canada announces new mandatory nutrition labelling to help Canadians make informed choices for healthy eating." News release, January 2, 2003. Ottawa: Health Canada. Available at **www.hc-sc.gc.ca/english/media/releases/2003/2003_01.htm**. Accessed March 13, 2003.

Lowry, R., D.A. Galuska, J.E. Fulton, H. Wechsler, L. Kann, and J.L. Collins. "Physical Activity, Food Choice, and Weight Management Goals and Practices Among U.S. College Students." *American Journal of Preventive Medicine* 18, 1 (2000): 18–26.

Makrides, L., P. Veinot, J. Richard, R. McKee, and T. Gallivan. "A Cardiovascular Health Needs Assessment of University Students Living in Residence." *Canadian Journal of Public Health*, 89, 3 (1998): 171–175.

Quinn, T.J., and M. Jenkins. "Nutritional Profiles of Selected College Females in a 15-Week Exercise and Weight-Control Class." *Health Values,* 15, 3 (1991): 34–41.

Statistics Canada. "Food Consumption in Canada." Catalogue No. 32-229-XPB, Part 1, 1997.

Statistics Canada. Food Consumption in Canada 2001, Part 1. "Food Consumption Highlights." Available at **www.statcan.ca/english/ads/23FOOD/XCB/highlight.htm**. Accessed March 6, 2003.

The Journal of NIH Research 7 (1995): 42.

Troyer, D., I.H. Ullrich, R.A. Yeater, and R. Hopewell. "Physical Activity and Condition, Dietary Habits, and Serum Lipids in Second-Year Medical Students." *Journal of American College Nutrition* 9 (1990): 303–307.

U.S. News & World Report (May 13, 1996), p. 93.

Lab Activity 8.1

Estimating Caloric Expenditure

INSTRUCTIONS: *The energy needs of your body depend on three factors: (1) body size, (2) age, and (3) the type and amount of your daily physical activity. Your basal metabolic rate (BMR) and caloric expenditure in normal daily activities combine to represent your required energy needs. Complete these steps to estimate your total caloric expenditure. Locate your height on scale 1 and then your weight on scale 2 in Table A. Using a straight edge, connect the appropriate points on scales 1 and 2. The intersection of this line with scale 3 is your body surface area.*

Table A ✦ Body Surface Area

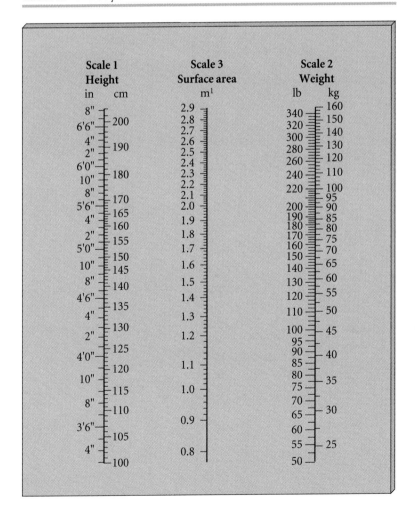

Lab Activity 8.1 *(continued)*
Estimating Caloric Expenditure

✦ Identifying BMR

Locate your BMR according to the values in Table B.

Table B ✦ Basal Metabolic Rate by Age and Gender

AGE	MEN	WOMEN
10	47.7	44.9
11	46.5	43.5
12	45.3	42.0
13	44.5	40.5
14	43.8	39.2
15	42.9	38.3
16	42.0	37.2
17	41.5	36.4
18	40.8	35.8
19	40.5	35.4
20	39.9	35.3
21	39.5	35.2
22	39.2	35.2
23	39.0	35.2
24	38.7	35.1
25	38.4	35.1
26	38.2	35.0
27	38.0	35.0
28	37.8	35.0
29	37.7	35.0
30	37.6	35.0
31	37.4	35.0
32	37.2	34.9
33	37.1	34.9
34	37.0	34.9
35	36.9	34.8
36	36.8	34.7
37	36.7	34.6
38	36.7	34.5
39	36.6	34.4
40–44	36.4	34.1
45–49	36.2	33.8
50–54	35.8	33.1
55–59	35.1	32.8
60–64	34.5	32.0
65–69	33.5	31.6
70–74	32.7	31.1
75+	31.8	

✦ Determining Activity Levels

To your BMR, you must add the caloric cost for your daily activities. It would be impractical to try to calculate your daily energy needs exactly every day, but you can arrive at a close estimate. Select the figure, from the following list, that best describes your activity level.

40%	Sedentary activities—limited to walking and sitting
50%	Semisedentary activities—standing, walking, and recreational activities
60%	Labourer or limited physical exercise
70%	Heavy worker—regular participation in sports and other physical activities
80%	Engaged in intercollegiate sports or in a vigorous daily physical-fitness program

✦ Calculating Total Energy Expenditure

Enter the values indicated and perform the necessary calculations.

1. Body surface area (from Table A) _____

2. BMR factor (from Table B) × _____

3. BMR/hour at rest (step 1 × step 2) = _____

4. Number of hours in a day (24) × _____

5. BMR/day at rest (step 3 × step 4) = _____

6. Activity level (enter .40, .50, .60, .70, or .80) × _____

7. Activity calories (step 5 × step 6) = _____

8. BMR/day at rest (enter number from step 5) + _____

Total energy expenditure (total kcal/24 hours) = _____

Lab Activity 8.2

Estimating Your Daily Fibre Intake

INSTRUCTIONS: *Record all the fibre-containing foods you eat for a period of three days in the space provided. Remember that you must keep records only of the amount and portion size of all fruits, vegetables, and grains eaten.*

To help you estimate the grams of fibre in each food item consumed, see Table 8.2. Now record the number of grams of dietary fibre you consume in each food daily in the last column. Divide the total grams by 3 to determine your average daily intake.

✦ **Record of Daily Fibre Intake**

DAY	FOOD ITEM	SIZE OR AMOUNT	GRAMS OF FIBRE
1	Fruits: _____	_____	_____
	Vegetables: _____	_____	_____
	Grains: _____	_____	_____
2	Fruits: _____	_____	_____
	Vegetables: _____	_____	_____
	Grains: _____	_____	_____
3	Fruits: _____	_____	_____
	Vegetables: _____	_____	_____
	Grains: _____	_____	_____

Total grams of dietary fibre in three days _____

Average grams per day _____

Recommended daily intake = 35 g

Additional daily fibre needed _____

- Are you consuming at least 35 g of dietary fibre daily? _____ Yes _____ No

- If you responded No, on the reverse side of this sheet list three or four ways you can alter your meal and snacking to increase fibre intake.

9

Exploring Weight and Fat Management

CHAPTER OBJECTIVES

By the end of this chapter, you should be able to:

1. Differentiate between weight loss and fat loss.

2. Evaluate and determine your ideal weight and percentage of body fat.

3. Define overweight, overfat, and obesity.

4. Describe a sound, long-term fat-loss program.

5. Discuss the role of exercise in weight and fat management.

6. Differentiate between anorexia nervosa and bulimia.

7. Identify the key behaviours linked to weight and fat loss, and describe how to use several behaviour modification techniques to achieve your desired weight.

SUSAN HAS ALWAYS been preoccupied with her weight. As far back as she can remember, she was too fat. For years, she considered it purely a genetic problem. After all, her father is obese and her mother is stocky. She thinks perhaps the cards are stacked against her. As an adult, she has tried every diet described in *Chatelaine* or that appeared on the bestseller list. Perhaps there is nothing she can do about it. According to the literature, diets don't work, and she hates to exercise. Why diet for a lifetime when you need to lose only 4–5 kilograms?

Is there any hope for people like Susan? This chapter provides the answers to these and other questions about weight and fat control.

TRENDS IN WEIGHT CONTROL

During the late nineteenth century, human muscle power provided 33 percent of the energy needed to run the farms, homes, and factories. Today, muscular effort contributes less than 1 percent of the energy. Most people work in office-bound, service-oriented jobs and use machines, computers, and pens and pencils to accomplish their tasks. The jobs we do and the types of energy needed for those jobs have changed over the past 100 years. The human body has remained the same as we became victims of a technology-oriented lifestyle. As a result, more and more people of all ages are overfat or obese. In 1998/99, about half of Canadians aged 15 or older were in the acceptable weight range and only 3 percent were underweight. Statistics Canada Health Reports (2001) show that almost one-third of Canadians were assessed (using body mass index measures) as overweight and 14 percent were considered obese. Furthermore, a higher percentage of men (42 percent) than women (24 percent) were overweight. With specific reference to children, the Canadian Medical Association has noted that in the age range of 7 to 13 years, between 1981 and 1996, overfatness increased from 15 to 33 percent and obesity at least tripled during the same time frame. Data on overfatness and obesity using the percentage of body fat rather than weight charts reveal similar findings. The increased number of overfat children will result in a significantly higher number of overfat adults in the future. With each passing decade, the typical adult also accumulates additional excess fat and loses some lean muscle tissue until, by middle age, 50 percent of adult men and women in Canada are overfat or obese.

At all ages, we are growing several kilograms heavier each decade. Although our average height is also increasing, the majority of this weight gain is fat, not muscle. This trend must be brought under control because obesity is associated with a number of disorders such as atherosclerosis, hypertension, diabetes, heart/lung difficulties, early heart attack, and numerous other chronic and degenerative diseases and disorders (see Table 9.1). The death rate for obese men ages 15–69 is 50 percent higher than that of normal-weight persons and 30 percent higher than for those classified as merely overweight. For every 10 percent a person is above normal weight, it is estimated that lifespan is decreased by one year. Unfortunately, the quality of life also declines dramatically in obese individuals.

This chapter examines critical aspects related to the management of body composition: causes of obesity, assessment, safe fat-loss methods, the role of exercise in weight and fat management, underweight and eating disorders, and the role of behaviour modification techniques in helping young people to manage body weight and fat during the late teenage and early adult years.

CAUSES OF OBESITY

Inactivity and overeating are the two most common causes of obesity and overfatness. Physical activity can do much to offset weight gain and regulate the tendency to put on unwanted weight. Weight gain of genetically obese mice, for example, is drastically reduced by treadmill exercise. In humans, extremely high caloric intake can also be offset by a vigorous exercise program and result in little or no weight gain.

Social, genetic, and psychological factors also result in overeating and obesity. It has been found that in only a small percentage of cases are glandular or other physiological disorders related to weight problems although many obese people blame these factors. Sedentary living and excessive eating are the two greatest perpetuators of obesity; both can be controlled.

Table 9.1 ✦ Health Problems Associated with Excess Body Fat, Grouped by Relative Risk*

SLIGHTLY INCREASED RISK (1–2)	MODERATELY INCREASED RISK (2–3)	GREATLY INCREASED RISK (>3)
Breast cancer (1.31)	Endometrial cancer (2.19)	Type 2 diabetes (4.37)
Coronary Artery disease (1.72)	Hypertension (2.51)	
Colorectal cancer (1.16)	Pulmonary embolism (2.39)	
Gallbladder disease (1.85)		
Hyperlipidemia (1.41)		
Stroke (1.14)		

* Relative risk is a statistical association in which values between 1 and 2 indicate a slight correlation, values between 2 and 3 indicate a moderate correlation, and values greater than 3 indicate a strong correlation.

Source: Based on C. Laird Birmingham, Jennifer L. Muller, Anita Palepu, John J. Spinelli, and Aslam H. Anis, "The Cost of Obesity in Canada," *Canadian Medical Association Journal,* February 23, 1999.

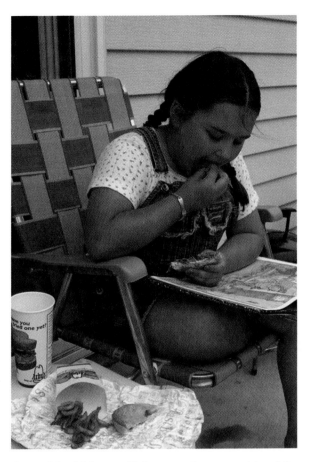

Overweight children are likely to grow into overweight adults.

Early Eating Patterns

Most experts agree that the eating habits formed in infancy and childhood carry over into the adult years. Rats who are exposed to unlimited milk, for example, continue to eat much more and exercise less after they are weaned than rats who receive only limited milk. In other words, rats who are overfed prior to weaning become sedentary adult rats who overeat, become fat, and suffer from early cardiorespiratory disease. In contrast, rats who eat less prior to weaning continue to eat less, exercise more, live longer, and experience less cardiorespiratory disease. The response in humans is similar. Children who are inactive and who overeat are also more likely to continue these behaviours later in life and become overfat adults.

Environmental forces appear to influence eating patterns more than physiological forces such as hunger. Negative eating behaviour may begin in infancy. Some experts feel that bottle feeding, for example, may predispose infants to obesity. Approximately three times more bottle-fed than breast-fed babies are overfat. Bottle feeding fails to provide the solace of breast feeding and tends to produce anxiety, which may provoke overeating. Breast-fed babies also learn to stop feeding when the richest portion of the milk gives way to more watery milk. The bottle does not provide such a natural mechanism, so bottle-fed babies require more calories to satisfy their hunger.

Perhaps a more important problem is feeding babies solid foods too early, which may contribute to the production of excess fat cells. Experts recommend that parents start feeding their infants solid foods at the age of 5 months rather than earlier, except for cases of very large or fast-developing babies. This is no easy task for sleep-deprived mothers who long for the day the baby sleeps through the night without waking for a feeding.

There is little danger that growing children will be obese if they themselves decide when to stop eating at a meal. Forcing children to clean the plate is a mistake and is the same as forcing them to overeat. Making sweets plentiful, using them as rewards, and placing emphasis on the fat baby also compounds the problem, shortens the life span, encourages premature heart disease, creates undesirable eating habits, and destines the child to a life of restricted eating because of the high number of fat cells formed in early life. A lean child with a great deal of energy and vitality is healthier and more likely to be healthy later in life.

There is no stage in life when excess fat is desirable; however, the earlier in life a child is obese, the greater the chance that the child will eventually be of normal weight. The later in life a child is obese, the less likely it is that he or she will ever return to normal weight. It is estimated that an obese adolescent, for example, has approximately a 1 in 16 chance of returning to normal weight as an adult. The fatter you are at any age, the less likely it is that you will ever return to normal weight. It is therefore advisable to start children off right and avoid overfeeding them. If their mechanism for moving away from the table when they are full is undermined, they are certain to need plenty of aerobic movement in the adult years to control weight.

Fat Cells

Our fat cells are formed early in life and increase in both size and number until the end of adolescence. Calorie restriction will decrease only the size of fat cells, not the number. With a large number of fat cells formed, a return to an overfat condition is quite easy. This partially explains why adults who were fat babies often have difficulty keeping their weight down. These extra adipose cells also affect metabolism and result in the need for fewer calories to maintain normal weight than are needed by someone who generally remains at normal weight. Unlike muscle, fat requires little energy to maintain, and additional fat weight will not increase metabolic rate.

The number of fat cells in the human body grows rapidly during three stages of development: (1) the last trimester of pregnancy (in the unborn child), (2) the first year of life, and (3) the adolescent growth spurt. Fat is acquired by an increase in the size of existing adipose cells (**hypertrophy**) and by new fat-cell formation prior to adulthood (**hyperplasia**). It is doubtful that new fat cells are formed after age 21 (approximately) unless someone becomes extremely obese.

There is a wide variation in the number of fat cells in different people. A nonobese person has approximately 25–30 billion fat cells while an extremely obese person may have as many as 260 billion. A formerly obese adult may never be cured because weight loss does not reduce the number of existing cells; it only reduces their size.

◼ Genetics

It is now quite clear that the genes we inherit influence our body weight and the amount and disposition of fat. Children of overfat or obese parents, particularly the biological mother, are much more likely to develop fat–weight problems. Twin studies also support the influence of genetics on overfatness and obesity. Heredity may be tied to weight and fat problems in a number of other ways, such as a predisposition to consuming sweet, high-fat foods, impaired hormonal functions (insulin and cortisol), a lower basal metabolic rate, differences in kilocalories used during the metabolism of food, inability of nutrients to suppress the appetite control centre, differences in the ability to store fat and burn calories during light exercise, and a tendency to develop more fat cells.

Ongoing research on the presence of a so-called fat gene and the development of drugs to permanently control hunger may offer hope for overweight individuals in the future. It is important to keep in mind, however, that environment is still critical. Genetics may merely predispose individuals or provide them with the tendency to become fat—a problem that regular exercise and proper nutrition can help overcome.

◼ Environmental Factors

Although heredity plays an important role, environment is also critical. Sound exercise and eating and drinking habits can overcome the genetic tendency to be either thin or fat.

One of the clearer causes of obesity and overfatness in children is watching television. People on TV programs eat about eight times per hour, and commercials generally advertise high-calorie, high-fat foods. TV watchers pick up on these cues and tend to eat more often and to consume more high-fat, high-calorie foods. In addition, television is a passive activity. Almost

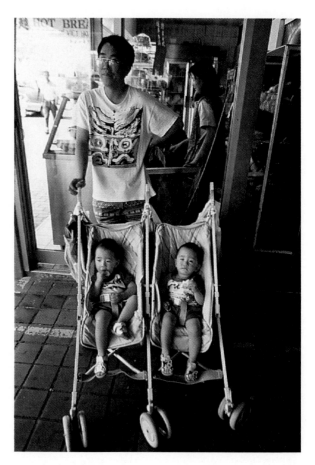

Genetics play a major role in determining body weight and fat.

any other activity will burn more calories. Although it is a good idea to restrict the number of TV-watching hours for all children and teenagers, it is absolutely necessary to do so for the overfat child.

Other environmental influences, such as eating and exercise habits of parents, food availability, and nutritional knowledge, may not be as important as was once believed. Experts feel that genetic influences account for about 70 percent of the differences in body mass index (BMI) that are found later in life and that childhood environment has less influence than was once thought. This does not mean that environment has no influence on obesity. Nongenetic factors are important determinants of body fat. These factors are reversible and capable of overcoming some of the genetic factors that make us fat.

◼ Metabolic Factors

Even small changes in metabolic rate translate into large increases in body fat and weight. A 10 percent decline in metabolism, for example, could result in an annual weight gain of about 6.8 kilograms for the average individual. Aerobic exercise increases metabolic rate both during and after the exercise session. The afterburn continues for from 20 minutes to several hours, depending on the duration and intensity of the workout. Coffee, tea, cocoa, colas, other caffeine-containing foods and drinks, and amphetamines and other drugs increase metabolic rate. In midafternoon, metabolism tends to slow, making this an excellent time for aerobic exercise to boost metabolic rate. As one ages, metabolism also slows; by age 50, metabolic rate may have decreased by as much as 15–25 percent in a sedentary individual. In those who have remained active through a combination of aerobic exercise and strength training, metabolic rate slows only slightly. Loss of muscle mass is one of the leading causes of reduced metabolic rate with aging. Thus, increasing muscle mass at all ages is important in increasing or maintaining an optimal metabolic rate.

SET-POINT THEORY

The human body regulates its own functions with tremendous precision. Body weight is one of these functions. Each individual appears to have an ideal biological weight (the **set point**) and will defend it against pressure to change. Those who do succeed in losing or gaining weight generally return to their set-point weight in a few months or years. Within 24 hours of beginning a very-low-calorie diet, for example, the dieter's metabolic rate (amount of calories burned at rest) slows by 5–20 percent as a means of conserving energy, making it more difficult to lose weight. The body is convinced it is starving, and the caloric conservation is a way of hanging on to the energy for a longer period of time. In addition, once excess fat cells become depleted, they signal the central nervous system to alter feeding behaviour by increasing caloric intake so that the set point can be maintained. In other words, some experts feel that an internal thermostat regulates body fat and weight and triggers an increase in food intake when fat and weight are lowered too much. Overcoming the set point is difficult. Will power and other factors that aid in tolerating the discomfort of hunger are a poor defence against a computerlike system that never quits.

Research suggests that one of the ways to take it off and keep it off may be to lower the thermostat. *Yo-yo* dieting (the cycle of losing and regaining fat and weight) may have the opposite effect and actually result in a higher setting on the thermostat, with the body then defending an even higher weight. This may explain why people who complete several cycles of losing and regaining 5 kilograms find it nearly twice as hard to lose weight and twice as easy to gain weight on their next attempt. With each yo-yo cycle, the individual also acquires extra body fat and loses some muscle mass.

Regular aerobic exercise four to five times a week combined with a sound nutritional plan appears to lower the thermostat over time and allows loss of weight and maintenance of that lower weight.

BODY COMPOSITION

Many people have an ideal body image that they would someday like to achieve. For some, such an image may be unrealistic. Regardless of your motivation to change, several methods derived from research or actuarial tables may help you set realistic goals for a better-looking body.

A simple method of estimating proper body weight is to use the Metropolitan Life Insurance height–weight standards. Charts of so-called ideal weight for men and women are based on data associating average weights by height and age with long life. Prior to 1980, figures indicated that those who weighed less than their recommended weight on the charts lived up to 20 percent longer than other people. The charts, which became the national guide for determining overweight and obesity for the general public, worked on the theory that "the greater the weight, the greater the risk of death." The validity of such data is now being questioned because it is evident that less-than-average weights may involve health risks even greater than those associated with overweight and that our preoccupation with slimness may not be much of a health advantage.

Authorities do not dispute that people who are much heavier than average (more than 20 percent above ideal weight) obtain health benefits from fat reduction. Even small amounts of fat loss, for example, may aid the diabetic patient. For those in normal health who are at average or near average fat, there are fewer benefits associated with losing fat. The key factor that determines what is too much or too little is body fat, not total body weight.

Determining Ideal Body Weight from Height–Weight Charts

Most people place far too much emphasis on height–weight charts as a measure of their desirable

Hypertrophy of fat cells The enlargement of existing fat cells.

Hyperplasia of fat cells New fat-cell formation.

Set point A theory postulating that each individual has an ideal weight (the set point) and that the body will attempt to maintain this weight against pressure to change it.

DIVERSITY ISSUES

Fat Control

Fat is the primary energy reserve of the body. The natural distribution and amount of fat varies considerably between men and women. Some experts identify the appropriate body fatness in women as 20–27 percent compared to 12–15 percent in men. Achieving a body-fat level below the level of essential fat represents no health advantage for either sex and may actually be detrimental to health.

Weight and fat management is a much more difficult task for women than for men because about 12 percent of fat in women is essential fat (as opposed to 4–7 percent in men), which includes an extra 5–9 percent of sex-specific fat in the breasts, pelvic region, and thighs. The childbearing role and the fact that women generally possess smaller bodies requiring fewer calories also make it much more difficult for a woman to lose fat and weight than for a man.

Fat accumulates in different sites on men and women. In general, men tend to possess fat receptors in the abdominal area and fat inhibitors in the buttocks, hips, and upper legs. This partially explains why most men develop the beer belly and rarely accumulate fat in other areas. Women tend to possess fat receptors in the hips, buttocks, and thighs and often have fat inhibitors in the abdomen. Various patterns of obesity exist in both sexes, with most obese individuals distributing fat throughout the body. Android (excessive fat in the lower body) and gynoid (excessive fat in the abdomen) obesity may result in both men and women. The so-called pear (fat accumulation in the hips and lower body common in women) and apple (fat accumulation in the abdominal area common in men) shapes have also been examined by researchers. Apple shapes with large fat accumulation around the midsection and chest may impose a greater risk for heart disease than the pear shape.

Because most women need significantly fewer calories to maintain their lower body weight, it is more difficult for them to enter into a large negative calorie balance daily and lose weight rapidly. A 50-kilogram woman may need only 1700 calories daily, for example. A 1000-calorie deduction leaves only 800 calories to obtain adequate nourishment and energy—a nearly impossible task. A 100-kilogram man, however, may require as much as 3300 calories daily to maintain weight. A 1000-calorie daily deficit still leaves a total of 2000 calories—enough for sufficient nourishment and energy.

We all must become more tolerant of our bodies and accept the fact that our percentage of body fat will increase slightly with age and that aging will alter the shape and appearance of our bodies regardless of our best exercise and eating efforts. Overemphasis on thinness (a cultural emphasis often referred to as "the Thinderella syndrome") and on a youthful body is dangerous for both sexes, and often leads to self-concept problems and serious eating disorders. ✦

weight. Some experts feel that both the bathroom scale and height–weight charts should be thrown into the nearest garbage can. Body weight provides no indication of what is really important—not how much you weigh, but how much fat your body contains and how fit you are. There are several additional limitations with height–weight charts: non-Caucasians are underrepresented; age is not considered; and desirable weights are too high for young people and too low for the elderly (but correct for those in their 40s). Merely pinching body parts (if you "pinch an inch," it's too much fat in that area) provides ample information to alert you to the need to lose body fat, but not necessarily body weight.

■ Determining Percentage of Body Fat

A more important consideration in goal setting for a better-looking and healthier body involves not body weight but the amount of adipose tissue you possess. What is commonly called "weight control" is better and more accurately labelled "fat control," and measurement of body fat is essential in setting goals for your body.

The average percentage of body fat is approximately 22 percent for females and 15–18 percent for males. Individuals are considered obese if they possess more than 23 percent (men) or 28 percent (women) body fat.

Because about half of all body fat lies just beneath the skin, it is possible to pinch certain body parts, measure the thickness of the two layers of skin and the connected fat, and estimate the total percentage of fat on the body.

You can measure the thickness of skinfold sites with a caliper. Considerable practice is needed before accurate measurements can be taken. Take a moment to complete Lab Activity 9.1: Determining Your

Percentage of Body Fat at the end of this chapter to develop your skills and determine your estimated percentage of body fat.

Determining Body Mass Index (BMI)

Body mass index (BMI) provides a ratio between body weight and height and is quickly becoming the standard way of realistically understanding body composition in relationship to risk factors and defining obesity for the general public. Canadian guidelines suggest that people keep their BMIs under 25.

To determine your BMI, use BMI = weight (kg)/height^2 (m^2) or see Lab Activity 2.1: Your Physical Fitness Profile and Figure 2.6. Health Canada guidelines suggest a BMI < 20 means you are likely underfat/weight; a BMI from 20 to 24.9 means acceptable fat/weight; possibly overfat/weight means a BMI of 25–27; a BMI greater than 27 suggests you might be at considerable risk for health-related problems such as cardiovascular diseases.

How Canadians "Weigh" In

The 1998–99 National Population and Health Survey used adult self-reported heights and weights to calculate BMI. This data was utilized to determine underweight (BMI < 20), acceptable weight (BMI 20–24.9), possibly overweight (BMI 25–27), and overweight (BMI > 27) categories. Findings indicate that 42 percent of Canadians aged 20–64 (excluding pregnant women) were at an acceptable BMI level; 19 percent had some excess fat/weight; and 31 percent were classified as overweight (up slightly from the same survey four years earlier). Of younger adults (20–24), 71 percent had acceptable BMI measures compared with 37 percent of adults aged 55–64. It should be clear by now that the focus ought to be on losing fat, not weight, and that Canadians need to be better informed about the difference. Still, the BMI data show conclusively that adult Canadians as a whole are steadily moving toward higher BMI ranges in the possibly overweight and overweight categories. This could be attributed to several factors, including lifestyle choices and an aging population in general.

There are other methods of estimating percent of body fat. **Electrical impedance** is a quick method. Electrodes are attached to your wrist and ankle. In less than 2 minutes, a printout provides your percentage of body fat, total amount of fat weight, ideal percentage of fat, and ideal body weight. It is necessary to follow certain nutritional and exercise rules for 24 hours before the test. **Hydrostatic weighing** is a fairly accurate method of estimating body fat. In this test, you sit on a scale in a tank of water, exhale as completely as possible, and then are submerged for approximately 10 seconds while your weight is recorded. The proportions of lean body mass and fat mass are determined from calculations that involve weight underwater, weight out of water, and known densities of lean and fatty tissues.

SAFE WEIGHT-LOSS PROCEDURES

Hunger and Appetite

Hunger is generally considered physiological, an inborn instinct, whereas **appetite** is a psychological, or a learned, response. This helps to explain why it is so common to have an appetite and eat when you are not hungry; conversely, some very thin people or those with eating disorders may experience hunger without appetite. Hunger is a passive experience, whereas appetite is active.

Satiety The feeling of fullness or satisfaction that prompts us to stop eating is called **satiety**, one of the key regulators of eating behaviour. Some experts feel that eating behaviour is always in operation except when the satiety signal turns it off. Just how that happens is unknown although a number of theories have been advanced. The **glucostatic theory** of hunger regulation suggests that blood-glucose levels and the exhaustion of liver glycogen may account for the starting and stopping of eating. The liver stores about 75 grams of glycogen, or 300-plus

---

Electrical impedance A quick, fairly accurate means of determining an individual's percentage of body fat that uses electrodes attached to the wrists and ankles to electronically determine the percentage.

Hydrostatic weighing A method of measuring body fat by submerging an individual in water.

Hunger A physiological response of the body involving unpleasant sensations indicating a need for food.

Appetite The desire to eat; pleasant sensations aroused by thoughts of the taste and enjoyment of food.

Satiety A state in which there is no longer a desire to eat.

Glucostatic theory A theory about hunger regulation suggesting that blood-glucose levels determine whether one is hungry or satiated through the exhaustion of liver glycogen.

energy units (calories). When liver glycogen levels fall significantly, feelings of hunger may occur. The **lipostatic theory** suggests that hunger is regulated in some way by the number of fat-storing enzymes on the surfaces of fat cells. The message that the cells send to the brain in this theory has not been identified. The **purinegic theory** is relatively new and untested and proposes that the circulating levels of purines, molecules found in DNA and RNA, govern hunger. Exactly where and how the brain receives these messages is also unknown. The **hypothalamus gland** appears to be important in regulating eating and satiety. Damage to this area can produce eating disorders and severe weight loss or gain.

Satiety appears to be controlled by other factors as well. Hormones secreted by the pancreas when blood-glucose levels rise too high (insulin) or drop too low (glucagon) also affect satiety and the desire to eat. Ingesting too many simple carbohydrates at one time by eating a candy bar, for example, will rapidly elevate blood-sugar levels and produce an insulin response that eventually drops blood glucose below normal levels, a condition sometimes referred to as "bonking." The faster the rate of entry of simple carbohydrates, the greater the release of insulin. Too much insulin is also responsible for driving sugar to the muscles and liver for storage as glycogen, amino acids to muscles, and fat to adipose tissue for storage. Rapid changes in blood-glucose levels produced by the ingesting of large amounts of concentrated sugars may be part of the puzzle that affects both satiety and energy levels. Although not scientifically proven, some experts feel that the ratio of dietary carbohydrates to protein controls the relative levels of insulin to glucagon every time you eat and helps maintain satiety. A sample meal may involve carbohydrate intake that contains no more than twice the calories as the protein consumed. Such a meal may contain 20 percent of calories from protein and no more than 40 percent from complex carbohydrates (fruits, vegetables, grains). Simple carbohydrates are kept to a minimum. This approach does increase the currently recommended daily intake of protein from 12–15 percent of calories to

20 percent and reduces complex carbohydrate intake from 48 percent to 40 percent. Avoiding anything but small amounts of simple carbohydrates in the form of concentrated sugars and increasing protein intake slightly can help prevent extreme fluctuations in blood-glucose levels that commonly occur during the day and help control your appetite by aiding satiety.

Still other hormones, such as endorphins, the body's natural painkillers, and cortisol, may affect satiety. Blood concentrations of digestive hormones such as cholecystokinin (CCK), secretin, gastrin, and others increase and combine with stomach distention to help control hunger.

Eating behaviour appears to occur in response to numerous signals. The possibility also exists that an inherited, internal regulatory defect is at least partially responsible for obesity, rather than its being a purely learned behaviour or genetically caused.

Obviously, there is much to be learned about the causes of obesity. An understanding of the difference between hunger and appetite and the factors suspected of controlling food intake will help you control your body weight and fat.

Controlling Appetite From the limited information available, we know that two basic approaches to controlling appetite are somewhat effective: (1) keeping the stomach full of low-calorie food and drink and (2) raising the body's blood-sugar level. Increasing your fluid intake (particularly your water consumption) and consuming complex carbohydrates such as raw fruits and vegetables both between meals and at mealtimes will keep the stomach relatively full. New raw-grain products are also available that are equally effective. Eating small amounts of candy, such as one or two chocolate squares, 20–30 minutes before a meal, or when you have the urge to snack, is another technique. Slow eaters (those taking 20 minutes or more) also experience this elevated blood-sugar level and are less likely to overeat.

Exactly how to control appetite remains somewhat of a puzzle. Modern researchers continue to examine areas such as appetite centres in the brain, feedback from centres outside the brain such as the liver and intestines, hormone actions, and the ratio of daily dietary protein to carbohydrates to unlock some of the mystery.

■ Drugs and Weight Loss

The search continues for a safe, effective drug, free of undesirable side-effects and potential for abuse, to aid in reducing body fat. Appetite-suppressant drugs (stimulants) such as Dexedrine and Benzedrine reduce appetite only a short time, and most users quickly develop tolerance to the drugs. These drugs also can be addictive and can cause nervousness, dizziness, weakness, fatigue, and insomnia.

Lipostatic theory A theory about hunger control suggesting that the size of fat stores signals us to eat.

Purinegic theory A theory about hunger suggesting that the circulating levels of purines, molecules found in DNA and RNA, govern hunger.

Hypothalamus gland A portion of the brain that regulates body temperature and other functions; thought to be important in the regulation of food intake.

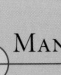

MANAGING YOUR WEIGHT

Managing your weight is not an easy task. To ensure success, you must make a real change in the way you eat and consider it a lifelong commitment rather than a diet. Analyzing where you are right now and then taking the steps outlined below will help you lose excess weight.

Making Decisions for You
The first step in managing your weight is an honest self-assessment of where you are. You don't need sophisticated fat-measurement techniques. What you need is a scale. Your university probably has a gym that has body-content assessment equipment available. Next you need to set a realistic goal. Ask yourself: Why do I want to meet this goal? What will I do when I reach this goal? Then set out a plan to reach your goal. Keep in mind what you enjoy doing. If you like taking walks, you might make walking part of your weight-loss program. If you absolutely love chocolate chip cookies, you might consider limiting yourself to two cookies per day.

Checklist for Change: Making Personal Choices
✓ *Design your plan for your needs.* Your plan must fit your personality, your priorities, and your work and recreation schedules. It should allow for sufficient rest and relaxation.

✓ *Plan for nutrient-dense foods.* Attempt to get the most from the foods you eat by selecting foods with high nutritional value.

✓ *Balance food intake throughout the day.* Although the evidence is inconclusive, research indicates that the body may burn calories more efficiently in small amounts than excessive quantities.

✓ *Plan for plateaus.* If you prepare yourself psychologically for plateaus you will be less likely to become discouraged. Exercise is probably the critical factor in getting past a plateau.

✓ *Chart your progress.* For many people, the daily "weigh-in" is a critical factor in maintaining their program. However, particularly for those who have reached a weight plateau, it may be necessary to think in terms of weekly weigh-ins to avoid frustration.

✓ *Chart your setbacks.* Rather than thinking in terms of failure and punishment, think in terms of temporary setbacks and how to accommodate them. By carefully recording your emotional states when eating, eating habits, environmental cues, and feelings, you may determine why you needed that ice cream cone or why you chose a pizza instead of a salad. Successful weight-loss plans may have to accommodate hormonal fluctuations as an influence on dietary habits.

✓ *Become aware of your feelings of hunger and fullness.* For many of us, eating is time-dependent, and we stop eating only when the food is gone (the "clean your plate" syndrome). Long years of "eating when it is time" instead of eating when it is necessary cost us the ability to tell when we really are hungry and when we really are full. By training yourself to become more aware of the eating process, by learning to recognize true hunger pangs and the first signals that you have eaten enough, you will be able to change your eating patterns.

✓ *Accept yourself.* For many people, this is the most important aspect of successful weight management. Although our culture can certainly oppress fat people, many overweight people are their own worst enemies. It is important to keep your weight in perspective. Unless you feel good about who you are inside, exterior changes will not help you very much.

✓ *Exercise, exercise, exercise.* Different people benefit from different types of activities. Just because your friends are into jogging or jazzercise does not mean that that type of exercise program is best for you. Select an exercise program that you consider fun, not a daily form of punishment for overeating. Variety may be the key here. Planning a program that includes friends and family may also improve your chances of success. It is important to remember that every little effort contributes toward long-term results.

Checklist for Change: Making Community Choices
✓ Identify volunteer organizations that provide physical fitness opportunities for teens.

✓ What opportunities for volunteering at nutrition- or weight-related programs does your campus provide?

Critical Thinking
Until university, your girlfriend Tami had taken ballet very seriously, practising several hours a day. Now that the time pressures of university, a part-time job, and your relationship are starting to get to her, Tami rarely has time to work out on the dance floor. You notice that she has consequently been more and more concerned about her weight. She rarely eats on your dates, but she says that that's because she wants the two of you to save money for a nice trip during spring break. When you find a laxative hidden under her pillow, she says, "Doesn't everyone get constipated now and then?" Then a mutual female friend tells you that she's heard Tami in the bathroom throwing up on several occasions after meals; Tami denies it.

Decide how you can approach Tami with your concern that she has an eating disorder. What help is available in your local area? Should you involve Tami's family? If Tami denies she has an eating disorder, what can you do?

Source: Adapted from Rebecca J. Donatelle, Lorraine G. Davis, Anne J. Munroe, and Alex Munroe, *Health: The Basics*, Canadian ed. (Toronto: Allyn and Bacon Canada, 1998), p. 200. Reprinted by permission of Pearson Canada.

There is still no magic bullet in the form of a pill that will safely and effectively reduce your appetite and control body weight and fat. Prescription medications may aid weight loss when you work with your physician or dietitian and combine medication with diet control, modifying problem behaviours and increasing physical activity.

Calorie Counting

If you are overfat according to the guidelines in this chapter, you may want to consider an exercise and diet regimen to lose body-fat weight. When you set goals for body-fat loss, you can expect to lose about 0.5 millimetres of body fat per week with an appropriate combination of diet and exercise. For example, if you are now classified as above-average fat, it is realistic to expect to reach the average-fat category after a ten-week program.

As a first step in losing body fat, turn to Lab Activity 9.2: Determining Your Caloric Needs at the end of the chapter to determine how many calories you need to maintain your present weight. These figures will help you decide how much to increase your daily energy expenditure and reduce your daily caloric intake to meet your weight- and fat-loss goals. You can then reduce your caloric intake and increase your exercise expenditure to produce slow, safe weight and fat loss.

How Exercise Helps

A pleasing side-effect that often accompanies weight losses of over 4–5 kilograms is enhanced self-concept and increased energy levels. Remember that the weight you choose as a target is one that, once reached, must be maintained for the rest of your life. It is not just weight loss per se, but the acceptance of a healthy lifestyle, that is most likely to keep your *thin self* going in the future. Regular vigorous exercise is an essential part of this healthy, holistic lifestyle.

If you expect to lose body fat and weight and then maintain this lower level, you need both to restrict your caloric intake and to engage in regular exercise. By remaining physically active, you will be able to consume more calories daily. The alternative is to remain mildly hungry most of your life. There are many other reasons both diet and exercise should be included in a weight-loss or weight-management program.

Exercise Depresses Appetite The amount of body weight and fat lost during an exercise program is greater than what can be attributed to the number of calories expended. This suggests that exercise acts on the body to further increase energy expenditure through changes in metabolism or to decrease energy intake through changes in appetite. It is also a well-established principle that physical activity decreases appetite. Physical inactivity and high body fat and decreases in appetite and regular aerobic exercise are all strongly associated. The food intake of elementary-school-age children has also been shown to decrease when the recess period is scheduled before, rather than after, lunch.

Exercise Maximizes Fat Loss and Minimizes Loss of Lean Muscle Tissue There is a critical difference between weight loss in terms of kilograms and fat loss in terms of adipose tissue. A reducing diet without exercise can result in about 70–80 percent fatty-tissue loss and 20–30 percent lean muscle loss. With the combination of exercise and diet, fatty-tissue loss can be increased to 95 percent and lean muscle loss kept to 5 percent or less of total weight loss.

Exercise Burns a High Number of Calories and Increases Metabolic Rate Exercise burns calories both during an exercise session and for 20 minutes to several hours after exercise ceases (afterburn). A 4.8-kilometre run or walk will expend 250–300 calories depending on the individual. For the next 20 minutes (for the walker) to several hours (for the jogger or runner), an additional 25–40 calories per hour will be burned due to an increase in metabolic rate. The total caloric benefit of a 4.8-kilometre run, then, may be as high as 500 calories. Four to five such workouts weekly would produce a body-weight/fat loss of about 1.4 kilograms per month, or 16.8 kilograms per year.

Strength-training programs involving weights add muscle mass and increase metabolism permanently. Keep in mind that fat is a dormant tissue and requires very few calories to maintain. Muscle tissue, on the other hand, requires considerable calories to maintain. It is estimated that for every 454 grams of muscle you add, metabolic rate increases 30–40 calories per 24-hour period. If you add 2.3 kilograms of muscle over a 6-month period, your metabolic rate may increase as much as 200 calories daily. This translates into about 6000 calories monthly and nearly 907 grams of fat (3500 kcal = 454 g of fat). This is obviously a very significant change.

The best system for controlling body fat is changing your eating habits and beginning an exercise program you enjoy and are likely to continue throughout life. If you change your behaviour in these two areas, you will go through life at your ideal body weight and fat. Body weight is carefully regulated by complex forces, but the formula for fat loss is simple. If you eat more calories than you burn through activity, a positive caloric balance exists and produces fat gain. If you burn up more calories than you eat, a negative caloric balance exists and fat loss will occur.

Walking, bicycling, swimming, dancing, jogging, and other aerobic activities are all effective means of exercise for weight loss. Some types of physical activity and sports are relaxing and enjoyable. Other activities are superior in terms of weight loss and aerobic benefits.

When you choose a particular exercise program, consider that:

- You are more likely to continue exercising in activities you enjoy.

- Activities that expend a moderately high number of calories per minute and allow you to continue exercise for 30–90 minutes are the best choices.

- Lifelong physical–recreational sports that provide heart–lung benefits are superior.

- The choice you make should allow you to start at your present fitness level and progress to higher levels later.

Exercise Brings Needed Calcium to the Bones As a result of normal aging and weight loss, bones lose calcium and other minerals and become brittle. You need adequate calcium in your diet (see Chapter 8) plus weight-bearing exercise (walking, jogging, running, aerobic dance) to increase the amount of calcium that reaches the bones and thereby helps prevent osteoporosis.

Exercise Changes the Way Your Body Handles Fats Exercise helps lower and maintain serum cholesterol (LDL) and triglycerides. HDL (high-density lipoprotein, the good cholesterol) increases, and the ratio of HDL to total cholesterol improves. High HDL counts and a high ratio of HDL to total cholesterol (1 to 4 or higher) have been associated with a lower incidence of heart attacks.

SPECIAL DIETS

There are many reasons the average diet lasts only 5–7 days: boredom, monotony, lack of energy, fatigue, depression, complicated or expensive meal planning and purchasing, and failure to lose weight and fat fast enough. These problems are less likely to occur with individuals on a sound, balanced diet based on *Canada's Food Guide*. Unfortunately, too many people choose diet magazines, books, or ads that promise some *secret,* easy method of shedding pounds and fat. These and practically all other diets simply do not work, are dangerous, and should be avoided. Safe, effective, and long-term management of body weight and fat involves a lifelong plan of proper nutrition and regular exercise. Quick weight-loss approaches provide only a temporary fix, with over 90 percent of those who try any of them regaining the lost weight within 6–12 months. In the meantime, the body may have been exposed to many health hazards.

Before you initiate any type of diet, complete Lab Activity 9.3: 10-Point Weight-Loss Program for a Sound, Safe Reducing Diet at the end of this chapter. If your approach does not adhere to the ten-point guidelines in the Lab, the diet is not safe and could have serious health consequences.

Snacking

Between-meal and late-evening snacking is a leading cause of overfatness. It is not uncommon to consume over 1000 calories between eight o'clock and midnight, or about 150 grams of fat. Yet it is unrealistic to expect people to avoid snacking altogether. In fact, planned snacking on the right foods can help you control hunger and eat less. Snacks likely to be low in calories are those that are thin and watery (tomato juice), crisp but not greasy (celery, carrots, radishes, cucumbers, broccoli, cauliflower, apples, berries, other fresh fruits and vegetables, and raw grains), and bulky (salad greens). Prepare a tray of these nutritious, low-calorie snacks and place it in the front of your refrigerator. Most snackers are compulsive and consume the first thing they see.

Characteristics of the Ideal Diet Plan

It is estimated that less than 5 percent of dieters who lose five or more kilograms are able to keep the weight off for a period of 12 months or more. Evidence clearly indicates that dieting does not work and does not produce lasting weight and fat loss. In addition, the type of dieting the majority of individuals resort to is not only dangerous but sometimes fatal. Unfortunately, the majority of people who are unhappy with their weight chase the same five kilograms of body fat throughout life. A mere five kilograms is responsible for the unhappiness of millions of individuals and inspires unsound, unsafe practices. For many of these individuals who are only slightly overfat, learning to accept their bodies would help them avoid considerable hardship and heartbreak.

The following ten-point program represents nothing more than sound nutrition and exercise advice, and it should be followed throughout life, including the period when you are involved in some type of diet:

1. Consume a minimum of 1200 calories daily.

2. Drink a minimum of 10 glasses of water daily when you diet.

3. Eat sufficient protein daily. Consult the recommended nutrient intake (RNI) table in Chapter 8 to determine your exact needs.

4. Eat at least 50–100 grams (200–400 kcal) of carbohydrates and 10 grams of fat (90 kcal) daily to spare protein. Unless your carbohydrate and fat intake is sufficient to meet your daily needs, some dietary protein and lean protein mass (muscle) will be converted to glucose to nourish the nervous system. Failing to spare protein for months at a time is not recommended. Fat is also very important for satiety.

5. Never skip a meal, even if you are not hungry. Choose a variety of foods (see Chapter 8).

6. Gear your program to a weight loss of 454–907 grams weekly and stay with it until you reach your goal.

7. Premeasure each food portion, keep records of your food and drink intake, identify problem areas, and take steps to change.

8. Avoid laxatives, stimulants, and diuretics, and use a multiple vitamin and mineral supplement daily.

9. Combine dieting with exercise in an activity or aerobic program you enjoy; exercise a minimum of three times weekly, for at least 30 minutes each time.

10. Plan to stay with your new eating and exercise routine for a minimum of 12 months.

In short, a lifetime plan for proper eating, regular exercise, and acceptance of your basic body type offers you the best chance of success, safety, and happiness.

UNDERWEIGHT CONDITIONS AND EATING DISORDERS

The problems of gaining weight are just as complex as those associated with weight loss. Hunger, appetite, and satiety irregularities, psychological factors, and metabolic problems can all cause dangerous underweight. For individuals who need additional weight and muscle for sports or who merely want to be and appear stronger, gaining a kilogram is just as difficult as losing a kilogram is for others.

◾ Gaining Weight

A drug-free muscle-weight-gain program requires considerable dedication to both diet and exercise. With a sound approach, individuals strive to add no more than 227 grams of muscle per week. This is about as quickly as the body can add lean muscle tissue. Faster approaches involving too many calories are almost certain to add adipose tissue.

A sound strength-training program, such as weight training, is an absolute must for muscle-weight gain (see Chapter 6). It may be necessary to train for several hours six times weekly, alternating muscle groups each workout.

The nutritional support for a sound weight-gain program involves an increase in food (about 400–500 additional calories daily) that provides high calories in as small volume as possible to keep you from getting uncomfortably full, a slight increase in total protein intake (14–15 percent of daily calories), and a slight reduction in total fat intake (18–20 percent of daily calories). Extra calories should come from complex carbohydrates (65–70 percent of daily calories) to provide long-term energy and for **protein sparing**. Using protein or amino acid tablets is hazardous and a waste of money. In the majority of cases, individuals consume more protein than they need already; adding more in the form of supplements is unnecessary.

◾ Eating Disorders

The current overemphasis on flat stomachs, lean thighs, firm buttocks, and slimness is at least partially responsible for aggravating two serious eating disorders that can lead to death: **anorexia nervosa** and **bulimia**. Both disorders are known only in developed nations and are most common in higher economic groups. The National Eating Disorders Information Centre estimates that in Canada 200 000 to 300 000 women aged 13-40 have anorexia nervosa and twice as many have bulimia (50 percent of anorexic women are also bulimic). These illnesses are fatal for 10–15 percent of those affected. Men are also afflicted by eating disorders, although research has mainly focused on females. According to the National Eating Disorders Information Centre, about one in every 10 people with an eating disorder is male.

Anorexia Nervosa The number of cases of anorexia nervosa is increasing and now occurs in nearly 1 in every 100 women, 19 in 20 of whom are young women. The disease is four to five times more common in identical than in fraternal twins, suggesting an inherited predisposition to the disease. Unfortunately, our culture encourages anorexia nervosa.

A typical case involves a young woman from a middle-class family who values appearance more than self-worth and self-actualization. Typically, family ties are strong and the young woman is efficient, eager to please her parents, and somewhat of a perfectionist. An absentee or distant father is also common. The characteristic behaviour of anorexia is obsessive and compulsive, resembling addiction. Anorexics may become obsessed with the idea that they are, or will become, fat. They may fear the transition from girlhood to womanhood resulting

WELLNESS HEROES

Mari Lisle

Mari Lisle had everything going for her as a young high school student living in Wingham, Ontario. An excellent student with top grades, Mari competed in track and field, basketball, and volleyball. By the end of Grade 9, she had won three Ontario Federation of Secondary School Association (OFSSA) gold medals in track and field events. By age 16, her self-perceived mounting pressure to excel became extreme. Her older sister was a national pole vaulting champion and that fact alone overwhelmed Mari and pressured her to be the best in everything. Somehow, her life had become a continuous cycle of long hours of training and schoolwork every day of the week. Gradually, she withdrew from her friends.

By the fall of her Grade 11 year, her training and competition regime became a fixation, along with subtle dietary changes. In the latter regard, she began to eat only minimal amounts of food. Within three months of that year, she dropped to 45.4 kilograms, an 18-kilogram loss from her muscular frame. Her mother, who had experienced anorexia in her teens, was the first to remark on Mari's weight loss and obsessive behaviours.

Mari denied everything, but in mid-January she was so weak that, extremely concerned, her parents took her to Toronto's Hospital for Sick Children. She was hypothermic and experiencing great fluctuations in blood pressure readings with even the smallest exertion.

Treatment was simple—"re-feeding" with Ensure for 7½ weeks. By spring, she was back home, and even won two more OFSSA medals, but the cycle of Mari's relentless quest for perfection started again and she was readmitted to the hospital.

By now, Mari knew she was depressed and so did the doctors, so Prozac was administered. This made her very sick. Her condition deteriorated to the point that in late October of her Grade 12 year, she took 66 Tylenol pills in an effort to kill herself. Her mother found her and rushed her to Wingham Hospital, where she felt such depression that she left on foot determined to walk until she dropped.

Fortunately, Mari was found and later taken to Homewood Centre in Guelph and admitted to its Eating Disorders Unit. There, Mari at last got the care she needed. Instead of merely focusing on anorexia as a disease, Homewood treated her as a whole person, providing training in self-esteem, leisure and body awareness activities, and so forth.

At the end of her first year of university, Mari was taking Effexor, an antidepressant, together with a mild medication to help her sleep. She made the intercollegiate track team and felt much more self-aware and self-accepting. Anorexia, Mari felt, had control of her; now, she feels in control of it. Mari Lisle will enter medical school in the fall of 2003.

Her own view and experience is that anorexia is not brought on by culture's deification of female thinness; rather, it is a coping mechanism for deeper issues—such as the quest for perfection. Mari's story and message need to be heeded: learn to love yourself for who you are; accept yourself and appreciate the wonder of your body and your life. ✦

Source: Personal interview with Mari Lisle.

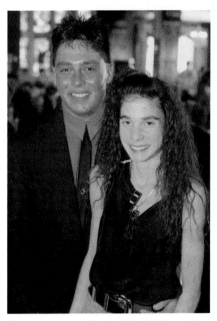

Former gymnast Christy Heinrich lost a long battle with eating disorders in 1994.

Protein sparing Consuming sufficient amounts of dietary carbohydrates and fat on a daily basis to prevent the conversion of dietary and lean muscle protein to glucose.

Anorexia nervosa An eating disorder that involves lack or loss of appetite to the point of self-starvation and dangerous weight loss.

Bulimia An eating disorder found most often in women involving some method of purging, and eating binges followed by self-induced vomiting or the use of laxatives to expel the unwanted food.

MYTH AND FACT SHEET

Myth	Fact
1. Overweight and obese people are always big eaters.	1. In both children and adults, studies show that the major cause of heaviness is inactivity followed by overeating. The major problem for the majority of overfat people is inactivity. A regular exercise program is still the best health insurance policy and the best approach to weight and fat loss.
2. The major part of excess weight and fat is water.	2. This is not true. Do not restrict your water intake in any way. Water is essential to the proper function of every body system. Fluid retention is common while dieting because water remains in the spaces freed by the disappearance of fat. This fluid generally remains for 2–3 weeks and often obscures actual weight loss. Drink water freely at all times, particularly when you are restricting your calories. The majority (about 80 percent) of excess weight is fat, not water.
3. There's nothing wrong with resorting to quick weight-loss diets.	3. You should lose weight at the rate of no more than 0.5–1 kilogram weekly. Very-low-calorie diets that produce rapid weight loss have a number of pitfalls: (1) they are dangerous and possibly life-threatening; (2) rapid weight loss is usually followed by rapid weight gain; (3) your percentage of body fat increases each time you lose and reacquire the weight; and (4) sufficient carbohydrates are often not consumed to spare protein resulting in lean-tissue loss even from the heart muscle itself. Sufficient cardiac tissue loss to the heart might cause serious rhythm problems.
4. Cellulite can be eliminated with special foods and exercise.	4. From a medical point of view, there is no such thing as cellulite as a particular form of fat. Fat is merely fat although the size and appearance of fat cells vary in different body parts and in different people. The lumpy, dimplelike deposits called cellulite tend to be most visible in women and often appear on the thighs, back of legs, and buttocks. These deposits are merely large fat cells that show through the somewhat thinner skin of women. Thicker-skinned males tend not to develop this appearance unless they become extremely fat. Prevention is easier than treatment and focuses on getting proper nutrition, maintaining normal weight and fat, and avoiding rapid-weight-loss attempts or yo-yo dieting.
5. It is better to remain fat than to lose weight and end up with wrinkled skin.	5. You are partially correct. It is better to stay somewhat fat than to lose and then regain body weight rapidly. If you lose weight and fat slowly through a combination of diet and exercise and lose only 5–7 kilograms, skin wrinkling is unlikely. It is also helpful to include weight training as part of your exercise routine. As your fat cells shrink, the added muscle mass will help your skin fit you better in some areas, such as the back of the arm. If you have more than 7 kilograms to lose, work with your physician on a 6-to-12-month program.
6. In the near future, everyone may be able to eat as much as they want of any type of food and never get fat.	6. The magic bullet is still a long way off and may never be found. Artificial fats, foods that taste good with only a small portion of the calories digested, so-called fat pills to increase energy expenditure or improve satiety, and a host of other approaches are being tested. All of these approaches are certain to have their limitations and even hazards. The best advice is still moderation, variation, and balance coupled with regular aerobic and strength-training exercise programs.

Myth	Fact
7. Sit-ups will remove fat from the stomach.	7. It requires reduced calories, regular exercise, and abdominal exercises to flatten your stomach. With calorie restriction, the fat cells in the stomach will shrink, and your stomach will get smaller. Your sit-up routine (see Chapter 6) will strengthen the underlying muscle tissue. Both adipose and muscle tissue need changing; you cannot convert fat tissue to muscle tissue, nor will muscle tissue change to fat when you become sedentary.
8. Laxatives help you lose weight.	8. The use of laxatives causes gastrointestinal trouble and can result in dehydration and undernourishment. It is better to be fat than to endanger your health. It is impossible to defecate away unwanted pounds safely.
9. Weight-reducing pills are a safe approach to depressing the appetite.	9. The use of drugs and drug combinations to depress appetite is dangerous and sometimes fatal. Drug usage is an attempt to cause weight loss by increasing metabolic rate, curbing the appetite, or causing fluid loss. Amphetamines and diuretics are the two most commonly used diet pills. Amphetamines toy with the thyroid gland, cause nervousness, speed up metabolism, and require increasingly stronger dosages as tolerance develops; diuretics result in rapid fluid loss. Both are dangerous, ineffective approaches to weight loss.
10. Reducing aids such as vibrators, body wraps, rubber suits, steam baths, and massages effectively remove fat from the body.	10. Each of these popular gimmick approaches to weight loss results in little calorie burning and is totally ineffective. To lose weight and fat, you must engage in exercise that burns a high number of calories, such as aerobics. You then achieve a negative caloric balance and lose weight and fat.

in a more curvaceous figure and become determined to stave it off by controlling their weight. This starvation approach is then carried to the extreme of undernourishment until total body weight is dangerously low. Even at that extreme, anorexics may still feel fat and continue to starve themselves, sometimes literally to death.

Young female anorexics generally develop **amenorrhea**. Females must reacquire 17–22 percent body fat before the menstrual cycle resumes. Thyroid hormone secretions, adrenal secretions, growth hormones, and blood-pressure-regulating hormones reach abnormal levels. The heart pumps less efficiently as cardiac muscle weakens, the chambers diminish in size, and blood pressure falls. Heart-rhythm disturbances and sudden stopping of the heart may occur due to lean-tissue loss and mineral deficiencies, producing sudden death in some patients. Other health problems include anemia, gastrointestinal problems, atrophy of the digestive tract, abnormal function of the pancreas, blood-lipid changes, dry skin, decreased core temperature, and disturbed sleep.

Early treatment is essential if permanent damage is to be avoided. Without treatment, about 10 percent of anorexics die of starvation. Forced feeding may temporarily improve health, but the condition can reappear unless proper psychological and medical therapy is initiated. Treatment is directed at restoring adequate nutrition, avoiding medical complications, and altering the psychological and environmental patterns that have supported or permitted the emergence of anorexia. About 5 percent of those in treatment eventually reach 25 percent of their desired weight, and 50–75 percent resume normal menstrual cycles. After treatment ends, about 66 percent fail to eat normally and 7 percent die. Thus, it seems that treatment that is merely diet/nutrition- or symptom-focused is only partially effective. More successful interventions—such as those provided to Wellness Hero Mari Lisle through Guelph's Homewood Centre—are ones that are more behaviour-oriented toward issues of self-esteem and body image. The National Eating Disorders Information Centre (NEDIC) a Toronto-based organization, was established in 1985 to

Amenorrhea Loss of at least three consecutive menstrual cycles when they are expected to occur.

VITALITY—FEELING GOOD ABOUT YOURSELF

VITALITY represents a shift in thinking about weight and its relationship to healthy living. There is nothing inherently wrong with pursuing a healthy body; but, after decades of the media's and the fashion, food, and fitness industries' glorification of unrealistic body images, many Canadians overidentify their body weight and size with attractiveness, success, happiness, and good health. The rigid pursuit of a standard size and shape inevitably fails for most people long-term. One- to two-thirds of lost weight is usually regained within a year, and almost all is regained within five years.

It was with these factors in mind that Health Canada initiated the VITALITY program—an integrated approach to healthy living that shifts the focus from rigid ideals, dieting, and prescriptive exercise toward an acceptance of a variety of body sizes and shapes and an emphasis on healthy eating, active living, and positive self- and body-image. Consider the differences between a "weight-centred" approach and the VITALITY approach:

Weight-Centred Approach	VITALITY Approach
Dieting	**Healthy Eating**
• Restrictive eating	• Take pleasure in eating a variety of foods
• Counting calories	• Enjoy lower-fat and complex carbohydrate foods more often
• Weight cycling (yo-yo diets)	
• Eating disorders	• Meet the body's energy and nutrient needs through a lifetime of healthy, enjoyable eating
	• Take control of how you eat by listening to your hunger cues
Exercise	
• "No pain, no gain"	**Active Living**
• Prescriptions such as three times per week within target heart rate zone	• Value and practise activities that are moderate in intensity and fun
• Burn calories	• Be active your way, every day
• High attrition rates for vigorous exercise programs	• Participate for the sheer joy of feeling your body move
	• Enjoy physical activity as part of your daily lifestyle
Dissatisfaction with Self	
• Unrealistic goals for body size and shape	**Positive Self and Body Image**
• Obsession and preoccupation with weight	• Accept and recognize that healthy bodies come in a range of weights, shapes, and sizes
• Fat phobia and discrimination against overweight people	• Appreciate your strengths and abilities
• Striving to be a "perfect 10" and to maintain an impossible "ideal" (thin or muscular) body size	• Be tolerant of a wide range of body sizes
• Accepting the fashion, diet, and tobacco industries' emphasis on slimness	• Relax and enjoy your unique characteristics
	• Be critical of messages that focus on unrealistic thinness (in women) and muscularity (in men) as symbols of success and happiness

Benefits of the VITALITY Approach

In its move away from dieting, prescriptive exercise, and body dissatisfaction, VITALITY offers a new approach that focuses on the integration of healthy eating, active living, and positive self- and body-image. The slogan

"Enjoy eating well, being active and feeling good about yourself—that's VITALITY" is designed to promote the spirit and meaning of this approach. The "eating well" component emphasizes a lifetime eating pattern based on *Canada's Food Guide to Healthy Eating*. Healthy eating conveys a sense of well-being and the opportunity to feel, look, and perform better. Former reduction-dieters can take control of their eating behaviour by learning to eat according to internal hunger cues and thereby decrease overeating and bingeing. The focus here is on meeting the body's energy and nutrient needs by enjoying healthy eating.

The "being active" component reflects the shift to active living, a way of life that values physical activity and makes it part of daily living. Active living is based on a sound, scientific rationale in which studies have shown that moderate, everyday activities such as walking, dancing, and yard work are important for health and longevity in the general population. Moreover, sustained, moderate energy expenditure is more effective than bouts of high-intensity exercise in managing body weight. Finally, VITALITY's "feeling good about yourself" message draws attention away from society's preoccupation with weight and negative body image. Self-respect and acceptance of others are shown as the ways to enhance enjoyment and family life rather than ends in themselves.

"The Vitality Approach—A Guide for Leaders" with explanatory materials and practical tools, together with materials with ideas on how you can use the concept at work, are available through the Health Canada Web site. See **www.hc-sc.gc.ca/hpfb-dgpsa/onpp-bppn/leaders_approach_e.html** ✦

Source: Adapted from *VITALITY: A Positive Approach to Healthy Living,* Health Canada Office of Nutrition Policy and Promotion Information, 2003. Available at **http://www.hc-sc.gc.ca/hpfb-dgpsa/onpp-ppn/leaders_approach_e.html**. Accessed March 14, 2003. Adapted and reproduced with the permission of the Minister of Public Works and Government Services. *Health Canada assumes no responsibility for any errors which may have occurred in the adaptation of its material.*

provide information and resources on eating disorders and weight preoccupation. Its very first premise is that reducing diets and diet fads are extremely harmful; one of its slogans is, "Scales are for fish, not people." Instead, the NEDIC holistic philosophy promotes healthy lifestyles and encourages clients to make informed choices based on accurate information.

Bulimia Bulimia is two times more common than anorexia nervosa and occurs in males as well as females. The typical profile of victims is similar to that of those suffering from anorexia nervosa, although bulimics tend to be slightly older and healthier, malnourished but closer to normal weight. The bulimic binge is generally not a response to hunger, and the food is not consumed for nutritional value. As the binge–purge cycle is repeated,

medical problems grow. Fluid and electrolyte imbalances may lead to abnormal heart rhythm and kidney damage. Infections of the bladder and kidneys may cause kidney failure. Vomiting results in irritation and infection of the pharynx, esophagus, and salivary glands, erosion of the teeth, and dental caries. In some cases, the esophagus or the stomach may rupture.

Bulimics are more cooperative and somewhat easier to treat than anorexic patients because they seem to recognize that the behaviour is abnormal. Most treatment programs attempt to help people gain control over their binge eating and encourage a minimum of 1500 calories daily. Lithium and other drugs have been shown to reduce the incidence of bulimic episodes by 75–100 percent. Most bulimics can also be helped by antidepressant medication.

SUMMARY

◼ Causes of Obesity

Overfatness and obesity are caused by a number of factors, with both genetics and environment playing key roles. Although it is a disadvantage to inherit the tendency to become fat, environment can overcome this

predisposition. Inactivity and overeating are still the two major behaviours associated with weight and fat gain.

The body appears to defend its biological weight, referred to as *set point*, by resisting attempts to lose weight. Lowering the set point requires regular aerobic exercise and reduced caloric intake for 6–12 months or until it is evident that the body is now defending the lower weight and fat levels.

Overeating in infancy, bottle-feeding instead of breast-feeding, and early consumption of solid foods prior to the age of five months may contribute to the development of excess fat cells and overeating later in life.

Fat cells increase in number only until growth ceases, at which time one becomes fat only through the enlargement of existing adipose cells. Adults who become obese may develop some new fat cells.

Small changes in metabolism result in large increases or decreases in weight over a period of 6–12 months. Only a small percentage of individuals with weight problems suffer from an underactive thyroid gland.

Body Composition

There are a number of ways to determine ideal body weight and percentage of body fat. Height–weight tables should only be used as a guide to ideal weight because they provide no indication of percentage of body fat, the key factor in determining health risks.

By measuring the thickness of two layers of skin and the underlying fat, you can secure an estimate of total body fat and identify ideal body weight. A number of different skinfold sites can be used. Electrical impedance and underwater weighing are more accurate techniques; however, special equipment is needed.

Safe Weight-Loss Procedures

Hunger is a physiological, inborn instinct designed to control food intake, whereas appetite is a psychological, learned response. Although numerous theories have been advanced to explain how food intake is controlled, the exact signals that cue us to consume food have not been positively identified.

Calories count, and the body handles the matter with computerlike precision, storing 500 grams of fat for every 3850 excess calories consumed.

Exercise is essential to the control of body weight and fat. Regular aerobic exercise depresses appetite, maximizes fat loss, minimizes the loss of lean muscle tissue, burns a high number of calories, brings needed calcium to the bones, and changes the way the body handles dietary fat.

Numerous new drugs to curb appetite, increase metabolic rate and exercise metabolism, deaden taste buds, and increase the burning of fat as energy are being tested and evaluated. The search for the magic pill that will help everyone attain ideal weight and body fat continues. Even if such a pill is developed, it will still be used in combination with a lifetime of sound nutrition and fitness practices.

Special Diets

The majority of special reducing diets fail, in many cases, within 5–7 days. Approximately 90 percent of those who succeed in losing weight will regain the weight within one year.

Reduction dieting is extremely dangerous and can prove fatal if certain nutritional guidelines are not followed. The best approach is to develop sound exercise and eating habits that can be followed throughout life and to avoid specialized reduction diets.

Underweight Conditions and Eating Disorders

Weight gain can be just as difficult as weight loss. A complete program of muscle-weight gain requires sound nutritional support and an organized weight-training program that involves up to six 2-hour workouts weekly.

The number of cases of anorexia nervosa and bulimia continue to increase in Canada. As long as society places such high value on slimness, this trend will continue. Both disorders are extremely difficult to treat and can produce numerous health consequences and even death.

STUDY QUESTIONS

1. What is the difference between losing weight and losing fat? Provide examples of each.

2. Discuss the ways most people become overfat.

3. How would you go about losing fat? How would you know how much fat to lose? How would you modify your behaviours in this process?

4. What are the best commercial diets?

5. One of your parents is sedentary, eats large meals, and feels that it is important to lose weight. What advice and assistance could you provide to help your parent?

6. What are the causes of eating disorders? What are the best ways to remedy these disorders?

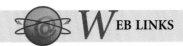

WEB LINKS

Body Composition
www.sport-fitness-advisor.com/bodycomposition.html

Methods of Determining Body Composition
www.gsu.edu/~wwwfit/bodycomp.html

Health Promotion On-line
www.hc-sc.gc.ca/

Calorie Counter Chart
www.caloriechart.org/

Canadian Fitness and Lifestyle Research Institute
www.cflri.ca

National Eating Disorders Information Centre
www.nedic.ca

REFERENCES

Anderson, R. "Obesity in Canadian Children." *Canadian Medical Association Journal* #164, 11 (2001): 1563–64.

Canadian Institute for Health Information data (unpublished).

Health Canada Web site facts and information (see Web links).

National Eating Disorder Information Centre Web site 2003. "Where Do Men and Boys Fit In." Available at **www.nedic.ca/qa.html**.

National Population and Health Survey, 2001 (unpublished and in rough draft).

Statistics Canada. *Health Reports*, vol 12, no. 30, 2001.

Name _____

Date _____

Lab Activity 9.1

Determining Your Percentage of Body Fat

INSTRUCTIONS: *One way to determine your percentage of body fat is to measure the thickness of several skinfolds. The procedure for measuring skinfold thickness is to grasp a fold of skin and subcutaneous (just under the skin) fat firmly with the thumb and forefinger, pulling it away and up from the underlying muscle tissue. Attach the jaws of the calipers 1 centimetre below the thumb and forefinger. All measurements should be taken on the right side of the body with the subject standing.*

Working with a partner, practise taking each other's measurements in the five areas described below:

For women, measure the triceps, suprailium, and thigh skinfold sites. For men, measure the chest, abdomen, and thigh sites.

Chest—Take a diagonal fold halfway between the nipple and the anterior axillary line (shoulder crease).
Abdomen—Take a vertical fold at a distance of 1 cm to the right of the umbilicus (navel).
Thigh—With the subject's weight resting on the left leg, take a vertical fold on the anterior midline of the right thigh, midway between the patella (kneecap) and inguinal crease of the hip.
Triceps—With the arm resting comfortably at the side, take a vertical fold parallel to the long axis of the arm midway between the tip of the shoulder and the tip of the elbow.
Suprailium—Just above the hip bone, take a diagonal fold following the natural line of the iliac crest.

Record the information below to complete your evaluation (for example, John is a 20-year-old who weighs 83.9 kilograms. His three skinfold measurements were 20, 37, and 33; follow his evaluation to help you understand the procedure):

1. Total of the three skinfold measures in millimetres
    (20, 37, 33 = 90 mm).   _____

2. Percentage of body fat based on this total from Table B on page 221.
    Moving down in the first vertical column to 90 and over to the <22 age
    group for males in column 2, we find that John has about 24.7 percent fat. _____

3. According to the percentage of body fat from Table C on page 222,
    John's ideal fat percentage is 14.9 percent or less.   _____

4. Percentage of fat to lose to reach the ideal percent from Table C on
    page 222. John has about 10 percent too much fat (24.7 – 14.9 = 10)
    and therefore needs to lose 10 percent of his body weight.   _____

5. Total fat loss needed to reach ideal weight
    (10% × 83.9 = 8.4 kg of fat).   _____

6. Ideal weight with 14.9 percent fat (high end of recommended ideal
    body fat for university-aged men) is 75.5 kg (83.9 – 8.4 = 75.5).   _____

Source: Definitions for chest, abdomen, and thigh skinfold measurements from "Common Skinfold Sites,"
Health/Fitness Assessment Tutorial: Body Composition, University of Massachusetts Web site information.
Available at **http://omega.cc.umb.edu/~umexcsci/index.html**. Accessed March 13, 2003.

(continued)

219

Lab Activity 9.1 *(continued)*
Determining Your Percentage of Body Fat

Table A ✦ Percent Fat Estimate for Women: Sum of Triceps, Suprailium and Thigh Skinfolds

SUM OF SKINFOLDS (mm)	AGE TO THE LAST YEAR								
	<22	23-27	28-32	33-37	38-42	43-47	48-52	53-57	>57
23-25	9.7	9.9	10.2	10.4	10.7	10.9	11.2	11.4	11.7
26-28	11.0	11.2	11.5	11.7	12.0	12.3	12.5	12.7	13.0
29-31	12.3	12.5	12.8	13.0	13.3	13.5	13.8	14.0	14.3
32-34	13.6	13.8	14.0	14.3	14.5	14.8	15.0	15.3	15.5
35-37	14.8	15.0	15.3	15.5	15.8	16.0	16.3	16.5	16.8
38-40	16.0	16.3	16.5	16.7	17.0	17.2	17.5	17.7	18.0
41-43	17.2	17.4	17.7	17.9	18.2	18.4	18.7	18.9	19.2
44-46	18.3	18.6	18.8	19.1	19.3	19.6	19.8	20.1	20.3
47-49	19.5	19.7	20.0	20.2	20.5	20.7	21.0	21.2	21.5
50-52	20.6	20.8	21.2	21.3	21.6	21.8	22.1	22.3	22.6
53-55	21.7	21.9	22.1	22.4	22.6	22.9	23.1	23.4	23.6
56-58	22.7	23.0	23.2	23.4	23.7	23.9	24.2	24.4	24.7
59-61	23.7	24.0	24.2	24.5	24.7	25.0	25.2	25.5	25.7
62-64	24.7	25.0	25.2	25.5	25.7	26.0	26.7	26.4	26.7
65-67	25.7	25.9	26.2	26.4	26.7	26.9	27.2	27.4	27.7
68-70	26.6	26.9	27.1	27.4	27.6	27.9	28.1	28.4	28.6
71-73	27.5	27.8	28.0	28.3	28.5	28.8	29.0	29.3	29.5
74-76	28.4	28.7	28.9	29.2	29.4	29.7	29.9	30.2	30.4
77-79	29.3	29.5	29.8	30.3	30.3	30.5	30.8	31.0	31.3
80-82	30.1	30.4	30.6	30.9	31.1	31.4	31.6	31.9	32.1
83-85	30.9	31.2	31.4	31.7	31.9	32.2	32.4	32.7	32.9
86-88	31.7	32.0	32.2	32.5	32.7	32.9	33.2	33.4	33.7
89-91	32.5	32.7	33.0	33.2	33.5	33.7	33.9	34.2	34.4
92-94	33.2	33.4	33.7	33.9	34.2	34.4	34.7	34.9	35.2
95-97	33.9	34.1	34.4	34.6	34.9	35.1	35.4	35.6	35.9
98-100	34.6	34.8	35.1	35.3	35.5	35.8	36.0	36.3	36.5
101-103	35.3	35.4	35.7	35.9	36.2	36.4	36.7	36.9	37.2
104-106	35.8	36.1	36.3	36.6	36.8	37.1	37.3	37.5	37.8
107-109	36.4	36.7	36.9	37.1	37.4	37.6	37.9	38.1	38.4
110-112	37.0	37.2	37.5	37.7	38.0	38.2	38.5	38.7	38.9
113-115	37.5	37.8	38.0	38.2	38.5	38.7	39.0	39.2	39.5
116-118	38.0	38.3	38.5	38.8	39.0	39.3	39.5	39.7	40.0
119-121	38.5	38.7	39.0	39.2	39.5	39.7	40.0	40.2	40.5
122-124	39.0	39.2	39.4	39.7	39.9	40.2	40.4	40.7	40.9
125-127	39.4	39.6	39.9	40.1	40.4	40.6	40.9	41.1	41.4
128-130	39.8	40.0	40.3	40.5	40.8	41.0	41.3	41.5	41.8

Source: Tables 5 & 6, pp. 85-86 reproduced, with permission, from Jackson, A.S., and Pollock, M.L.; "Practical Assessment of Body Composition." *The Physician and Sportsmedicine* 13, 5 (1985): 76-90. © The McGraw Hill Companies.

Table B ✦ Percent Fat Estimate for Men: Sum of Chest, Abdomen, and Thigh Skinfolds

SUM OF SKINFOLDS (mm)	AGE TO THE LAST YEAR								
	<22	23-27	28-32	33-37	38-42	43-47	48-52	53-57	>57
8-10	1.3	1.8	2.3	2.9	3.4	3.9	4.5	5.0	5.5
11-13	2.2	2.8	3.3	3.9	4.4	4.9	5.5	6.0	6.5
14-16	3.2	3.8	4.3	4.8	5.4	5.9	6.4	7.0	7.5
17-19	4.2	4.7	5.3	5.8	6.3	6.9	7.4	8.0	8.5
20-22	5.1	5.7	6.2	6.8	7.3	7.9	8.4	8.9	9.5
23-25	6.1	6.6	7.2	7.7	8.3	8.8	9.4	9.9	10.5
26-28	7.0	7.6	8.1	8.7	9.2	9.8	10.3	10.9	11.4
29-31	8.0	8.5	9.1	9.6	10.2	10.7	11.3	11.8	12.4
32-34	8.9	9.4	10.0	10.5	11.1	11.6	12.2	12.8	13.3
35-37	9.8	10.4	10.9	11.5	12.0	12.6	13.1	13.7	14.3
38-40	10.7	11.3	11.8	12.4	12.9	13.5	14.1	14.0	15.2
41-43	11.6	12.2	12.7	13.3	13.8	14.4	15.0	15.5	16.1
44-46	12.5	13.1	13.6	14.2	14.7	15.3	15.9	16.4	17.0
47-49	13.4	13.9	14.5	15.1	15.6	16.2	16.8	17.3	17.9
50-52	14.3	14.8	15.4	15.9	16.5	17.1	17.6	18.2	18.8
53-55	15.1	15.7	16.2	16.8	17.4	17.9	18.5	19.1	19.7
56-58	16.0	16.5	17.1	17.7	18.2	18.8	19.4	20.0	20.5
59-61	16.9	17.4	19.9	18.5	19.1	19.7	20.2	20.8	21.4
62-64	17.6	18.2	18.8	19.4	19.9	20.5	21.1	21.7	22.2
65-67	18.5	19.0	19.6	20.2	20.8	21.3	21.9	22.5	23.1
68-70	19.3	19.9	20.4	21.0	21.6	22.1	22.7	23.3	23.9
71-73	20.1	20.7	21.2	21.8	22.4	23.0	23.6	24.1	24.7
74-76	20.9	21.5	22.0	22.6	23.2	23.8	24.4	25.0	25.5
77-79	21.7	22.2	22.8	23.4	24.0	24.6	25.2	25.8	26.3
80-82	22.4	23.0	23.6	24.2	24.8	25.4	25.9	26.5	27.1
83-85	23.2	23.8	24.4	25.0	25.5	26.1	26.7	27.3	27.9
86-88	24.0	24.5	25.1	25.7	26.3	26.9	27.5	28.1	28.7
89-91	24.7	25.3	25.9	26.5	27.1	27.6	28.2	28.8	29.4
92-94	25.4	26.0	26.6	27.2	27.8	28.4	29.0	29.6	30.2
95-97	26.1	26.7	27.3	27.9	28.5	29.1	29.7	30.3	30.9
98-100	26.9	27.4	28.0	28.6	29.2	29.8	30.4	31.0	31.6
101-103	27.5	28.1	28.7	29.3	29.9	30.5	31.1	31.7	32.3
104-106	28.2	28.8	29.4	30.0	30.6	31.2	31.8	32.4	33.0
107-109	28.9	29.5	30.1	30.7	31.3	31.9	32.5	33.1	33.7
110-112	29.6	30.2	30.8	31.4	32.0	32.6	33.2	33.8	34.4
113-115	30.2	30.8	31.4	32.0	32.0	33.2	33.8	34.5	35.1
116-118	30.9	31.5	32.1	32.7	33.3	33.9	34.5	35.1	35.7
119-121	31.5	32.1	32.7	33.3	33.9	34.5	35.1	35.7	36.4
122-124	32.1	32.7	33.3	33.9	34.5	35.1	35.8	36.4	37.0
125-127	32.7	33.3	33.9	34.5	35.1	35.8	36.4	37.0	37.6

Source: Tables 5 & 6, pp. 85-86 reproduced with permission, from Jackson, A.S., and Pollock, M.L.; "Practical Assessment of Body Composition." *The Physician and Sportsmedicine* 13, 5 (1985): 76-90. © The McGraw Hill Companies.

(continued)

Lab Activity 9.1 *(continued)*
Determining Your Percentage of Body Fat

Table C ✦ Fatness Ratings of University-Aged Men and Women

RATING	BODY FAT (PERCENTAGE)	
	Men	*Women*
Very low fat	5–7.9	12–14.9
Low fat	8–10.9	15–17.9
Ideal fat	11–14.9	18–21.9
Above ideal fat	15–17.9	22–24.9
Overfat	18–22.9	25–27.9
High fat	23+	28+

Lab Activity 9.2

Determining Your Caloric Needs

INSTRUCTIONS: *Complete each of the following steps carefully to identify how many calories you need daily to attain and maintain your ideal weight as determined in Lab Activity 9.1: Determining Your Percentage of Body Fat.*

1. Rate your level of physical activity from the list below by honestly estimating your activity level.

ACTIVITY PATTERN	CALORIES NEEDED PER KILOGRAM
Very inactive (sedentary, never exercise)	28.6
Slightly inactive (occasional physical activity)	30.8
Moderately active (fairly active on the job; engage in aerobic exercise twice weekly)	33.0
Relatively active (almost always on the go; engage in aerobic exercise three to four times a week)	35.2
Frequent strenuous activity (daily aerobic exercise for an hour or more)	37.4

2. Multiply your rating (calories per kilogram) by your actual weight. A sedentary 18- to 21-year-old female who weighs 59.0 kilograms, for example, would need 1687 calories per day ($59 \times 28.6 = 1687$). In theory, if she is consistently eating more than 1687 calories daily, she is gaining weight.

3. Multiply your physical activity rating by your ideal weight from Lab Activity 9.1. This figure is the number of calories needed per day to maintain your ideal weight. The ideal weight in the example in Lab Activity 9.1 is 75.5 kilograms. Because John is sedentary, he needs only 28.6 calories per kilogram and 2159 calories daily to maintain this weight ($75.5 \times 28.6 = 2159$).

Once you determine your ideal weight, you can eventually reach it by consuming only the number of calories necessary to maintain that weight. This is a common, sound approach to weight and fat loss. Weight loss that occurs slowly and safely is much more likely to be maintained in the future.

Lab Activity 9.3

10-Point Weight-Loss Program for a Sound, Safe Reducing Diet

INSTRUCTIONS: *Although most people are aware that fad diets are an unwise choice for safe, permanent weight and fat loss free from the risk of illness, millions continue to try practically any new, highly publicized diet on the market. Quick-weight-loss programs boasting some secret, easy method of rapidly shedding pounds are often hard to resist. Unfortunately, unsound dieting is dangerous and can result in permanent negative health consequences and even death.*

1. Before you even consider using a "gimmick" diet, consult your physician about your personal health concerns and ask your dietitian to evaluate the entire program.

2. Compare the fad diet to the 10-point weight-loss program by completing the following chart. Study the fad diet carefully and put Yes or No in the column to the right of each of the criteria for a sound, safe diet.

3. If you put No in the right-hand column, even in one area, the diet is suspect and possibly unsafe if used longer than a few days. If you put No in the right-hand column in two or more areas, don't consider its use, even for a day.

(continued)

Lab Activity 9.3 *(continued)*
10-Point Weight-Loss Program for a Sound, Safe Reducing Diet

Name _____ Date _____ Weight _____ % Body Fat _____

Weight/Fat-Loss Objective _____ Time Period _____
(454–907 grams weekly only)

Week (circle) 1 2 3 4 5 6 7 8 9 10

M	T	W	T	F	S	S	Daily Requirements	Yes/No
☐	☐	☐	☐	☐	☐	☐	1. 12+ 227-millilitre glasses of water	_____
☐	☐	☐	☐	☐	☐	☐	2. One multiple vitamin/mineral	_____
☐	☐	☐	☐	☐	☐	☐	3. A minimum of 15.4 calories per kilogram of your ideal weight (ideal weight × 15.4 = _____)	_____
☐	☐	☐	☐	☐	☐	☐	4. Three meals daily (no skipping)	_____
☐	☐	☐	☐	☐	☐	☐	5. Sufficient fat intake for satiety and essential fatty acids	_____
☐	☐	☐	☐	☐	☐	☐	6. Servings from the five food groups (bread, cereal, grains, pasta: 6–11; vegetables: 3–5; fruits: 2–4; milk, yogurt, cheese: 2–3; meat, fish, poultry, dry beans, eggs, nuts: 2–3)	_____
☐	☐	☐	☐	☐	☐	☐	7. Sufficient carbohydrates (simple and complex) to spare protein and prevent ketosis (50–120 g [200–480 cal] depending on body weight)	_____
☐	☐	☐	☐	☐	☐	☐	8. 25–35 grams of dietary fibre	_____
☐	☐	☐	☐	☐	☐	☐	9. 30 min of aerobic exercise	_____
☐	☐	☐	☐	☐	☐	☐	10. Recordkeeping of food/fluid intake	_____

Note: Weigh yourself no more than once weekly at the same time, under the same conditions. Pinch fatty areas the first 14 days; no weighing.

10

Stress Management and Physical Fitness

CHAPTER OBJECTIVES

By the end of this chapter, you should be able to:

1. Define stress, stressor, and stress reactivity.
2. List sources of stress and differentiate between distress and eustress.
3. Describe the bodily changes that occur when a person experiences stress.
4. Manage stress by using coping mechanisms at various levels of the stress response.
5. Use time-management techniques to free up time for regular exercise.
6. Detail the role of exercise in the management of stress.

EMILIO'S WIFE DIED last year, and he grieved long and hard for her. He felt that her death was unfair (she was such a kind person), and a sense of helplessness crept over him. Loneliness became part of his days, and tears became the companions of his late evening hours. There were those who were not even surprised at Emilio's own death just one year after his wife's. They officially called it a heart attack, but his friends know he died of a broken heart.

You probably know some Emilios—people who have died or become ill from severe stress with seemingly little physically wrong with them. That is what stress can do. In this chapter, you will learn how stress can actually change your body to make you susceptible to illness and disease or other negative influences. Contrary to what some people might tell you, it is not all in your mind. And you will learn how you can prevent these negative consequences from occurring, including the role of exercise in that process.

STRESS-RELATED CONCEPTS

Even the experts do not agree on the definition of **stress**. Some define it as the stimulus that causes a physical reaction (such as being afraid to take a test), while others view it as the reaction itself (for example, increases in blood pressure, heart rate, and perspiration). For our purposes in this text, we define stress as a combination of the cause (**stressor**) and the physical reaction (**stress reactivity**). The significance of these definitions is not merely academic. It is important to consider a stressor as having the potential to result in stress reactivity but not necessarily to do so.

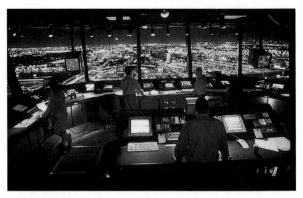

A demanding, fast-paced job can cause a great deal of stress if you let it.

Common Stressors

There are biological stressors (toxins, heat, cold), sociological stressors (unemployment), philosophical stressors (deciding on a purpose in life), and psychological stressors (threats to self-esteem, depression). Each has the potential to result in a stress reaction.

We all encounter stressors in our daily lives. The Canadian Health Promotion Survey recently found that almost half of all Canadians lead "fairly" stressful lives, and an additional 12 percent lead "very" stressful lives. You may have stressors associated with school (getting good grades, taking exams, having teachers think well of you), with work (too much to do in a given amount of time, not really understanding what is expected of you, fear of a company reorganization), with family (still being treated as a child when you are an adult, arguing often, lack of trust), or with your social life (making friends, telephoning for dates). Even scheduling exercise into your already busy day may be a stressor.

Stress Reactivity

When a stressor leads to a stress response, several changes occur in the body. The heart beats faster, muscles tense, breathing becomes rapid and shallow, perspiration appears under the arms and on the forehead, and blood pressure increases. These and other changes prepare the body to respond to the threat (stressor) by either fighting it off or running away. That is why stress reactivity is sometimes called the **fight-or-flight response**. Although many people consider the fight-or-flight response harmful, it is only bad for you if it is inappropriate to fight or run away—that is, when it is inappropriate to do something physical. For instance, if you are required to present a speech in front of your class, you cannot run from the assignment (you will fail the class if you do so) and you cannot strike out at the instructor or your classmates. It is

in these situations, when you do not or cannot use your body's preparedness to do something physical, that the stress reaction is unhealthy. Your blood pressure remains elevated, more cholesterol roams about your blood, your heart works harder than normal, and your muscles remain tense. That, in turn, can lead to various illnesses, such as coronary heart disease, stroke, and hypertension. At this point, pay attention to your body, particularly to your muscle tension. If you think you can drop your shoulders, that means your muscles are unnecessarily raising them. If your forearm muscles can be relaxed, you are unnecessarily tensing them. This wasted muscle tension—wasted because you are not about to do anything physical—is the result of stress and can cause tension headaches, backaches, or neck and shoulder pain. Lab Activity 10.1: Experiencing Stress Reactivity at the end of this chapter will help you identify how your heart reacts to stress.

Psychosomatic Disease

When built-up stress products (for example, increased heart rate and blood pressure) are chronic, go unabated, or occur frequently, they can cause illness and disease. These are called **psychosomatic**, from the Greek words *psyche* (the mind) and *soma* (the body). That does not mean these conditions are all in the mind; instead, it means that there is a mind–body connection causing the illness. An example is the effect of stress on allergies. Stress results in fewer white blood cells in the immunological system, which, in turn, can lead to an allergic reaction (teary eyes, stuffy nose, itchy throat). That is because it is the white blood cells that fight off *allergens* (the substances to which people are allergic); fewer of them will make a person more susceptible to an allergic reaction.

To determine to what degree you experience physical symptoms of stress, complete Lab Activity 10.2: The Physical Stress Symptoms Scale. If your score indicates excessive physical stress symptoms, pay particular attention to the stress-management techniques described later in this chapter.

A MODEL OF STRESS

Stress can be better understood by considering the model depicted in Figure 10.1. The model begins with a *life situation perceived as distressing*. Once it is perceived this way, *emotional arousal* (anxiety, nervousness, anger) occurs that, in turn, results in *physiological arousal* (increased heart rate, blood pressure, perspiration). That can lead to negative *consequences* such as psychosomatic illness, low grades at school, or arguments with family and friends.

Now let us see how the model operates in a stressful situation. Imagine you are a university student and that all you need in order to graduate this semester is to pass a physical-fitness class. Imagine further that you fail this class (life situation). You might say to yourself, "This is terrible. I will not be able to start work. I must be a real dummy. What will all my friends and relatives think?" In other words, you view the situation as distressing (perceived as distressing). That can result in fear and insecurity about the future, anger at the physical-fitness instructor, or worry about how you will obtain your degree (emotional arousal).

Figure 10.1 ✦ A Model of Stress

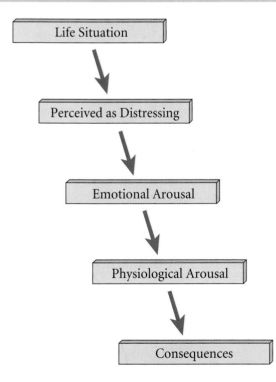

DIVERSITY ISSUES

Stress and the Family

Stress is often the result of specific life events, such as those involving school, work, or family. Greater sources of stress include loss of job, divorce, physical illness, or death in the family. An increasingly common stressor is the dual-career family. When both husband and wife work, whether the reasons are financial or career-oriented, they face such stress as how best to care for the children, how to find time to get the household chores done, and how to find enough quality time to spend as a family. When family responsibilities conflict with work requirements, such as when a child is sick and a parent needs to stay home, stress can build up.

There are no easy answers for alleviating dual-career family stressors. Sometimes, the demands of work and family are severe and need to be resolved creatively. Outlets for reducing stress include physical activity, relaxation, and time-management techniques. By working a combination of these stress relievers into their schedules, dual-career families can work their way toward a happier, healthier, lower-stress family life. ✦

These emotions can lead to increased heart rate, muscle tension, and the other components of the stress response (physiological arousal). As a result, you can develop a tension headache or an upset stomach (consequences).

Stress The combination of a stressor and stress reactivity.

Stressor A stimulus that has the potential to elicit stress reactivity.

Stress reactivity The physical reaction to a stressor that results in increased muscle tension, heart rate, blood pressure, and so forth.

Fight-or-flight response A physiological reaction to a threatening stressor; another name for stress reactivity.

Psychosomatic Illnesses or diseases that either are worsened or develop in the first place because of body changes resulting from an interpretation of thoughts.

It is as though a road winds its way through the towns of Life Situation, Perceived as Stressful, Emotional Arousal, Physiological Arousal, and Consequences. And that means that, as with any road, a roadblock can be set up that interferes with travel. Remember, a stressor only has the potential to lead to stress. A roadblock can prevent that stressor from proceeding to the next "town." This is the very essence of stress management—that is, setting up roadblocks on the stress model to interfere with travel to the next level.

Using the example of failing a physical-fitness class again, imagine that your reaction was, "It's not good that I failed this course, but I still have my health and people who love me. They'll help me get through this." In this case, the life situation is not perceived as distressing. Consider this change in perception a roadblock preventing emotional arousal. Without emotional arousal, there will be no physiological arousal and no negative consequences. In fact, there might even be positive consequences. Maybe failing the course will result in your studying extra hard the next time with the benefit of learning much more about physical fitness and becoming more fit than you would have been otherwise. In that instance, rather than experience distress, you have experienced **eustress**, stress that results in personal growth and positive outcomes.

*E*XERCISE'S UNIQUE CONTRIBUTION TO STRESS MANAGEMENT

Exercise is a unique stress-management intervention because it can be plugged in at many levels on the stress model. It is a life-situation intervention when you give up stressful habits (for example, cigarette smoking) because they interfere with your exercising. When you make friends through participating in a training program, you may also be using exercise as a life-situation intervention because loneliness and social isolation may be remedied.

Exercise can be a perception intervention as well. The brain produces neurotransmitters (endorphins) during exercise, and their euphoric, analgesic effect serves to relax the brain and the rest of the body. That relaxed state helps us perceive stressors as less stressful.

Exercise is also an emotional-arousal intervention. During exercise, we focus on what we are doing, not on our problems and stressors. It can therefore be relaxing to engage in physical activity. Furthermore, numerous research studies have found that exercise enhances well-being. It reduces feelings of depression and anxiety while increasing the sense of physical competence. The result is a higher level of self-esteem. And exercise can use up the built-up stress by-products and the body's preparedness to do something physical. Consequently, it can also be a physiological-arousal intervention.

Most Canadians know that physical activity reduces stress, but not all Canadians who are stressed engage in physical activity. The Canadian Fitness and Lifestyle Research Institute (CFLRI) advocates participation in physical activity for alleviating emotional distress because it promotes relaxation, acts as a timeout, provides a psychological distraction, enhances mood, self-esteem, and feelings of competence, provides time to process and work through problems, and generally acts to regulate emotional and psychological reactions to a stressful event. Of particular importance for exercise to reduce anxiety, CFLRI notes that exercises should be aerobic activities lasting 20–40 minutes, and should be included in long-term programs lasting 15 weeks or longer. Regular physical activity, especially aerobic activity, not only alleviates the buildup of distress but also helps prevent it.

It is because of its unique ability to be plugged into all the different levels of the stress model that exercise is particularly useful as a means of managing stress. Be careful, however, to exercise in ways recommended in this book. Although exercise is an excellent stress-management coping mechanism, if done incorrectly it can result in injury or discomfort. In that case, it will be a stressor rather than a stress reliever. And if exercise in itself is not your cup of tea but you participate anyway because you know it is good for you, you can still make it more pleasant.

One of the tenets of Health Canada's Active Living movement is that active people have more energy; they cope with stress better, and experience improved well-being and an enhanced quality of life. While Active Living is anchored in physical activity, it is sensitive to ensuring that it does not foster added stress but rather helps to relieve it. It includes a wide variety of activity choices such as: walking to work; gardening; joining in outdoor activities and recreational games; participating in exercise classes at school, through the workplace, or in the community; expressing feelings through dance; and competing in high-performance sport.

Stress and Athletic Injuries

There is a good deal of research demonstrating the relationship between stress and subsequent athletic injuries. One explanation for this relationship is the stress–injury model developed by Anderson and Williams (1988). According to this model, when people are put into stressful sports situations (for example, an important competition or tournament), three factors may contribute to a stress response: (1) a history of stressors (previous stressful events, past injuries, daily hassles), (2) personality characteristics (trait anxiety, external locus of control), and (3) coping resources (support of others, communication skills). Someone with a history of stressors, a personality that often interprets situations as anxiety-provoking, and few resources with which to cope with these perceptions is likely to have a stress response. Such individuals—those with high stress—experience increased muscle tension, narrowed fields of vision, and increased distractibility. It is because of these variables that stressful people are prone to athletic injury. Imagine trying to move out of the way of a baseball travelling toward you at a high speed if you are distracted or if your field of vision is narrowed. Or imagine trying to avoid muscle strains, sprains, or other musculoskeletal injuries when fatigue or a lack of flexibility results from the muscle tension associated with stress. And it is not only sports injuries that are involved. Traffic accidents can occur when a driver is distressed and therefore not as alert or able to react as quickly to another car running a red light.

Recognizing the relationship between stress and injury, some athletic programs have begun teaching their athletes stress-management techniques, with the result being fewer injuries. If you are interested in reading more about the stress–injury model and the research supporting its validity, see the 1996 article by Jean M. Williams in the *International Journal of Stress Management* entitled "Stress, Coping Resources, and Injury Risk" (vol. 3, no. 4, pp. 209–221).

Managing Stress

To manage stress, you need to set up roadblocks at each level of the stress model.

◣ The Life-Situation Level

At the life-situation level, you can make a list of all your stressors, routine ones that occur regularly and unusual ones that are often unanticipated. Then go through the list trying to eliminate as many of them as you can. For example, if you jog every day but find jogging stressful, try a different aerobic exercise or vary exercises from day to day. If you commute on a crowded highway and often become distressed about the traffic and construction slowdowns, try taking a different route. If you often argue with a friend and the associated stress interferes with your work, see the friend less often or not at all. There are probably many stressors that you tolerate by habit but that can be eliminated, thereby decreasing the stress in your life.

◣ The Perception Level

Stressors that cannot be eliminated can be handled by interpreting them as less distressing. One way to do that is through **selective awareness**. In every situation, there is some good and some bad. Choosing to focus on the good while not denying the bad will result in a more satisfying and less distressing life. For example, rather than focusing on the displeasure of standing in line at the checkout counter, you can choose to focus on the pleasure of being able to do nothing when your day is usually so hectic.

Consider the story about a female university student who writes her parents that she is in the hospital after having fallen out of her third-floor dormitory window. Luckily, she continues, she landed in some shrubs and was only temporarily paralyzed on her right side (that explains why her handwriting is so unclear). In the hospital, she says, she met a janitor and fell in love with him, and now they are planning to elope. She explains that the reason for eloping is that he is of a different religion, culture, and ethnic background, and she suspects her family might object to the marriage. She goes on to say she is confident that the marriage will work because her lover learned from his first marriage not to abuse his spouse and the jail term he served reinforced that lesson. She concludes the letter as follows: "Mom and Dad, I am not really in a hospital, have not fallen out of any window, and have not met someone with whom I am planning on eloping. However, I did fail chemistry, and I wanted you to be able to put that in its proper perspective." Now that is a lesson in selective awareness for the parents.

Eustress Stress that results in personal growth or development, so that the person experiencing it is better for having been stressed.

Selective awareness A means of managing stress by consciously focusing on the positive aspects of a situation or person.

The Emotional-Arousal Level

An excellent way to control your emotional responses to stress is to engage regularly in some form of relaxation. Some of the more effective ways of relaxing are described in this section.

There is no research to allow us to diagnose which relaxation technique is best for you. The only way to determine that is to try several and evaluate their ability to make you feel relaxed. To help you do that, we have provided a relaxation technique rating scale (see Table 10.1). Use it after you try each of the relaxation techniques.

Progressive Relaxation With **progressive relaxation**, you first tense a muscle group for ten seconds, all the while paying attention to the sensations that are created. Then relax those muscles, paying attention to that

Table 10.1 ✦ The Relaxation Technique Rating Scale

To determine which is most effective for you, try each relaxation technique presented in this chapter and evaluate it by answering these questions, using this scale:

1 = Very true   4 = Somewhat untrue

2 = Somewhat true   5 = Very untrue

3 = I'm not sure

1. It felt good.
2. It was easy to fit into my schedule.
3. It made me feel relaxed.
4. I handled my daily chores better than I usually do.
5. It was an easy technique to learn.
6. I was able to shut out my surroundings while I was practising this technique.
7. I did not feel tired after practising this technique.
8. My fingers and toes felt warmer after trying this relaxation technique.
9. Any stress symptoms I had (headache, tense muscles, anxiety) before practising this relaxation technique disappeared by the time I was done.
10. Each time I concluded this technique, my pulse rate was much lower than it was when I began.

Now sum up the values you responded with for a total score. Compare the scores of all the relaxation techniques you try. The lower the score, the more appropriate a particular relaxation technique is for you.

Source: Jerrold S. Greenberg, *Comprehensive Stress Management,* 5th ed. (Dubuque, IA: Brown and Benchmark, 1996), p. 134.

sensation. The idea is to learn what muscular tension feels like so you will be more likely to recognize it when you are experiencing it and to be familiar with muscular relaxation so that when you are tense, you can relax those muscles. It is called *progressive* because you progress from one muscle group to another throughout the body.

Autogenic Training **Autogenic training** involves imagining that your arms and legs are heavy, warm, and tingly. When you are able to imagine that, you are increasing the blood flow to those areas. This precipitates the relaxation response. After your body is relaxed, think of soothing images (a day at the beach, a park full of trees and green lawn, a calm lake on a sunny day) to relax your mind.

Body Scanning Even when you are tense, there is some part of your body that is relaxed. It may be your thigh or your chest or your hand. The relaxation technique called **body scanning** requires you to search for a relaxed body part and transport that feeling to the tenser parts of your body. That can be done by imagining the relaxed

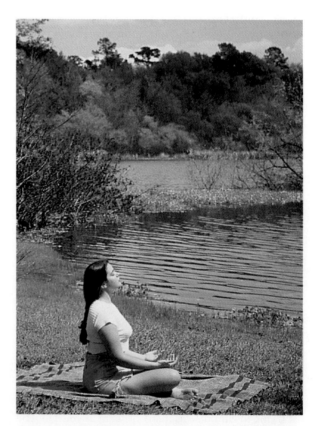

Progressive relaxation, meditation, autogenic training, and body scanning are effective relaxation techniques for people who typically find it difficult to relax.

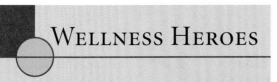

Hans Selye

Dr. Hans Selye (1907–82) is internationally acknowledged as "the father of the stress field" and, as such, is a Canadian resource to the world. On the basis of protracted experiments on animals in Montreal, Selye developed his theory and model of stress, the General Adaptation Syndrome (GAS). This three-stage syndrome of alarm–resistance–exhaustion was conceived as a biologic, bodily reaction to any stress. Selye's definition of *stress* as "the nonspecific response of the body to any demand" suggested that the demand can be positive and energizing (*eustress*) or negative and draining (*distress*).

After publishing in 1936 the first scientific paper to identify and define stress, Selye wrote more than 1700 more scholarly papers and 39 books on the subject. At the time of his death in 1982, his work had been cited in more than 362 000 scientific papers and countless popular magazine stories, in most major languages and in all countries worldwide. He is still by far the most frequently cited author on topics of stress.

Dr. Selye earned three doctorate degrees (MD, PhD, DSc) and was awarded 43 honorary doctorate degrees. He was an elected member of several dozen of the world's most recognized medical and scientific associations. He gained respect not only for his scientific innovations, but equally for his commitment to sharing the practical benefits of his work with everyday people. Two of his books, *The Stress of Life* and *Stress Without Distress*, were unrivalled bestsellers (the latter in 17 languages). His collaborative research with Dr. Richard Earle resulted in two final contributions to the literature on stress, *Stress and the Workplace* and *Your Vitality Quotient*. While his theory of the GAS has been refined and revised—even called into question—his pioneering contribution to the whole field has been profound. ✦

Sources: F. J. McGuigan, *Encyclopedia of Stress* (Toronto: Allyn and Bacon, 1999); various Internet sources.

part as a fiery, hot ball that you roll to the tenser parts of your body. The more you practise this technique, the more effective you will become with it. This is true with all relaxation techniques.

Biofeedback This technique involves the use of an instrument to mirror what is going on in the body and to report the results back to the individual. Biofeedback instrumentation can measure and *feed back* to the person numerous physiological parameters: temperature, blood pressure, heart rate, perspiration, breathing rate, muscle tension, brain waves, and many others. Interestingly, individuals can control these responses—previously thought to be involuntary—once the measure has been reported back to them. The physiological parameters already enumerated in this paragraph can be increased or decreased with biofeedback training. Because the body and the mind are connected, changes in either can effect changes in the other. Consequently, when a person is taught to decrease heart rate and muscle tension, for example, the psychological states of anxiety and nervousness may also be decreased.

Lab Activity 10.3: How to Meditate is another effective relaxation technique. Complete this Lab Activity to experience and determine the effectiveness of meditation for you.

■ The Physiological-Arousal Level

This is the point at which your body is already prepared to do something physical. To manage stress at this level requires engaging in some physical activity, which can range from the obvious to the obscure. Running around the block as fast as you can will use the stress by-products and do wonders for your disposition. Dribbling a basketball up and down the court mimicking fast breaks, serving 30 tennis balls as hard as you can, biking as fast as you can, or swimming several laps at breakneck speed, as well as other tiring exercises, can also relieve stress. Still, you need not engage in formal sports activities to relieve stress at this level on the model. You can simply punch your mattress or pillow as hard and as long as you can. You will not hurt them or yourself, but you will feel better.

Progressive relaxation A relaxation technique in which you contract, then relax, muscle groups throughout the body.

Autogenic training A relaxation technique in which you imagine your arms and legs are heavy, warm, and tingly.

Body scanning A relaxation technique in which you identify a part of your body that feels relaxed and transport that feeling to another part of your body.

TYPES A AND B BEHAVIOUR PATTERNS AND THE EXERCISER

Researchers have discovered a **behaviour pattern (Type A)** related to the subsequent development of coronary heart disease. Type A people are aggressive and competitive, never seem to have enough time, do two or more things at once (this is called being *polyphasic*), are impatient, and become angry easily. In contrast, the **Type B behaviour pattern** seems to protect against the development of coronary heart disease. Type B people exhibit no free-floating hostility, always seem to have enough time to get things done and do not fret if they don't, are more cooperative than competitive, and are concerned with quality rather than quantity (it is not how fast they run but whether they enjoy their run).

Recent research has clarified the relationship between Type A behaviour and coronary heart disease. Apparently, hostility is the trait of major concern. People who tend to become angry and/or cynical easily are more apt to develop coronary heart disease than are others.

Our friend Jorge, mentioned toward the beginning of Chapter 3, characterizes the Type A exerciser. If you remember, on a sunny, windless day, Jorge was playing tennis when he hit one too many errant backhands. Losing control, he threw his racquet over the fence, over several trees, and into the creek alongside the court. As the racquet floated downstream, Jorge was at a loss about what to berate more severely: his tennis skills or his temper. This aggressiveness and hostility are classic characteristics of Type A behaviour.

Type A exercisers are aggressive (they may smack their golf clubs into the ground when they hit a shot off target), hostile (they may accuse their opponents of cheating), competitive (they may not be able to bear losing), and numbers-oriented (they evaluate themselves on how many matches they won rather than whether they played well or had fun participating). If you see yourself as a Type A, think about a change. Use the behavioural change techniques and strategies presented in Chapter 3 to become more Type B. You may be healthier, and you will probably be happier.

TIME MANAGEMENT: FREEING UP TIME TO EXERCISE

To manage stress, you need to set aside time. To exercise regularly, you also need to set aside time. Because stress can sap your attention, energy, and time, it can interfere with your exercise regimen. After all, stress can be a threat to your physical self and your self-concept. Who can blame you for postponing or cancelling exercise to

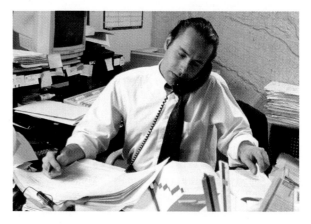

Adopting time-tested time-management techniques will help you to better control your use of time.

manage that threat? But you can organize your time better so there is plenty of time for exercising, managing stress, and doing the myriad of other things you need, and choose, to.

To be serious about using time-management strategies, you need to realize several things:

- Time is one of your most precious possessions.
- Time spent is gone forever.
- You cannot save time. Time moves continually, and it is used, one way or another. If you waste time, there is no bank where you can withdraw the time you previously saved to replace the time wasted.
- To come to terms with your mortality is to realize that your time is limited. None of us will live forever, and none of us will be able to do everything we would like to do.

You can *invest* time to free up (not to save) more time than you originally invested. Then you will have sufficient time to use the stress-management techniques presented in this chapter and plenty of time to participate in a regular exercise program. The techniques we will now describe will help you to do that. As you read the following suggestions for better managing your limited time, try to make direct application of these techniques to your situation. Most of these techniques you will want to incorporate into your lifestyle; others you will decide are not worth the effort or the time.

▪ Assessing How You Spend Time

As a first step, analyze how you spend your time now. To do this, divide your day into 15-minute segments. Record what you are doing every 15 minutes. Review this time diary and total the time spent on each activity throughout the day. For example, you might find you spent 3 hours socializing, 4 hours eating meals, 3 hours watching television, 1 hour doing homework, 2 hours shopping, 2 hours listening to music, 6 hours sleeping, and 3 hours on the telephone, as shown in the example in Table 10.2. Evaluate this use of time as shown in Table 10.2, and note in the adjustment column that the adjustments would free up 6½ hours a day. That would leave plenty of time to exercise. A good way to actually make the changes you desire is to draw up a contract with yourself that includes a reward for being successful. Refer to Chapter 3 for the most effective way to develop such a contract.

Prioritizing

One important technique for managing time is to prioritize your activities. Not all of them are of equal importance. You need to focus on those activities of major importance to you and only devote time to other activities after the major ones are completed. One of the major activities for which you should prioritize your time is exercise.

To prioritize your activities, develop A, B, and C lists. On the A list, place those activities that *must* get done, that are so important that not to do them would be very undesirable. For example, if a term paper is due tomorrow and you have not typed it yet, that goes on your A list.

On the B list are those activities you would like to do today and need to get done. If they don't get done today, however, it would not be too terrible. For example, if you have not spoken to a close friend and have been meaning to telephone, you might put that on your B list. Your intent is to call today, but if you don't get around to it, you can always call tomorrow or the next day.

On the C list are those activities you would like to do if you get all the A- and B-list activities done. But if the C-list activities never get done, that is no problem.

For example, if a department store has a sale and you would like to go browse, put that on your C list. If you do all of the As and Bs, you can go browse.

In addition, make a list of things *not* to do. For example, if you tend to waste your time watching television, you might want to include that on your not-to-do list. In that way, you will have a reminder not to watch television today. Other time wasters should be placed on this list as well.

Other Ways to Free Up Time for Exercise

There are many other time-management strategies you can use to make time for exercise.

Say No Because of guilt, concern for what others might think, or a real desire to engage in an activity, we often have a hard time saying no. Creating A, B, and C lists and prioritizing your activities will help you identify how much time remains for other activities and make saying no easier.

Delegate When it is possible, get others to do things that need to be done but that do not need your personal attention. Conversely, avoid taking on chores that others try to delegate to you. This does not mean that you use other people to do work you should be doing or that you do not help out others when they ask. What it means is that you should be more discriminating regarding delegation of activities. In other words, don't hesitate to seek help when you are short on time or overloaded. And help others when they really need it and when you have the time available to do so.

Give Tasks the Once-Over Many of us will open our mail, read through it, and set it aside to act on later. This is a waste of time. If we pick it up later, we have to familiarize ourselves with it once again. As much as possible, look things over only once.

Table 10.2 ✦ Summary of Daily Activities

Activity Needed	Total time spent on activity (hours)	Adjustment
Socializing	3	1 hour less
Eating meals	4	1 hour less
Watching television	3	1½ hours less
Doing homework	1	1 hour more
Shopping	2	1 hour less
Listening to music	2	1 hour less
Sleeping	6	None
Talking on telephone	3	2 hours less

Type A behaviour pattern A combination of behaviours that makes individuals susceptible to coronary heart disease, including hostility, cynicism, aggression, and overly competitive tendencies.

Type B behaviour pattern A combination of behaviours that seems to protect people from contracting coronary heart disease, such as: lack of hostility, anger, and aggression; cooperativeness; and the ability to focus on one task at a time.

MYTH AND FACT SHEET

Myth	Fact
1. Stressful events of necessity cause stress and a stress reaction.	1. Stressful events only have the potential to cause a stress reaction. They need not do so if they are interpreted as nonstressful.
2. There is really nothing you can do about stress—it is simply a normal part of life.	2. There are many ways to manage stress so it does not make you ill or interfere with the satisfaction you derive from life.
3. Exercise is stressful because of the toll it takes physically.	3. Exercise is an excellent way of managing stress because it relates to every level of the stress model.
4. You should try to eliminate all stress from your life.	4. There is an optimal level of stress that results in joy and stimulation and encourages your best performance. Therefore, you need some stress to make life worth living.

Use the Circular File How many times do you receive junk mail that is obvious from its envelope and yet still take the time to open it and read the junk inside? You would be better off bypassing the opening and reading part and going directly to the throwing-out part. That would free up time for more important activities, such as exercise.

Limit Interruptions Throughout the day, you will be interrupted. Recognizing this fact, you should actually schedule in times for interruptions. That is, don't make your schedule so tight that interruptions will throw you into a tizzy. On the other hand, try to keep these interruptions to a minimum. There are several ways you can accomplish this. You can accept phone calls only between certain hours. You can also arrange to have someone take messages so you can call back later, or you can use an answering machine. Do the same with visitors. Anyone who visits should be asked to return at a more con-

venient time. If you are serious about making better use of your time, you will adopt some of these means of limiting interruptions.

Recognize the Need to Invest Time The bottom line of time management is that you need to invest time initially in order to free it up later. We often hear people say, "I don't have the time to organize myself the way you suggest. That would put me further in the hole." This is an interesting paradox. If you are so pressed for time that you believe you do not even have sufficient time to get yourself organized, that in itself tells you that you are in need of applying time-management strategies. The investment in time devoted to organizing yourself will pay dividends by allowing you to achieve more of what is really important to you. After all, what is more important than your health and wellness? And what better way is there to achieve health and wellness than freeing up time for regular exercise?

BEHAVIOURAL CHANGE AND MOTIVATIONAL STRATEGIES

There are many things that might interfere with your ability to manage stress. Here are some barriers (roadblocks) and strategies for overcoming them.

Roadblock	Behavioural Change Strategy
You may have a lot to do with little time to get it all done. Term papers are due, midterm or final exams are approaching, you are invited to a party, you are expected to attend a dinner celebrating your sister's birthday, your team is scheduled for an intramural game, and your professor is holding a study session.	When responsibilities are lumped together, they often appear overwhelming. Use the behaviour change strategy of *divide and conquer*. Buy a large calendar, and schedule the semester's activities by writing on the calendar when you will perform them, when you will do library research for term papers, when you will begin studying for exams, and when you will read which chapters in which textbooks. Do not forget to include nonacademic activities as well. For example, write your intramural team's schedule and times of parties or dinners to attend on the calendar. You will soon realize that you have plenty of time. You simply need to get organized. That realization will go a long way in relieving unnecessary stress.
You are not accomplishing your fitness objectives, and because of that you feel distressed. You are not running as fast as you would like to run, nor are you lifting the amount of weight you would like to lift, doing the number of repetitions you would like to do, losing the amount of weight you would like to lose, or participating in aerobic dance classes.	Use the *goal-setting* strategies outlined in Chapter 3. Set realistic fitness goals, give yourself enough time to achieve them, and make your workout fun. If you are distressed because your goals seem elusive, perhaps they are. Maybe they are too difficult to achieve, at least in the amount of time you have allotted. If you are injuring yourself regularly, perhaps your fitness program is too difficult or too intense. Use *gradual programming* and *tailoring* to devise a program specific to you and to the level of fitness you presently possess.
You try to relax but cannot. Your thoughts seem nonstop. You become fidgety. You are anxious to move on to do something that needs doing. Finding the time to engage in a relaxation technique is impossible. You are simply too busy.	Use *material reinforcement* to encourage the regular practice of relaxation. Every time you set aside time to relax, reward yourself with something tangible. You might put aside a certain amount of money or buy a healthy snack. Another behavioural change technique that could help is *boasting*. Be proud of taking time to relax and share that feeling of pride with friends. That will make you feel good and more likely to engage in that relaxation technique again. You will also need to assess your relaxation method periodically. Use Table 10.1 to help you perform this assessment. You will find that some relaxation techniques are more effective for you than others, so you will learn which ones to use regularly.
List roadblocks interfering with your ability to manage stress.	Cite behavioural change strategies that can help you overcome the roadblocks you just listed. If you need to, refer back to Chapter 3 for behavioural change and motivational strategies.
1. _____	1. _____
2. _____	2. _____
3. _____	3. _____

SUMMARY

Stress-Related Concepts

Stress can be defined as a combination of the cause (stressor) and the physical reaction (stress reactivity). A stressor has the potential to result in stress reactivity, but it does not necessarily do so. Whether it does depends on how the stressor is perceived or interpreted. Stressors can take a variety of forms: biological (toxins, heat, cold), sociological (unemployment), philosophical (deciding on a purpose in life), or psychological (threats to self-esteem, depression).

When a stressor leads to a stress response, several changes occur in the body. The heart beats faster, muscles tense, breathing becomes rapid and shallow, perspiration appears under the arms and on the forehead, and blood pressure increases. These and other changes make up the fight-or-flight response.

When built-up stress products (for example, increased heart rate and blood pressure) are chronic, go unabated, or occur frequently, they can cause illness and disease. These are called *psychosomatic*. That means these conditions stem from a mind–body interaction that causes the illness or makes an existing disease worse.

A Model of Stress

A model to better understand stress and its effects begins with a life situation occurring that is perceived as distressing. Once the situation is perceived this way, emotional arousal occurs (anxiety, nervousness, anger), which, in turn, results in physiological arousal (increased heart rate, blood pressure, muscle tension, perspiration). This can lead to negative consequences such as psychosomatic illness, low grades at school, or arguments with family and friends. The essence of stress management is to set up roadblocks on the stress model to interfere with travel to the next level.

The goal, however, is not to eliminate all stress. Certainly, some stress (distress) is harmful. On the other hand, some stress is useful because it encourages peak performance; this type of stress is called eustress.

Exercise's Unique Contribution to Stress Management

Exercise is a unique stress-management intervention because it can be plugged in at many levels on the stress model. It is a life-situation intervention when you give up stressful habits because they interfere with exercising. It is a perception intervention when your brain produces neurotransmitters during exercise that make you feel relaxed. It is an emotional-arousal intervention when you focus on the physical activity and ignore problems and stressors. And it is a physiological-arousal intervention when you use the built-up stress by-products by doing something physical.

Managing Stress

Managing stress involves interventions at each of the levels of the stress model. At the life-situation level, you can assess routine stressors and eliminate them. At the perception level, you can use selective awareness. At the emotional-arousal level, you can do progressive relaxation, autogenic training, body scanning, biofeedback training, and meditation, and at the physiological level, you can exercise regularly.

Types A and B Behaviour Patterns and the Exerciser

People who are aggressive and competitive, never seem to have enough time, do two or more things at once, are impatient, and become angered easily exhibit Type A behaviour patterns. Type A people are prone to coronary heart disease, with the most harmful characteristic being free-floating hostility. Type B people—who exhibit no free-floating hostility, always seem to have enough time to get things done, are more cooperative than competitive, and are concerned with quality rather than quantity—seem to be protected from developing coronary heart disease.

Time Management: Freeing Up Time to Exercise

Time cannot be saved, but you can free up time by being more organized. Some effective time-management strategies include assessing how you spend time so you can make sensible adjustments, prioritizing your activities, learning to say no so you do not take on too many responsibilities, delegating tasks to others, looking things over only once, avoiding spending time on junk mail, and limiting interruptions. Time invested in applying time-management strategies will pay off in terms of freeing up time for such important activities as regular exercise.

STUDY QUESTIONS

1. Define a stressor and give examples from your own life experiences.

2. How did Dr. Selye contribute to our understanding of stress and its impact on the body?

3. Describe three stress-management techniques you could utilize effectively to manage your stress.

4. What negative emotions and behaviour types are known to provoke a stress response?

5. How can exercise alleviate stress? Give examples.

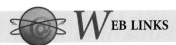 WEB LINKS

Centre of Balance
www.centerofbalance.com

Mindfulness Based Stress Reduction
www.mbsr.com

Blue Ridge Mindbody Institute
www.ne-mindbody.com

Modern Life Guide
www.modlife.com

10 Ways to Reduce Stress on the Job
www.smartbiz.com/sbs/arts/bly61.htm

Are You Suffering from Hidden Stress?
www.smartbiz.com/sbs/arts/mos70.htm

Mind Tools
www.bazis.nl/personal/rvermey/selfhypn.html

Work Out Your Stress
www.cflri.ca/LT/95LT/LT95_07.html

Stress Reduction with Exercise Study
www.pslgroup.com/dg/23236.htm

The Canadian Institute of Stress
www.stresscanada.org/

The American Institute of Stress
www.stress.org/

Stress Management Techniques
www.mindtools.com/smpage.html
www.imt.net/~randolfi/StressLinks.html

Stress and Anxiety Research Society
www.star-society.org/

Stress and Exercise
www.holistic-online.com/stress/stress_exercise.htm

REFERENCES

Anderson, M. B., and J. M. Williams. "A Model of Stress and Athletic Injury: Prediction and Prevention." *Journal of Sport and Exercise Physiology* 10 (1988): 294–306.

Greenberg, J. S. *Comprehensive Stress Management,* 5th ed. Dubuque, IA: Brown and Benchmark, 1996.

Seaward, Brian L. *Managing Stress: Principles and Strategies for Health and Well Being,* 3rd ed. Toronto: Jones & Bartlet, 2002.

Williams, Jean M. "Stress, Coping Resources, and Injury Risk." *International Journal of Stress Management* 3, 4 (1996): pp. 209–221.

Lab Activity 10.1

Experiencing Stress Reactivity

INSTRUCTIONS: *While seated in a comfortable position, determine how fast your heart beats at rest using one of these methods. (Use a watch that has a second hand.)*

1. Place the first two fingers (index and middle finger) of one hand on the underside of your other wrist, on the thumb side. Feel for your pulse and count the number of pulses for 30 seconds.

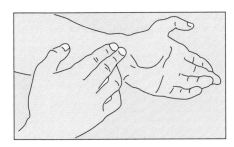

2. Place the first two fingers of one hand on your lower neck, just above the collarbone; move your fingers toward your shoulder until you find your pulse. Count the pulse for 30 seconds.

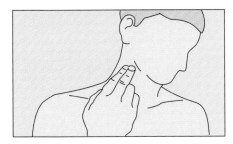

3. Place the first two fingers of one hand in front of your ear; move your fingers until you find a pulse. Count the pulse for 30 seconds.

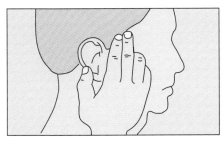

(continued)

Lab Activity 10.1 *(continued)*
Experiencing Stress Reactivity

Multiply your 30-second pulse count by two to determine how many times your heart beats each minute while you are at rest. Now close your eyes and think of either someone you really dislike or some situation you experienced that really frightened you. If you are recalling a person, think of how that person looks and smells and what he or she does to incur your dislike. Really feel the dislike, do not just think about it. If you recall a frightening situation, try to place yourself back in that situation. Sense the fright, be scared, vividly recall the situation in all its detail. Think of the person or situation for one minute and then count your pulse rate for 30 seconds, as you did earlier. Multiply the rate by two and compare your first total with the second.

Most people find that their heart rates increase when they are experiencing stressful memories. This increase occurs despite a lack of any physical activity; the very thoughts increase heart rate. This demonstrates two things: the nature of stressors and the nature of stress reactivity.

Source: Jerrold S. Greenberg, *Comprehensive Stress Management*, 5th ed. (Dubuque, IA: Brown and Benchmark, 1996), p. 10.

Name Angela Chaffey

Date 13/03/06

Lab Activity 10.2

The Physical Stress Symptoms Scale

INSTRUCTIONS: *Indicate how often each of the following effects happen to you either when you are experiencing stress or following exposure to a significant stressor. Respond to each item with a number between 0 and 5, using the scale that follows:*

0=NEVER   2=EVERY FEW MONTHS   4=ONCE OR MORE EACH WEEK

1=ONCE OR TWICE A YEAR   3=EVERY FEW WEEKS   5=DAILY

1. Cardiovascular Symptoms

___4̶ 3 Heart pounding   ___3 Heart racing or beating erratically

___4 Cold, sweaty hands   ___4 Headaches (throbbing pain)   Subtotal 14

2. Respiratory Symptoms

___4 Rapid, erratic, or shallow breathing   ___3 Shortness of breath

___1 Asthma attack   ___2 Difficulty speaking because of poor breathing control   Subtotal 10

3. Gastrointestinal Symptoms

___3 Upset stomach, nausea, or vomiting   ___2 Constipation

___2 Diarrhea   ___2 Sharp abdominal pains   Subtotal 9

4. Muscular Symptoms

___3 Headaches (steady pain) ___4 Back or shoulder pains

___3 Muscle tremors or hands shaking   ___0 Arthritis   Subtotal 10

5. Skin Symptoms

___0 Acne   ___0 Dandruff

___4 Perspiration   ___1 Excessive dryness of skin or hair   Subtotal 5

(continued)

Lab Activity 10.2 *(continued)*
The Physical Stress Symptoms Scale

6. Immunity Symptoms

_3_ Allergy flare-up   _1_ Common cold

_0_ Influenza   _0_ Skin rash   Subtotal _4_

7. Metabolic Symptoms

_3_ Increased appetite   _4_ Increased craving for tobacco
or sweets

_34_ Thoughts racing or   _4_ Feelings of anxiety or
difficulty sleeping   nervousness   Subtotal _15_

Overall Symptomatic Total (add all seven subtotals) _67_

What Does Your Score Mean?

0–35 Moderate physical stress symptoms
A score in this range indicates a low level of physical stress manifestations, hence minimal overall probability of encounter with psychosomatic disease in the near future.

36–75 Average physical stress symptoms
Most people experience physical stress symptoms within this range. It is representative of an increased predisposition to psychosomatic disease but not an immediate threat to physical health.

76–140 Excessive physical stress symptoms
If your score falls in this range, you are experiencing a serious number and frequency of stress symptoms. It is a clear indication that you may be headed toward one or more psychosomatic diseases sometime in the future. You should take deliberate action to reduce your level of stress.

Source: Roger J. Allen and David Hyde, *Investigations in Stress Control* (Minneapolis: Burgess, 1980), pp. 101–105.

Lab Activity 10.3

How to Meditate

There are many ways to meditate. The following is a description of a classic meditation that uses mantras and is simple and easy.

Mantras

A mantra is a sound, word, or phrase that is repeated to yourself. It can be spoken aloud as a chant, or silently as in meditation. Many people think that the best mantras are sounds that have no clear meaning and are used as a way of displacing your usual thoughts and moving your awareness inward. There are many mantras, using words taken from anywhere from Hindu Sanskrit to Christian scripture (especially when "saying the rosary," where the repetition is meditative). If you do not already know of a good mantra to use, use the sound "hamsa." This is a natural mantra, being the sound one makes when breathing, with "ham" (h-ah-m) on inhalation and "sa" (s-ah) on exhalation.

Directions for the Hamsa Meditation

- Sit comfortably. A quiet place is preferred, but not required.

- Close your eyes. Breathe naturally. Sit for about one minute before you begin thinking the mantra to allow your heart and breathing to slow.

- Gently bring your attention to your breath and begin to think the mantra, gently and easily. Just let it come, do not force it. Think "ham" on the inhale and "sa" on the exhale. Allow yourself to be absorbed in it.

- Allow your thoughts and feelings to come and go with detachment. Do not try to control them in any way. Just note them, and when you realize that you are not repeating the mantra, gently return to the mantra. Do not try to force yourself to think the mantra to the exclusion of all other thoughts. You may experience a deep state of relaxation but it is all right if you do not.

- Meditate in this way for 20 minutes.

- When done, take about a minute to slowly return to normal awareness. Be gentle with yourself when opening your eyes or coming to stand after a meditation. It is not good for your heart to get up quickly after the state of deep rest that is often a result of meditation.

Note: You may glance at a clock to time the meditation, but do not use an alarm timer.

Source: Adapted from Gabriel Zappia, "How to Meditate," 1995, off *Meditation: The Feldenkrais Method* Web page, accessed April 21, 1999 **www.alternative-medicine.net/meditation/english.html**

11

How Chemicals Affect Physical Fitness

CHAPTER OBJECTIVES
By the end of this chapter, you should be able to:
1. Differentiate between drug use, misuse, and abuse and give examples of each.
2. Describe the prevalence of alcohol on campus and make suggestions for drinking responsibly.
3. Cite methods taken by universities to control alcohol use on campus.
4. Describe the prevalence of tobacco use and its effects on the body.
5. Describe strategies to quit smoking and/or to make smoking less harmful.
6. List drugs used to enhance athletic performance and discuss their safety and effectiveness.

THE THOMAS AND CHEN families both experienced a very difficult year. Glenn Thomas was diagnosed with angina (pain in the chest due to constricted coronary arteries) and started taking nitroglycerin pills periodically. His wife, Barbara, contracted a sinus infection in February and was prescribed antibiotics. In May her gynecologist recommended she begin regular doses of estrogen to replace her body's decreased production of estrogen caused by menopause. Their son, Clark, was diagnosed with attention deficit disorder, and his pediatrician put him on the drug Ritalin.

The Chens were no more fortunate. Jeff decided that he needed assistance to stop smoking and was encouraged by his doctor to wear a nicotine patch. Mary Chen was diagnosed with high blood pressure and instructed to take hypertension medication daily. And Kelly, the Chens' teenage daughter, was found to be anemic and began taking an iron supplement each day.

More than ever before, drugs—prescription and nonprescription—are available to treat medical and psychological conditions, thereby improving the quality of our lives. Without these drugs, the Thomases and the Chens would not feel as well each day and would probably live shorter lives and/or have their activities limited.

You, too, are a drug user; we all are. In fact, Canada is a drug-taking society. And, in many respects, it is fortunate that we are. Think about the important drugs we use:

- Vaccines that provide protection from diseases that can wipe out whole societies
- Antibiotics that control previously fatal bacterial diseases
- Oral contraceptives that help some people plan families and that have a profound, though controversial, effect on our society
- Tranquilizers and antidepressants that allow people with mental illness to function

For all the good that has come from drugs, many people believe that Canadian society has become too reliant on medication and mood-altering substances. Too often, the remedy for anxiety is a tranquilizer, the response to a headache is an aspirin or some other painkiller, the answer to a problem is alcohol, and the driving force of a social occasion is some illegal drug.

DRUG USE, MISUSE, AND ABUSE

You will soon see that differentiating between drug use, misuse, and abuse is not as easy as it at first appears. Start this section by listing the last ten times you can remember taking a drug.

Drug Use

Your list probably includes an occasion when you were ill and took either a drug prescribed by your physician or one available over the counter. Perhaps you had a strained muscle from exercising and took aspirin or ibuprofen to control the inflammation and pain. If you used this drug properly, it probably helped you overcome your malady. In fact, this drug might have been so important to your health that if you had not used it, your condition might have worsened. For example, if you contracted pneumonia and did not take the antibiotic prescribed for you, you might die. This is **drug use**—that is, when drugs are used as they are recommended to be used and for the purposes for which they were recommended.

Drug Misuse

Unfortunately, some people ruin a good thing. They take too many aspirin tablets in too short a period of time or ingest ibuprofen without drinking enough fluids. The result could be intestinal problems such as a bleeding stomach caused by damage to stomach tissue. When a legal drug is used inappropriately, it is **drug misuse**.

Drug Abuse

When an illegal drug is used or when a legal drug is used for purposes other than for what it was intended, that is **drug abuse**. Typical abused drugs include marijuana, cocaine, heroin, anabolic steroids, and amphetamines. These drugs are often taken for the euphoria they produce rather than for any medical or physiological reason. Legal drugs that are sometimes abused include Demerol (meperidine), Dilaudid (hydromorphine), and Darvon (propoxyphene). These drugs are prescription pain relievers that are sometimes sold illicitly for their narcotic effects. It has been estimated that drug abuse costs Canadian taxpayers, corporations, and other agencies nearly $85 billion annually (Single et al., 1996).

Drugs That Are Difficult to Categorize

Although the differentiation between drug use, misuse, and abuse may at first appear clear, there are a number of drugs and drug usages that are difficult to categorize. For example, how would you classify tobacco products? They are legal but cause the body harm. What about alcoholic beverages? In this case, the amount of drug used (the dosage) might dictate its categorization. And in which category would you place over-the-counter diet remedies? They, too, can be taken in excessive amounts or in place of changes in eating and exercise habits.

Space dictates that we limit our discussion of drugs and fitness and the effects of drugs on health and wellness. Consequently, we have chosen to discuss only the more prevalent drugs or those with direct application to physical fitness.

ALCOHOL

Canada's Alcohol and Other Drugs Survey in 1996/1997 found that 74 percent of women and men aged 12 years and older—about 18.1 million Canadians—consume alcohol. This is an increase of 2 percentage points since the 1994 National Alcohol and Other Drugs Survey. However, provincial variations exist, as shown in Table 11.1.

Table 11.1 ✦ Current Drinking in Canada and the Provinces (%)

	1989	1994
Canada	**77.7**	**72.3**
Newfoundland	67.6	71.4
Prince Edward Island	63.7	67.2
Nova Scotia	71.2	72.1
New Brunswick	68.0	67.8
Quebec	76.4	73.9
Ontario	77.6	69.4
Manitoba	79.3	73.6
Saskatchewan	78.4	73.0
Alberta	81.9	76.4
British Columbia	82.9	75.6

Source: Health Canada, Minister of Supply and Services, *Canada's Alcohol and Other Drugs Survey*, 1995, Catalogue No. H39-338/1995E. Adapted and reproduced with the permission of the Minister of Public Works and Government Services Canada, 2003. *Health Canada assumes no responsibility for any errors or omissions which may have occurred in the adaptation of its material.*

Fewer women are current drinkers than men (66.7 percent versus 78.1 percent), and women are almost twice as likely as men to report never drinking (16.7 percent versus 8.9 percent). In terms of the maximum number of drinks per occasion, men report an average of 7.4 drinks and women 4.2. Among women, the rate of current drinking is highest in the 18–19-year-old age group (79.1 percent) and among men in the 20–24 group (90.9 percent).

People drink for many reasons: to relax, to be sociable, to have something to do with their hands during social occasions, and to decrease inhibitions and become less shy. When drinking is limited, alcohol-related problems usually do not occur. When too much alcohol is ingested in too short a period of time, is taken with other drugs or medications, or is combined with events requiring coordination and speedy reflexes (such as driving an automobile), however, serious consequences can result.

Alcohol's Effects

Alcohol affects the body in many different ways. It results in blood vessels in the head dilating, which can lead to headaches. It also increases heart rate and blood pressure while at the same time constricting (narrowing) the blood vessels supplying the heart. And when the liver is subjected to excessive doses of alcohol over a period of time, it, too, can be damaged. **Cirrhosis** of the liver is a condition to which alcoholics are prone; it is irreversible and sometimes leads to death. Malnutrition, cancer (of the

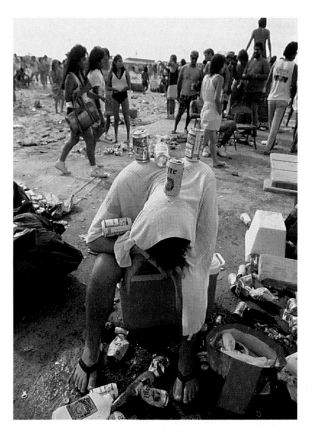

Alcohol is the drug most frequently used by both high school and university students, and too often vandalism and other troublesome acts are a consequence.

liver, esophagus, nasopharynx, and larynx), endocrine and reproductive problems, neurological disorders, and mental illness are but a few other potential effects of alcohol abuse.

How to Take Control of Your Drinking

Alcohol can significantly impair your physical functioning (see Table 11.2). To be physically fit, remain healthy, and possess a high level of wellness all require either abstaining from ingesting alcohol or drinking responsi-

Drug use The proper use of a drug.

Drug misuse The inappropriate use of a legal drug.

Drug abuse The use of an illegal drug or the use of a legal drug for purposes other than those it was intended for.

Cirrhosis A scarring of cells of the liver that is associated with the excessive use of alcohol.

Table 11.2 ✦ Effects of Alcohol Consumption

BAC	GENERAL PHYSICAL EFFECTS
.02–.03	No observable effects. Slight euphoria and loss of shyness.
.04–.06	Feeling of well-being, relaxation, lower inhibitions, sensation of warmth. Sociable, talkative. Euphoria. Some impairment of reasoning and memory, lowering of caution.
.07–.09	Impairment of balance, speech, vision, attention span, reaction time and hearing.
.10–.12	Significant impairment of motor coordination and loss of judgment.
.13–.15	Gross motor impairment and lack of physical control. Blurred vision and major loss of balance. Euphoria is reduced and anxiety and restlessness begin.
.16–.20	Drinker appears to be "sloshed." Staggering gait. Becomes more anxious and may be nauseated.
.21–.25	Needs assistance walking, confused, restless, anxious. Likely to vomit, may be incontinent.
.26–.30	Stupor. Most people will black out at some point after entering this stage.
.31–.44	Entry into a coma. Risk of death due to respiratory arrest.
.45+	Death from respiratory arrest.

Source: Weinrath, Michael; Kaplan, Gerry. *A Summary of Research Findings on Alcohol's Effects on Driving, and the Relationship Between Fatal Crash Risk and Blood Alcohol Concentration.* Addictions Foundation of Manitoba. August, 1999. p. 23.

bly. That means limiting the amount of alcohol ingested to no more than one drink containing no more than 17 millilitres of alcohol per hour (the amount your liver can metabolize in an hour), drinking only when it is appropriate and never when you are driving, and refraining from drinking when you need good judgment.

And yet, saying no to alcohol is often easier said than done. Imagine that your friends drink alcohol every time you socialize. Either they go to a bar near campus, bring in beer and sit around and drink, or attend a party where alcohol is available. If you do not drink, they will think you are strange. You fear they might not want anything more to do with you. What can you do?

You can adopt any of the following strategies:

1. Take one drink and nurse it for a long time to limit the amount of alcohol you ingest.

2. Tell your friends you are taking medication that prohibits you from drinking.

3. Invite someone else to join you who also does not want to drink. With company, it will be easier to withstand peer group pressure.

4. Practise refusal skills in which you assertively tell your friends that you prefer not to drink. Do so without turning them off by not being judgmental. For example, you might say, "You can drink if you like but I would prefer not to." You might have to say this several times for your friends to believe that you mean it, but once they do, they will usually accept your decision.

If you do decide to drink, however, follow these guidelines:

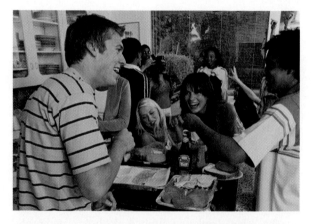

More and more, we are becoming aware of alcohol's potential negative effects, resulting in more designated drivers, alcohol-free parties, and pressure on people to control their drinking behaviour.

1. Drink in moderation.

2. Never drink on an empty stomach. Food in your stomach will slow down the absorption of the alcohol.

3. Never drink when you are taking medication.

4. Never ingest alcohol in combination with other drugs.

5. Drink slowly.

6. Dilute your drinks with water or a mixer.

7. Do not drink and eat salty or spicy foods at the same time. The salts and spices will make you thirsty, and you will drink more.

DIVERSITY ISSUES

Alcohol and Harm in Canada

In Canada's Alcohol and Other Drugs Survey, the vast majority of both current and former drinkers (79.2 percent) felt their own consumption of alcohol had not harmed them. On the other hand, 73.4 percent of all Canadians, drinkers and nondrinkers alike, say they have been harmed somehow at some point in their lives by others' drinking.

Nearly half of all Canadians (49.4 percent)—some 11 million people—had been insulted or humiliated by someone else's drinking; 34 percent had been a passenger with a drinking driver; 33.8 percent had had serious quarrels; 30.3 percent had been pushed or shoved; 18 percent had had family or marriage problems; and 15.4 percent had been physically assaulted. Alcohol abuse occurs at all age ranges and between both sexes, but in general young adults are at higher risk for alcohol-related harm.

Young adults aged 15 to 24 years are more likely to report insults, arguments, and being pushed or hit, and being a passenger with a drinking driver, than older adults. Approximately one in five current drinkers (20.3 percent) admits to driving after consuming two or more drinks, and men are almost three times as likely as women to drive after drinking. The pressures to consume large quantities of alcohol, often leading to dangerous or irresponsible behaviours, are overwhelming for some young adults, especially those in university who struggle with the transition to their new-found freedom from parental scrutiny.

With media ads often presenting alcohol consumption as the social norm, practised by successful, sophisticated, and sexually adventurous adults, accusations have been made that deliberate efforts are made to "prime" young people for a drinking lifestyle before they even reach the legal drinking age. By beguiling young people with the things they desire most in life—good times, social acceptance, and sex—it seems that the advertisers' aim is to have them slip almost unawares into an adult world where alcohol consumption is accepted as a natural and normal part of living. ✦

Sources: Adapted from: Health Canada, Minister of Supply and Services, *Canada's Alcohol and Other Drugs Survey*, 1995, Catalogue No. H39-338/1995E; J. Mintz [Chief of Marketing and Communications, Health Promotion Directorate], *The Marketing of Alcohol in Canada ... a Sobering Thought* (Ottawa: Health and Welfare Canada), quoted in *Health Education*, Summer 1984. Adapted and reproduced with the permission of the Minister of Public Works and Government Services Canada, 2003. *Health Canada assumes no responsibility for any errors or omissions which may have occurred in the adaptation of its material.*

Too many have a problem with alcohol. To determine whether you are one of these people, complete Lab Activity 11.1: Compare Your Drinking to That of Other Canadians at the end of this chapter.

◼ Alcohol on Campus

A number of strategies have been developed in response to the problems created by alcohol on university campuses. These include, but are not limited to, the following:

- Some universities have offered dry bars, that is, bars that only serve nonalcoholic beverages. Here, students can gather and meet as they do at alcoholic bars but with neither the pressure nor the opportunity to ingest alcohol.

- Some universities have offered hangover-free Friday night gatherings that include music and dancing.

- A national organization has formed to educate students about how to drink responsibly, how to prevent friends who have been drinking from experiencing problems (such as driving drunk), and how to control their own drinking. This organization, funded by the alcohol industry, is called BACCHUS (Boost Alcohol Consciousness Concerning the Health of University Students) and is now present on many campuses across Canada.

- University theatre groups have presented skits educating students regarding responsible use of alcohol.

- On many campuses, university administrators have prohibited beer kegs at parties and require that food and soft drinks be served where beer is available.

What is your campus doing to respond to both the pressure to drink and the problems resulting from the consumption of alcohol? If you decide to become proactive, you can obtain assistance from the organizations listed in Table 11.3.

*T*OBACCO

Another too-prevalent drug is tobacco and its products, including cigarettes, cigars, pipes, and chewing tobacco. The Canadian government estimates that tobacco use is responsible for over 45 000 deaths in Canada each year, which accounts for 21 percent of all deaths in Canada, and is the most preventable cause of death and disease in our society. Tobacco use is the major risk factor for: heart and blood diseases; chronic bronchitis and emphysema;

Table 11.3 ✦ Alcohol-Related Groups, Organizations, and Programs

Canadians for Safe and Sober Driving (CSSD)/Against Drunk Driving (ADD) National Office P.O. Box 397, Station "A" Brampton, ON L6V 2L3 Telephone: 905.793.4233 Fax: 905.793.7035 www.add.ca	**Alcoholics Anonymous Canada** **A.A. Central Office, Ontario** 807 Main Street West Unit B Hamilton, ON L8S 1A2 Telephone: 905.522.8399 www.aa.org	**Comité permanent de lutte à la toxicomanie** 970, rue de Louvain Est Montréal, PQ H2M 2E8 Téléphone: 514.389.6336 Télécopieur: 514.389.1830 www.msss.gouv.qc.ca/fr/organisa/organism/index.htm
Addiction Centre, Foothills Medical Centre 1403 29 Street South West Calgary, AB T2N 2T9 Telephone: 403.670.2025 Fax: 403.670.2056	**Centre for Addiction and Mental Health** 33 Russell Street Toronto, ON M5S 2S1 Telephone: 416.595.6000 www.camh.net	**Drug and Alcohol Registry of Treatment** 232 Central Ave. London, ON N6A 1M8 Telephone: 1.800.565.8603 www.dart.on.ca
Alcohol Policy Network, Ontario Public Health Association 468 Queen St. E. Suite 202 Toronto, ON M5A 1T7 Telephone: 416.367.3313 ext. 23 or 27 Fax: 416.367.2844	**Canadian Medical Association** 1867 Alta Vista Drive Ottawa, ON K1G 3Y6 Telephone: 613.731.9331 www.cma.ca	**Ontario Prevention Clearinghouse** 180 Dundas St. Suite 1900 Toronto, ON M5G 1Z8 Telephone: 1.800.565.8603 www.opc.on.ca
	Canadian Centre on Substance Abuse 75 Albert Street Suite 300 Ottawa, ON K1P 5E7 Telephone: 613.235.4048 Fax: 613.235.8101 www.ccsa.ca/	

cancers of the lung, larynx, pharynx, oral cavity, esophagus, pancreas, and bladder; and other problems such as respiratory infections and stomach ulcers. Smoking exacts both a personal and an economic toll. In 1991, the estimated economic costs of smoking to Canadian society totalled approximately $15 billion. This figure included 4 million days in hospital, 3.3 million doctor visits, 1.3 million prescriptions, and 28 million missed work days. As well, the over 45 000 deaths translates into approximately $10.6 billion in lost future income (Health Canada, 1997). Recently, a number of Canadian cities have implemented strict tobacco regulations that stipulate no smoking in workplaces and restaurants. Many business owners have been concerned and convinced that these strict regulations would reduce revenues due to decreased patronage and employee productivity. Researchers have since found that there is actually no reason for these concerns and state that "policy makers should discount industry claims that smoking regula-

tions impose undue economic hardship" (Cremieux and Ouellette, 2001, p. 33).

Smoking Rates

An estimated 21.5 percent of Canadians smoke daily (Statistics Canada, 2002). Men have a somewhat higher rate of smoking than women (23.5 percent versus 19.4 percent, respectively). In 2000/2001, Canadians aged 35–44 reported the highest levels of daily smoking (27.1 percent) followed by the 20-34-year-olds (26.1 percent), and the 45-64-year-olds (24.9 percent). Fortunately, there appears to have been a reduction in the smoking levels of teenagers (18.3 percent of 15-19-year-olds) from years past when rates were reported as high as 37 percent. It is critical that smoking rates continue to decline in all age groups; smoking is associated with mortality and a wide variety of morbidities, which makes the associated human and financial costs a continued concern for all Canadians.

DIVERSITY ISSUES

Clove and Herbal Cigarettes

Over the years, clove and herbal cigarettes have become increasingly popular. Many people are under the impression that these products are healthier alternatives to smoking tobacco. However, the smoke from any plant products—such as marijuana—may contain toxins capable of causing long-term damage to the airways and lung tissues. (Some studies show marijuana contains cancer-causing tars.) The only safe alternative is not to smoke at all.

Many people believe clove cigarettes to be tobacco-free and harmless, but studies have shown that they contain between 60–70 percent tobacco and 30–40 percent cloves. Clove cigarettes produce higher levels of tar, nicotine, and carbon monoxide than regular all-tobacco cigarettes and pose the same danger to health. There have been several reports of individuals hospitalized with life-threatening respiratory illnesses shortly after smoking clove cigarettes.

Herbal cigarettes' contents vary, depending on the manufacturer, but they may contain herbs such as red clover, and none contain tobacco or nicotine. Consequently, they are often advertised as aids to stop smoking. But, although little is known about what herbal cigarettes contain, their packages often report tar and carbon monoxide values, and the inhalation of these substances from any burning material is hazardous to health. As well, manufacturers' claims that smoking herbal cigarettes may help people to quit or reduce consumption of regular tobacco cigarettes are unproven. ✦

Source: Inventory of Canadian Tobacco Cessation Programs and Resources, Health Canada, 2000. Adapted and reproduced with the permission of the Minister of Public Works and Government Services Canada, 2003. *Health Canada assumes no responsibility for any errors or omissions which may have occurred in the adaptation of its material.*

Smokeless Tobacco

Smokeless tobacco includes primarily moist or dry snuff and chewing tobacco; many young Canadian adults, especially young men, use it. The rate of use is significantly higher among men than women. Smokeless tobacco users are quite susceptible to oral cancer, long-term snuff users being 50 times more likely to develop such cancer than nonusers. Adolescent males make up the great majority of the new users. They may see their favourite athlete (usually a baseball player) chew tobacco and emulate that behaviour.

Tobacco's Effects on the Body

Of the 45 000 people who will die this year in Canada due to tobacco use, more than 1000 will be non-smokers. Nonsmokers who live with a smoker experience severe physiological damage that puts them at elevated risks of dying from heart disease and suffering from other smoking-related diseases as well (de Groh and Morrison, 2002).

Tobacco affects the body in many ways. The nicotine in tobacco stimulates the central nervous system and therefore increases the heart rate. Tobacco use also constricts blood vessels, increases blood pressure, destroys air sacs in the lungs, and increases the production of hydrochloric acid in the stomach. The result is: shortness of breath; upset stomach; cold and clammy fingers and toes; the development of heart disease, hypertension, stroke, emphysema, and/or digestive disorders; and lung and other cancers.

Why People Use Tobacco Products

Before reading further, complete Lab Activity 11.2: Why Do You Smoke? at the end of this chapter. If you are not a smoker, complete the Lab by guessing how most smokers would respond to the statements presented.

The purpose of tobacco advertising is to sell tobacco products—and advertisers do a pretty good job of it, as the statistics just presented suggest. In our search to be desirable, envied, "cool," and admired, we are taught to emulate the people depicted in the tobacco product ads. They are handsome and pretty, they are smiling and obviously happy, and they appear wealthy enough to have fine furniture and expensive clothing.

There are other reasons people use tobacco products. They provide something to do with the hands. Best friends or parents may smoke, so their behaviour is copied. It is *anti-authority* (schools and workplaces disallow it and parents often object) and therefore "cool" to do. It relieves boredom and is psychologically relaxing for some people, in spite of it being a central nervous system stimulant. It substitutes for food and can be used to control weight.

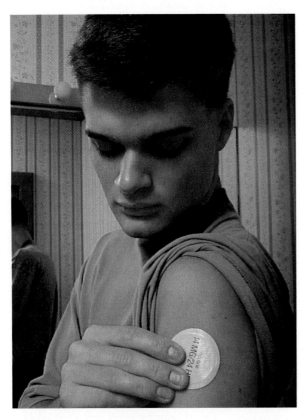

There are many methods available to smokers who truly want to quit, ranging from the nicotine patch, to nicotine gum, to a host of smoking cessation programs.

How to Quit

Researchers have found that the best way to quit smoking is simply to quit. That might sound simplistic, but what usually happens is that smokers try to quit when they are not really committed to doing so. Eventually, they reach the point at which they are well motivated and during that next attempt are successful. That is why it is difficult to cite any one program that is better than another. The key ingredient in any program is the motivation and seriousness of the smoker wishing to quit.

Imagine you smoke cigarettes and cannot seem to quit. They relax you after dinner and give you something to do with your hands during social occasions. You have tried to quit many times without any success. Do not give up. There are strategies you can employ that are effective.

You can write a *contract* using the form in Chapter 3 with the goal being to decrease the number of cigarettes you smoke progressively over several weeks until you quit altogether. The contract can be witnessed by a friend or relative who will check on your progress at predetermined intervals.

You can also use *chaining*. With this approach, you want to increase the links in the chain leading to smok-

ing. For example, you can take your pack of cigarettes and place it in a sweat sock. Then wrap the sock with masking tape and place it in a locked drawer as far away from where you usually smoke as possible (perhaps upstairs if you tend to smoke downstairs). Next, take the key to the drawer and place it in the other sock, wrap it with masking tape, and deposit it in a drawer far away from the drawer in which the pack of cigarettes is located. Now, to smoke, you have to go through a bunch of inconveniences. Compare this to simply reaching into your pocket or pocketbook and lighting up almost without thinking.

Here are some other suggestions that can help motivated smokers stop smoking or at least lessen the harm to which they expose themselves:

1. Smoke only one cigarette per hour and eventually taper down.

2. Smoke exactly half as many cigarettes each week as you did the week before.

3. Inhale less and with less vigour, avoiding deep inhalation.

4. Smoke each cigarette only halfway.

5. Remove the cigarette from your mouth between puffs.

6. Smoke slowly.

7. Smoke brands with low tar and nicotine content.

8. Place unlighted cigarettes in your mouth when you have the urge to smoke.

9. Switch to a brand you dislike.

10. Put something else in your mouth when you want a cigarette (for example, chewing gum, fruit, hard candy).

11. Exercise regularly so you do not smoke out of boredom.

12. Develop the sense of wanting to do well by your body.

13. Spend time in places where smoking is prohibited.

14. Brush your teeth directly after every meal.

15. Alter your behaviour pattern. For example, avoid friends who smoke for several weeks after quitting and substitute another activity for smoking after dinner.

16. Remind yourself frequently why you quit smoking.

17. Use the other behavioural change techniques discussed in Chapter 3 to quit smoking.

18. Speak to your physician about nicotine replacement therapy.

DRUG-TAKING TO ENHANCE ATHLETIC PERFORMANCE

Athletes are competitive by nature. They try hard to beat someone else in their sport or, competing against themselves, strive to do better than they have ever done before. It stands to reason they would want whatever edge they can get. This desire to perform at their best has led some athletes to a search for drugs that can enhance performance. Among these drugs are anabolic steroids, caffeine, amphetamines, and cocaine.

Anabolic Steroids

So you want to be strong? So you want to run faster than you ever thought you could? Well, forget about all the work of weight training or exercise that makes you perspire. Try steroids. In today's quick-weight-loss, quick-fitness, quick-everything society, why not engage in quick bulking up? As we will soon see, the reason not to is simple: anabolic steroids are quite dangerous.

Anabolic steroids made the news when Olympic world record holder Ben Johnson was disqualified from receiving a gold medal for winning the 100-metre sprint at the 1988 Olympic Games. When he was routinely tested just after the race, Johnson tested positive for a steroid. The death of former professional football player Lyle Alzado of cancer, which was attributed to anabolic steroid use in an attempt to gain strength, also fuelled publicity about these drugs.

Anabolic steroids are derivatives of the male sex hormone testosterone. They are prescribed as treatment for anemia and growth problems and as an aid in recovery from surgery. A black market has developed, however, and steroids are illegally used to increase body weight and muscle mass, gain power, and increase strength.

Steroids can be taken in pill form or injected directly into the bloodstream. It is not unusual for steroid users to take more than one steroid at a time, believing that the effect will be hastened or enhanced. This is called *stacking*.

Steroid users place themselves at risk for liver cancer, high blood pressure, heart disease, and sterility. In men, steroid use can lead to atrophied testicles, prostate cancer, and breast growth. In women, it can result in menstrual irregularities, deepening of the voice, decreased breast size, baldness, and facial hair growth. In both men and women, anabolic steroid use can lead to clogging of the arteries, eating compulsions, and increased aggressiveness, and hostility.

The *Physician's Desk Reference* (p. 2122) states that "anabolic steroids have not been shown to enhance athletic ability." Still, a recent study found that as many as 83 000 young Canadians between the ages of 11 and 18 have used steroids in the past year. Fifty-four percent of male users say they use steroids to be better in sports and almost half say that they use steroids to improve their looks (Health Canada, Nutrition Web page).

Suppose, in the gym in which you work out, there are many men and women your age who look fantastic. The men are chiselled. Their muscles are round and hard, and they do not have a gram of fat on them—or so it seems. And the women are curved to perfection.

WELLNESS HEROES

Dying to Win

Dr. Bob Goldman, former world-class athlete, leading steroid expert, chair of Athletes Against Drug Abuse Canada, and author of the *Death in the Locker Room* books exposing steroid use in Olympic-level athletics, is perhaps most famous for one thing. Every two years since 1982 he has conducted an informal survey asking world-class athletes the following question: "If I had a magic drug that was so fantastic that if you took it once you would win every competition you would enter, from the Olympic decathlon to Mr. Universe, for the next five years, but it had one drawback—it would kill you five years after you took it—would you take the drug?" When he posed this question to 198 athletes in 1984 before the Summer Olympics, the results were shocking: Of those asked, 103 (52 percent) said yes. Winning was so attractive that they would not only be willing to achieve it by taking a pill (in other words, through an outlawed, unfair method—in effect, cheating), but also give their lives to do it. ✦

Source: Bob Goldman, 1987. Cited in J. Le Clair, *Winners and Losers: Sport and Physical Activity in the 90s* (Toronto: Thomson Educational Publishing, 1992), p. 288; T. Blair and R. Usher, "May the Best Drug Win," *Time*, August 1998, 152 (6).

Anabolic steroids Drugs that are derivatives of the male sex hormone testosterone; sometimes used illegally by those desiring to increase their body size, speed, or strength.

MYTH AND FACT SHEET

Myth	Fact
1. Beer will not get you as drunk as hard liquor will.	1. It is the alcohol that is responsible for inebriation. You can ingest just as much alcohol from beer as you can from other sources.
2. Drinking alcohol is relaxing.	2. A small amount of alcohol initially acts as a stimulant. Larger amounts depress the central nervous system. The feeling of relaxation, however, arises because the brain is deadened. The price paid is that other bodily functions are depressed as well, such as the ability to think clearly or be coordinated. The result can be accidents or poor decisions that lead to injury or ill health.
3. The use of marijuana, cocaine, and similar drugs is the major "drug problem" on university campuses.	3. Alcohol is both the most prevalent and frequently abused drug on university campuses. Alcohol intoxication can lead to vandalism, fights, and other behaviours resulting in suspension or expulsion from school, not to mention the legal consequences.
4. Being physically fit and possessing a high level of wellness means never using drugs.	4. We all use drugs. We take prescribed antibiotics, we buy over-the-counter cold remedies, and we ingest aspirin or ibuprofen when our muscles ache. The key is to use safe drugs safely, as they were intended to be used.

They have muscles in all the right places and are round where they should be round. But you learn that they take steroids. Without the drugs, you are told, they would not look so good. You would love to look like they do and are tempted to try these drugs. How can you overcome this temptation?

You can always use *selective awareness*. Instead of focusing on how good you could look if you took steroids, concentrate on their potential effect on your liver, your sexual organs (atrophied or shrunken testicles if you are a male and menstrual irregularities if you are a female), and the threat they pose to your life. Imagine yourself as a perfectly chiselled corpse.

You could also use *covert modelling*. After watching someone weight-train who looks good and does not take steroids, close your eyes and imagine you are doing just what you observed the other person doing. Smell the smells, hear the noise, see the sights, and so forth. Make it vivid. Refer back to Chapter 3 for other ways to take charge of your behaviour.

Caffeine

Caffeine is a stimulant drug that appears in coffee, tea, chocolate, and soft drinks. It can activate the brain, decreasing drowsiness and fatigue, and it increases heart and breathing rates. In addition, caffeine stimulates skeletal muscles and enables the body to use fatty acids for energy. The result is an increase in physical-work output. That is why caffeine has been suggested as an aid to physical fitness and athletic activities.

Caffeine consumption as an adjunct to physical activity, however, is not recommended because caffeine can have serious side-effects. Depending on the dosage, caffeine can result in irregular heart beat, hyperactivity, headaches, insomnia, an increase in low-density lipoprotein (LDL), which is associated with coronary heart disease, and low birth weight when consumed by pregnant women.

Amphetamines

Amphetamines are drugs that stimulate the central nervous system. They result in increased heart rate, blood pressure, rate of breathing, and blood sugar and in high arousal levels. It is this psychological-arousal effect, along with the physiological-arousal effects, that disguises muscle fatigue so greater work output can occur.

Amphetamines should not be used to increase work output for several reasons. First, there is no evidence that their use enhances athletic performance. In fact, they may even interfere with athletic performance by increasing

BEHAVIOURAL CHANGE AND MOTIVATIONAL STRATEGIES

There are many things that might interfere with your healthy use of chemical substances. Here are some barriers (roadblocks) and strategies for overcoming them.

Roadblock	Behavioural Change Strategy
You want to quit smoking but are afraid you will gain weight. Your looks are important to you. Therefore, you decide not to stop smoking in order to look better.	Many smokers say they continue to smoke because they are afraid of gaining weight. And yet most smokers do not gain weight when they quit. In fact, only one-third gain weight, another one-third stay the same weight, and the rest actually lose weight. Even when weight gain does occur, it is usually minimal and certainly worth the health benefits of not smoking.
Weight gain is only one of the excuses smokers use for not quitting. Others include "The air is polluted anyway, I might as well smoke" and "It's too late to quit, I've been smoking too long."	Knowledge can go a long way in dispelling these myths. The truth is that even in heavily polluted urban areas, the concentration of pollutants in the air is tiny in comparison with the concentrations in cigarette smoke. Regarding smoking for a long time, it is never too late to prevent a serious disease. After you quit, your chances of dying from smoke-related diseases gradually decrease until they are close to those of people who have never smoked.
You have an important exam next Tuesday so you plan to stay up all Monday night studying. Around one o'clock Tuesday morning, however, you start feeling drowsy, so you think about drinking a large amount of caffeine to keep going.	Of course, the best strategy is to plan to study for several nights rather than pulling an all-nighter. But, given that you did not follow this advice, you can use selective awareness to focus on the benefits you will derive from getting some sleep. It will make your learning more efficient because you will not be drugged; it will be healthier; and you will be more alert during the exam. A few hours of sleep can do wonders for your performance. You can also focus on the negative aspects of ingesting a lot of caffeine. After all, who wants to subject themselves to heart problems? A bad grade on an exam is preferable to a bad electrocardiogram (ECG).
List roadblocks interfering with your using chemicals appropriately. 1. _____ 2. _____ 3. _____	Now cite behavioural change strategies that can help you overcome the roadblocks you just listed. If you need to, refer back to Chapter 3 for behavioural change and motivational strategies. 1. _____ 2. _____ 3. _____

hyperactivity when more-controlled physical responses are needed. Second, amphetamine users often become dependent on these drugs and resort to taking barbiturates to come down from an amphetamine high. This yo-yo drugging effect can be quite dangerous. Not enough people know that barbiturates are extremely addictive and that withdrawing from them without medical supervision can be deadly.

Caffeine A stimulant drug present in coffee, tea, and colas and other soft drinks that have not been decaffeinated.

Amphetamines Drugs that stimulate the central nervous system, increasing heart rate, blood pressure, and other body processes.

Cocaine

Cocaine is another drug people take to improve physical performance or for "recreational" reasons, though less than 1 percent of Canadians currently use it. Cocaine can be snorted through the nose, smoked as crack, or

> **Cocaine** A drug that stimulates the central nervous system and that can cause tremors, rapid heartbeat, and harmful psychological effects.

injected. It, too, can increase work output by the nature of its stimulating effect on the central nervous system. It also produces a euphoria that disguises fatigue.

However, not only is cocaine illegal, but it can result in dire health consequences. It can cause tremors and rapid heartbeat, raise blood pressure dangerously high to the point of threatening stroke, lower the effectiveness of the immune system, and decrease appetite resulting in malnutrition. In addition, it can cause acute anxiety, confusion, and depression. In a few cases, *cocaine psychosis* has occurred in heavy users, leading to delusions and violence.

SUMMARY

Drug Use, Misuse, and Abuse

When drugs are used as they are recommended and for the purposes for which they were recommended, that is drug use. When a legal drug is used inappropriately, that is drug misuse. When an illegal drug is used or a legal drug is used for purposes other than those for which it was intended, that is drug abuse.

Alcohol

Alcohol is the most prevalent drug on university campuses. It dilates blood vessels in the head, causing headaches; narrows the blood vessels supplying the heart; damages cells in the liver; often leads to malnutrition, endocrine, and reproductive system problems; and can cause cancer at several body sites.

Drinking responsibly means not getting inebriated by limiting the amount of alcohol ingested to no more than one average-sized drink (17 mL of alcohol) an hour, drinking only when appropriate, never drinking and driving, and refraining from drinking when good judgment is needed. To control drinking, drink in moderation, never drink on an empty stomach, never drink when taking medication, never ingest alcohol in combination with other drugs, drink slowly, dilute drinks, and do not eat salty or spicy foods when drinking.

Tobacco

Tobacco use is the most preventable cause of death in Canada. It is the major risk factor for heart and blood diseases; chronic bronchitis and emphysema; cancers of the lung, larynx, pharynx, oral cavity, esophagus, pancreas, and bladder; and other problems such as respiratory infections and stomach ulcers. These health concerns are true for smokers and for those exposed to secondhand smoke.

Tobacco use constricts blood vessels, increases blood pressure, destroys air sacs in the lungs, and increases the production of hydrochloric acid in the stomach. The results are shortness of breath; upset stomach; cold and clammy fingers and toes; the development of heart disease, hypertension, stroke, emphysema, and digestive disorders; and lung and other cancers.

To quit, or cut down on, smoking, smoke only one cigarette an hour, smoke only half the cigarette, inhale less, smoke slowly, smoke brands you dislike, place unlighted cigarettes in your mouth when you get the urge, exercise regularly as a diversion, and spend time in places where smoking is prohibited.

Drug-Taking to Enhance Athletic Performance

Among the drugs taken in an attempt to improve on athletic performance are anabolic steroids, caffeine, amphetamines, and cocaine. All of these drugs present a serious threat to health.

Anabolic steroids place the user at increased risk for liver cancer, high blood pressure, heart disease, and sterility. In men, it can lead to atrophied testicles, prostate cancer, and breast growth. In women, it can result in menstrual irregularities, a deepening of the voice, decreased breast size, baldness, and facial hair growth. In both men and women, anabolic steroid use can lead to clogging of the arteries, eating compulsions, and increased aggressiveness and hostility.

Caffeine is a stimulant. It increases heart and breathing rates, enables skeletal muscles to use fatty acids for energy more efficiently, and decreases fatigue and drowsiness. Caffeine, however, can have serious side-effects depending on the amount ingested: irregular heartbeat, hyperactivity, headache, insomnia, an increase in LDL (associated with coronary disease), and low birth weight when consumed by pregnant women.

Amphetamines and cocaine are also stimulants. They can create feelings of psychological and physiological arousal. However, they are drugs on which people can become dependent, and they can cause serious cardiac problems that can even result in death.

STUDY QUESTIONS

1. What are the effects of alcohol and tobacco on the body?

2. What strategies can you employ to drink responsibly and/or to avoid drinking when you feel pressured into doing so?

3. How have strict smoking regulations impacted the profit margins of restaurants and businesses and

what is being recommended to policymakers because of this effect?

4. What risks are associated with exposure to second-hand smoke?

5. What suggestions would you offer to help someone who wants to quit smoking?

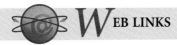

WEB LINKS

Health Canada
www.hc-sc.gc.ca

Quit For Life
www.quit4life.com/

Physicians for a Smoke-Free Canada
www.smoke-free.ca/

Against Drunk Driving Canada
www.add.ca

Canadian Centre on Substance Abuse
www.ccsa.ca

World Health Organization Programme on Substance Abuse
www.who.int/psa/

REFERENCES

Cremieux, P., and P. Ouellette. "Actual and Perceived Impacts of Tobacco Regulation on Restaurants and Firms." *Tobacco Control* 10, 1 (2001): 33–7.

De Groh, M., and H. Morrison. "Environmental Tobacco Smoke and Deaths from Coronary Heart Disease in Canada." *Chronic Diseases in Canada* 23, 1 (2002).

Health Canada, Health Protection Branch, Laboratory for Disease Control. *Heart Disease and Stroke in Canada,* 1997.

Health Canada, Minister of Supply and Services, *Canada's Alcohol and Other Drugs Survey,* 1995, Catalogue No. H39-338/1995E.

Health Canada, Ministry of Supply and Services. *National Population Health Survey Highlights; Smoking Behaviour of Canadians,* cycle 2, 1996/97. January 1999.

Physician's Desk Reference: PDR. Oradell, N.J.: Medical Economics Co., 1974–2003.

PRIDE. *Press Release: Student Use of Most Drugs Reaches Highest Level in Nine Years—Most Report Getting "Very High, Bombed, or Stoned."* Atlanta: PRIDE, September 25, 1996.

Single, E., L. Robson, X. Xiaodi, and R. Jürgen. [In collaboration with R. Moore, B. Choi, S. Desjardins, and J. Anderson, *The Costs of Substance Abuse in Canada; Highlights of a major study of the health, social and economic costs associated with the use of alcohol, tobacco and illicit drugs.* Canadian Centre on Substance Abuse (1996).

Statistics Canada, CANSIM II, table 105-0027 and Catalogue no. 82-221-X1E. January 2002.

Substance Abuse and Mental Health Services Administration. *Preliminary Estimates from the 1995 National Household Survey on Drug Abuse.* Rockville, MD: Substance Abuse and Mental Health Services Administration, August 1996.

U.S. Department of Health and Human Services. *Prevention Resource Guide: College Youth.* Washington, DC: DHHS, 1991. Pub. No. (ADM) 91-1803.

U.S. Department of Health and Human Services. *Healthy People: National Health Promotion and Disease Prevention Objectives.* Washington, DC: U.S. Government Printing Office, 1991. Pub. No. (PHS) 91-50212.

Name _____

Date _____

Lab Activity 11.1

Compare Your Drinking to That of Other Canadians

Take this simple test to find out how your drinking habits compare with those of other Canadians.

◆ **1. What was your drinking like during a typical week in the past year?**

List roughly how many drinks you had on each day of a typical week and add up the total:

Monday _____

Tuesday _____

Wednesday _____

Thursday _____

Friday _____

Saturday _____

Sunday _____

TOTAL _____

Be sure to estimate the number of "standard" drinks you usually have. Each of the drinks on the chart below have the same amount of alcohol in them and will all affect you in the same way.

One standard drink is:

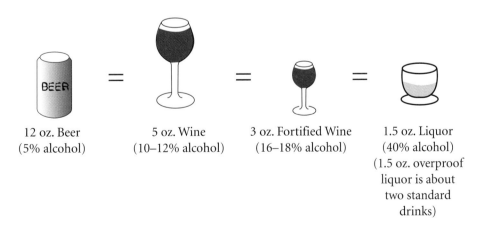

12 oz. Beer
(5% alcohol)

5 oz. Wine
(10–12% alcohol)

3 oz. Fortified Wine
(16–18% alcohol)

1.5 oz. Liquor
(40% alcohol)
(1.5 oz. overproof
liquor is about
two standard
drinks)

(continued)

Lab Activity 11.1 *(continued)*
Compare Your Drinking to That of Other Canadians

✦ **2. Now compare your weekly total to that of other Canadians.**

How does your weekly average compare? Look at the pie charts below to find where your drinking fits with the rest of the adult population. For example, if you are a male who drinks 15 standard drinks per week, you drink more alcohol than 90 percent of other men in Canada do.

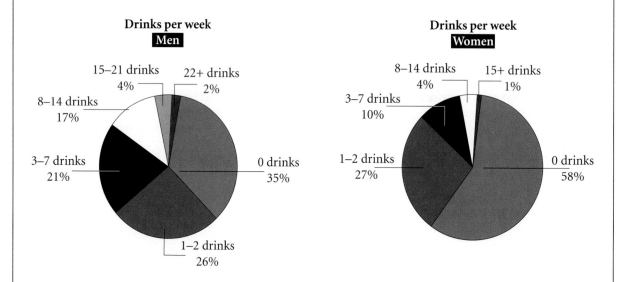

✦ **3. Risky drinking.**

A recent national survey looked at how much people drank in a week and how their drinking was affecting different areas of their lives. People were asked about their physical health, outlook on life, friends/social life, relationships with their spouses or partners and children, home life, financial position, and work or studies. Not surprisingly, the results showed that the more people drank in a week, the greater the chance that the drinking was affecting more and more areas of their lives.

How likely are you to have problems as a result of your drinking? Look at the chart below to see where you fit.

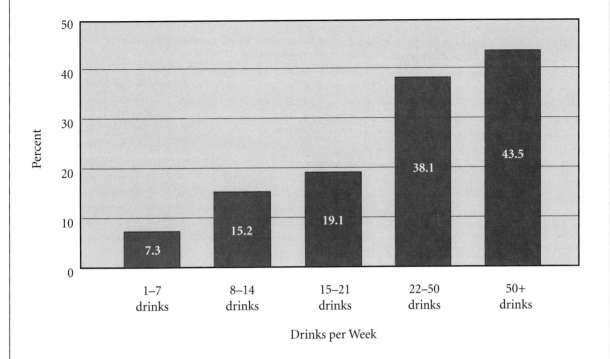

Drinks per Week

Your choices about drinking

Are you concerned about your drinking? Take a look at the options below to see if there is anything you would like to do right now. It is your choice.

- My drinking is fine for now. I will continue to watch how much I drink.

- I will think about changing my drinking. Did you know that 75 percent of people change their drinking on their own?

- I will reduce my drinking to a low-risk level. This means I will drink no more than two drinks a day, with a weekly maximum of 14 drinks for men and nine drinks for women. Most people watch their drinking—they put limits on how much, when and where they drink. To avoid intoxication, they drink slowly, waiting at least one hour between drinks. They have food and non-alcoholic drinks along with alcohol. They have at least one or two days a week without any alcohol. And they don't drive or operate heavy equipment after drinking. Women who are pregnant, trying to conceive, or are breast-feeding are encouraged not to consume any alcohol.

(continued)

Lab Activity 11.1 *(continued)*
Compare Your Drinking to That of Other Canadians

- I will contact the Drug and Alcohol Registry of Treatment (DART) to find out about other programs and groups that can help me or someone that I am concerned about. (Call toll free 1-800-565-8603.)

For more information on addiction and mental health issues, or a copy of this brochure, please contact the Centre for Addiction and Mental Health's 24-hour Information Line:

Ontario toll-free: 1-800-463-6273
Toronto: 416-595-6111

Source: Reprinted with permission by the Centre for Addiction and Mental Health © 2002. Available at **www.camh.net/ addiction/pims/evaluate_your_drinking.html**. Accessed March 14, 2003

Lab Activity 11.2

Why Do You Smoke?

INSTRUCTIONS: *Here are some statements made by people to describe what they get out of smoking cigarettes. If you are a smoker, how often do you feel this way when smoking cigarettes? If you are not a smoker, how often do you think smokers feel this way when they smoke? Perhaps responding to these questions, even if you do not smoke cigarettes, will help you better understand why other people smoke. Circle one number for each statement.* **Important: Answer all statements**.

	Always	Frequently	Occasionally	Seldom	Never
A. I smoke cigarettes in order to keep myself from slowing down.	5	4	3	2	1
B. Handling a cigarette is part of the enjoyment of smoking it.	5	4	3	2	1
C. Smoking cigarettes is pleasant and relaxing.	5	4	3	2	1
D. I light up a cigarette when I feel angry about something.	5	4	3	2	1
E. When I have run out of cigarettes, I find it almost unbearable until I can get them.	5	4	3	2	1
F. I smoke cigarettes automatically without even being aware of it.	5	4	3	2	1
G. I smoke cigarettes to stimulate myself, to perk myself up.	5	4	3	2	1
H. Part of the enjoyment of smoking a cigarette comes from the steps I take to light it up.	5	4	3	2	1
I. I find cigarettes pleasurable.	5	4	3	2	1
J. When I feel uncomfortable or upset about something, I light up a cigarette.	5	4	3	2	1
K. I am very much aware of it when I am not smoking a cigarette.	5	4	3	2	1
L. I light a cigarette without realizing I still have one burning in the ashtray.	5	4	3	2	1
M. I smoke cigarettes to give myself a "lift."	5	4	3	2	1
N. When I smoke a cigarette, part of the enjoyment is watching the smoke as I exhale it.	5	4	3	2	1

(continued)

	Always	Frequently	Occasionally	Seldom	Never
O. I want a cigarette most when I am comfortable and relaxed.	5	4	3	2	1
P. When I feel "blue" or want to take my mind off cares and worries, I smoke cigarettes.	5	4	3	2	1
Q. I get a real gnawing hunger for a cigarette when I haven't smoked for a while.	5	4	3	2	1
R. I've found a cigarette in my mouth and didn't remember putting it there.	5	4	3	2	1

Scoring

1. Enter the numbers you have circled in the test questions in the spaces below, putting the number you have circled for question A over line A, for question B over line B, and so on.
2. Add the three scores on each line to get your totals. For example, the sum of your scores over lines A, G, and M gives you your score on Stimulation; lines B, H, and N give the score on Handling, and so on.

Scores	Totals	Comment
___ + ___ + ___ = A G M	_____ Stimulation	11 or above suggests you are stimulated by the cigarette to get going and keep going. To stop smoking, try a brisk walk or exercise when the smoking urge is present.
___ + ___ + ___ = B H N	_____ Handling	11 or above suggests satisfaction from handling the cigarette. Substituting a pencil or paper clip or doodling may aid in breaking the habit.
___ + ___ + ___ = C I O	_____ Pleasurable relaxation	11 or above suggests you receive pleasure from smoking. For this type of smoker, substitution of other pleasant habits (eating, social activities, exercise) may aid in eliminating smoking.
___ + ___ + ___ = D J P	_____ Crutch: tension reduction	11 or above suggests you use cigarettes to handle moments of stress or discomfort. Substitution of social activities, eating, or handling other objects may aid in stopping.
___ + ___ + ___ = E K Q	_____ Craving: psychological addictions	11 or above suggests an almost continuous psychological craving for a cigarette. "Cold turkey" may be your best method of breaking the smoking habit.
___ + ___ + ___ = F L R	_____ Habit	11 or above suggests you smoke out of mere habit and may acquire little satisfaction from the process. Gradually reducing the number of cigarettes you smoke may be effective in helping you to stop.

Scores can vary from 3 to 15. Any score of 11 or above is *high*; any score of 7 and below is *low*.

Source: Reproduced with permission of the Nova Scotia Department of Health.

12

Exploring, Preventing, and Treating Exercise and Physical-Activity Injuries

CHAPTER OBJECTIVES

By the end of this chapter, you should be able to:

1. Explain an 11-point injury-prevention plan for someone who is about to begin a new exercise program.

2. Describe the body's response to soft-tissue injury and the three stages of healing.

3. Discuss the correct use of cold, heat, and massage in the emergency treatment of exercise injuries.

4. Demonstrate the correct technique of PRICE therapy in the treatment of an ankle sprain and other soft-tissue injuries.

5. Describe the proper use of common over-the-counter and prescription drugs for the treatment of soft-tissue injuries.

6. Describe the proper emergency treatment for at least 25 common exercise injuries.

MOST OF LEE's friends exercise regularly. Some jog, cycle, and swim; others engage in aerobic exercise classes, or play sports such as tennis, racquetball, basketball, soccer, and touch football. At one time or other, it seems as if every one of them has experienced an injury of some sort. Sprained ankles, torn Achilles tendons, sore knees and backs, and inflamed shoulders and elbows are just a few of the complaints Lee hears. Lee feels good most of the time although her weight is creeping upward and she is generally tired by late afternoon. If it were not for the risk of injury, Lee would join her friends in an aerobic activity she enjoys.

This chapter presents a program designed to keep Lee injury-free while she receives the full benefits of an exercise program of her choice. Although there are no guarantees, the information in this chapter can significantly reduce Lee's risk of injury.

Entering into an exercise program involves a slight risk of injury or illness during the first month or so. Later, a key benefit of improved conditioning is the reduction in the incidence and severity of serious exercise-, job-, and home-related injuries. The danger of injury increases considerably when you fail to follow simple rules of training. For the "weekend athlete," exercise can be very dangerous. This chapter is designed to help you avoid common hazards and to make exercise a safe, enjoyable experience. It includes 11 steps for injury prevention for your body; discusses how tissue responds to injury; describes the proper use of cold, heat and massage; provides basic treatment procedures for common injuries and illnesses; and discusses the special injury-proofing problems of women.

PROTECTING YOUR BODY FROM INJURY AND ILLNESS

Common sense and the application of some basic conditioning concepts can eliminate the majority of risks in most exercise programs. The 11-point injury-prevention program that follows is designed to help minimize your risk of injury and initiate a sound, safe fitness program.

Analyze Your Medical History Before You Begin

If you are over 40 years of age, have been inactive for more than 2–3 years regardless of age, or are in a high-risk group (obese, hypertense, diabetic, high blood lipids), a thorough physical examination is recommended. A qualified personal or professional exercise trainer can also check your heart rate and blood pressure during exercise on a stationary bicycle to secure valuable information about how you will respond to a program. Although the chances of a serious problem are slight for young people, the adage "Better safe than sorry" still applies.

Competitive athletes, on the other hand, may need special attention. Although sudden death is rare (1 in 200 000 high school athletes dies while on the practice or playing field or arena), the occasional

tragedy does occur, and it always gets considerable media attention. It is nearly impossible to eliminate all potentially fatal conditions in spite of rigorous screening. If you suspect an inherited disorder or abnormality, ask your physician to secure a careful medical history from family members.

Improve Your General Conditioning Level

You need to be extra careful in the first month of a new exercise program when you are particularly vulnerable to muscle, joint, **ligament**, tendon, **cartilage**, and other **soft-tissue** injuries. Injuries of all types are also more likely to occur when you are generally fatigued because the blood supply to muscles is reduced, muscle fibres are somewhat devitalized and easily torn, and joint stability and muscle groups are weakened. A state of general fatigue is common during the early stages of an exercise program. Strengthening the injury-prone areas such as the ankles, wrists, knees, shoulders, lower back, and neck (see Chapter 6) before beginning a new program will help reduce the incidence of fatigue-related injuries.

Warm Up Properly Before Each Workout

Warming up is not the same as stretching. A warm-up raises your body temperature 1–2 degrees to prepare muscles, ligaments, and tendons for vigorous movement. A good rule of thumb for warm-up is to reach the point of just starting to sweat. A fast walk, a slow jog, or a mild form of exercise specific to your workout activity for 4–5 minutes to elevate core temperature, followed by several minutes of stretching, will help prevent muscle pulls, strains, sprains, and lower-back discomfort and reduce muscle soreness that may occur 8–24 hours later (see Chapter 7). In general, the closer the nature of the warm-up activity to the workout activity, the better for your body.

Cool Down at the End of Each Exercise Session

The cool-down is a key phase of the fitness workout that should be enjoyed rather than avoided. Experienced joggers or runners, for example, complete the final 0.8–1.6 kilometres at a slow, easy pace rather than with a kick or sprint. The final 3–5 minutes of any workout should also include several minutes of stretching as the body cools and slowly returns to a near-resting state (see Chapter 4). The cool-down will reduce the

Ligament Fibrous bands or folds that support organs, hold bones together, or help anchor muscles to the bones they act on.

Cartilage Fibrous connective tissue between the surfaces of movable and immovable joints.

Soft tissue Tissue other than bone.

incidence of injury during this fatigued state of your workout and decrease muscle soreness the next day.

Progress Slowly

It is wise to add only small increments to your workout each exercise session. Too much, too soon is a common cause of muscular injuries. Plan your program over a 3-to-6-month period to maximize enjoyment and minimize pain and the risk of injury.

Table 12.1 classifies runners, a group that typically tends to add extra distance too soon, according to mileage and pace and identifies the injuries common to each group. Within each category, injuries are often the result of excessive distance, intensive workouts, and a rapid increase in distance over a short time period. Compounding the problem is running surface (a soft, level surface is preferred); running up and down curbs, which increases shock to the legs, feet, and back; sloping or banked roads, which force the foot on the higher part of the slope to twist inward excessively; overstressing tendons and ligaments; or uphill (strains the Achilles tendon and lower-back muscles) and downhill (increases the force to the heel) running. Complete Lab Activity 12.1: Evaluating Your Potential for Foot and Leg Injuries at the end of this chapter. Also, regular checks of the soles of your running shoes are important; a sole worn even half a centimetre when multiplied by thousands of footfalls can have serious repetitive effects on joints and soft tissues.

In your workout you should also avoid increasing your heart rate to more than 60 percent of your maximum the first 2–4 weeks. After this acclimation period, you can train at higher heart rates more safely.

Alternate Light- and Heavy-Workout Days

Many people make the mistake of trying to exercise hard every day. The body then does not have adequate time to repair or rebuild, and the full benefit of each workout may not be realized. In addition, injuries, boredom, and peaking out early are much more likely to occur. The chance of an exercise-related injury can be reduced by alternating light- and heavy-workout days each week.

Avoid the "Weekend Athlete" Approach to Fitness

One sure way to guarantee numerous injuries and illnesses is to exercise vigorously only on weekends. The older "weekend athlete" is particularly susceptible to heart attack, while individuals of all ages increase their chances of soft-tissue injuries to muscles, tendons, and ligaments.

In the early spring of each year and during the first major snowfall, 25–50 men in Canada die of heart attacks. The early-spring victims are generally middle-aged men who recently purchased a pair of $200 running shoes and decided to get in shape in just one workout. The 8-kilometre run usually attempted is often the first time this person has exercised in the past year. Or the snow shovelling after the first major snowfall is the first exposure to exercise since the previous winter. For these individuals, who may already be at risk for disease, the result is often fatal. These deaths can probably be prevented by a few months of walking and light strength training as a means of preconditioning.

Occasionally death occurs after unaccustomed exertion in cold weather even though an autopsy reveals no

Table 12.1 ✦ Classification of Runners and Potential Injuries

CLASSIFICATION	DISTANCE	POTENTIAL INJURIES
Jogger or novice runner	4.8–32.2 kilometres per week at 9–12 minutes per kilometre	Shin splints, chondromalacia, runner's knee, soreness, hamstring strains, and lower back pain
Sports runner	32.2–64.4 kilometres per week, participant in fun runs and races of 4.8–9.7 kilometres	Achilles tendinitis, stress fractures
Long distance runner	64.4–112.7 kilometres per week at 4.4–5.0 minutes per kilometre; may compete in 10 000 metres (10.0 kilometres) or marathons (42.2 kilometres)	More serious injuries to thigh, calf, and back; sciatica and tendon pulls
Elite marathoner	112.7–321.9 kilometres per week at 3.1–4.4 minutes per kilometre	Stress fractures, acute muscle strain in the back, sciatica

Source: © 1986 Ciba-Geigy Corporation. Reprinted with permission from David M. Brody, MD, and Frank H. Netter, MD, "Running Injuries," *Clinical Symposia* 32 (1986) (4) illustrated by Frank H. Netter, MD.

signs of a heart attack. While this condition is rare, it is a possibility when men and women try to do it all in one weekend workout. Cold air constricts the blood vessels of the skin and increases blood pressure slightly. Vigorous exercise also increases blood pressure, heart rate, and the oxygen needs of the heart dramatically. Without proper warm-up and with the presence of hidden signs of heart disease, a heart attack may occur. If one exercises outdoors regularly, throughout the seasons, the body gradually acclimatizes to seasonal decreases in temperature. Assuming proper use of layers of clothing, the danger of freezing your lungs in cold Canadian weather is slight except under extreme conditions.

If the weekend is the only time you can exercise, avoid long bouts in extremes of hot or cold weather and strenuous exercise (jogging, running, racquetball, handball, tennis, basketball, soccer, rugby, and so on) unless you take frequent breaks. Consider supplementing your weekend routine with one other workout during the week. After one month, try increasing to two workouts during the week in addition to one on weekends. If you choose an aerobic activity and progress slowly for several months, you can minimize the risk of serious illness or injury. With a total of three workouts weekly, you have the foundation for a good conditioning program.

■ Pay Close Attention to Your Body Signals

Pain and other distress signals during exercise should not be ignored. Although some breathing discomfort and breathlessness is common and minor pain may be present in joints or muscles, severe, persistent, and particularly sharp pain is a warning sign to stop exercising. Also stop exercising immediately if you notice any abnormal heart action (pulse irregularity, fluttering, palpitations in the chest or throat, rapid heartbeats); pain or pressure in the chest, teeth, jaw, neck, or arms; dizziness; lightheadedness; cold sweat; or confusion.

Paying attention to your body can also help you detect the early onset of heat-related injuries that commonly occur in hot, humid weather during an exercise session. Early awareness and treatment can prevent heat exhaustion and heat stroke and the possible serious health consequences of these conditions. If you experience any of the symptoms described in Table 12.2, stop exercising immediately, begin the suggested treatment, and seek medical attention. A careful look at your diet, including fluid intake (water, juice, electrolyte drinks), may also help explain why a specific heat-related problem tends to recur and help you eliminate the problem in the future. Ingesting water (hydrating) and/or glucose

Table 12.2 ✦ Heat Injuries: Causes, Clinical Findings, and Treatment

HEAT INJURIES	CAUSES	CLINICAL FINDINGS	TREATMENT
Heat syncope	Excessive vasodilation; pooling of blood in the skin	Fainting, weaknesses, fatigue	Place on back in cool environment; give cool fluids
Heat cramps	Excessive loss of electrolytes in sweat; inadequate salt intake	Cramps	Rest in cool environment; ingest salt drinks; salt foods daily; get medical treatment in severe cases
Salt-depletion heat exhaustion	Excessive loss of electrolytes in sweat; inadequate salt intake	Nausea, fatigue, fainting, cramps	Rest in cool environment; replace fluids and salt by mouth; get medical treatment in severe cases
Water-depletion heat exhaustion	Excessive loss of sweat; inadequate fluid intake	Fatigue, nausea, cool pale skin, active sweating, rectal temperature lower than 40° C	Rest in cool environment; drink cool fluids; cool body with water; get medical treatment if serious
Anhidrotic heat exhaustion	Same as water-depletion heat exhaustion	Nausea, sweating stopped, dry skin, rectal temperature lower than 40° C	Same as water-depletion heat exhaustion
Heat stroke	Excessive body temperature	Headache, disorientation, unconsciousness, rectal temperature greater than 41° C	Cool body immediately to 38.9° C with ice packs, cold water; give cool drinks with glucose if conscious; get medical help immediately

beverages before, during, and after activity is always wise in order to avoid dehydration.

Exercise may also be inadvisable for some persons afflicted with certain medical conditions. Study Table 12.3 to identify the adjustments that you should make when you are ill, injured, or suffering from a medical condition that requires modifications. When you are obviously ill or not up to par, avoid exercise, rest a few days, and return to a lower level or an easier workout.

After each workout, let your body analyze the severity of your exercise session. The workout was probably too light if you did not sweat, and it was too heavy if you were still breathless 10 minutes after you stopped exercising, your pulse rate was above 120 beats per minute 5 minutes after stopping, prolonged fatigue remained for more than 24 hours, nausea or vomiting occurred, or sleep was interrupted. To remedy these symptoms in the future, exercise less vigorously and lengthen your cool-down period. Use the "talk test": if you cannot carry on a conversation while exercising, you are probably working out too hard.

Master the Proper Form in Your Activity

For all activities, correct form improves efficiency and reduces the risk of injury. Proper running form, for example, is important to most fitness programs. Joggers should avoid running on the toes, which produces soreness in the calf muscles. The heel should strike the ground first before rolling the weight along the bottom and out-side of the foot to the toes for the pushoff. A number of other running-form problems often produce mild muscle or joint strain.

Participants in racquet sports are also susceptible to numerous form-related injuries (elbow, shoulder, and wrist inflammation and lower-back problems) from faulty stroke mechanics such as elbow-led ground strokes, bent-elbow hits, muscles not firm at impact, and so on. A few professional lessons in your sport can help to reduce the risk of these types of injuries.

Dress Properly for the Weather

Weather extremes can also cause health problems during exercise. Consider the suggestions in Table 12.4 (p. 273) to reduce the risk of overheating on hot, humid days or over-exposure on cold days. It is also helpful to become familiar with the early symptoms and emergency treatment for heat- and cold-related injuries such as heat exhaustion, heat stroke, **hypothermia**, and **frostbite** (see Table 12.4).

If you are a runner, plan your jogging course to avoid being too far out on either a hot or a cold day in case you get symptoms of heat exhaustion or cold over-exposure. It is always wise to plan your cold-weather

Hypothermia Subnormal body temperature.
Frostbite Destruction of tissue by freezing.

Table 12.3 ✦ Disqualifying Conditions for Sports Participation

CONDITIONS	COLLISION[a]	CONTACT[b]	NONCONTACT[c]	OTHERS[d]
General health				
Acute infections: Respiratory, genitourinary, infectious mononucleosis, hepatitis, active rheumatic fever, active tuberculosis	×	×	×	×
Obvious physical immaturity in comparison with other competitors	×	×		
Hemorrhagic disease: Hemophilia, purpura, and other serious bleeding tendencies	×	×	×	
Diabetes, inadequately controlled	×	×	×	×
Diabetes, controlled	e	e	e	e
Jaundice	×	×	×	×
Eyes				
Absence or loss of function of one eye	×	×		
Respiratory				
Tuberculosis (active or symptomatic)	×	×	×	×
Severe pulmonary insufficiency	×	×	×	×

(continued)

Table 12.3 ✦ Disqualifying Conditions for Sports Participation *(continued)*

CONDITIONS	COLLISION[a]	CONTACT[b]	NONCONTACT[c]	OTHERS[d]
Cardiovascular				
Mitral stenosis, aortic stenosis, aortic insufficiency, coarctation of aorta, cyanotic heart disease, recent carditis of any etiology	×	×	×	×
Hypertension on organic basis	×	×	×	×
Previous heart surgery for congenital or acquired heart disease	f	f	f	f
Liver, enlarged	×	×		
Skin				
Boils, impetigo, and herpes simplex gladiatorum	×	×		
Spleen, enlarged	×	×		
Hernia				
Inguinal or femoral hernia	×	×	×	
Musculoskeletal				
Symptomatic abnormalities or inflammations	×	×	×	×
Functional inadequacy of the musculoskeletal system, congenital or acquired, incompatible with the contact or skill demands of the sport	×	×	×	
Neurological				
History of symptoms of previous serious head trauma or repeated concussions	×			
Controlled convulsive disorder	g	g	g	g
Convulsive disorder not moderately well controlled by medication	×			
Previous surgery on head	×	×		
Renal				
Absence of one kidney	×	×		
Renal disease	×	×	×	×
Genitalia				
Absence of one testicle	h	h	h	h
Undescended testicle	h	h	h	h

[a]Football, rugby, hockey, lacrosse, and so forth.

[b]Baseball, soccer, basketball, wrestling, and so forth.

[c]Cross-country, track, tennis, crew, swimming, and so forth.

[d]Bowling, golf, archery, field events, and so forth.

[e]No exclusions.

[f]Each individual should be judged on an individual basis in conjunction with his or her cardiologist and surgeon.

[g]Each patient should be judged on an individual basis. All things being equal, it is probably better to encourage a young boy or girl to participate in a noncontact sport rather than a contact sport. However, if a patient has a desire to play a contact sport and this is deemed a major ameliorating factor in his or her adjustment to school, associates, and the seizure disorder, serious consideration should be given to letting him or her participate if the seizures are moderately well controlled or the patient is under good medical management.

[h]The Committee approves the concept of contact sports participation for youths with only one testicle or with an undescended testicle(s), except in specific instances such as an inguinal canal undescended testicle(s), following appropriate medical evaluation to rule out unusual injury risk. However, the athlete, parents, and school authorities should be fully informed that participation in contact sports with only one testicle carries a slight injury risk to the remaining healthy testicle. Fertility may be adversely affected following an injury. But the chances of an injury to a descended testicle are rare, and the injury risk can be further substantially minimized with an athletic supporter and protective device.

Source: Daniel D. Arnheim, *Modern Principles of Athletic Training* (St. Louis: Times Mirror/Mosby College Publishing, 1989), pp. 51–52. Reproduced with permission of The McGraw-Hill Companies.

Table 12.4 ✦ Preventive Techniques on Hot and Cold Days

HOT, HUMID WEATHER	COLD WEATHER
1. Listen to weather reports and avoid vigorous exercise if the temperature is above 32° C and the humidity is above 70 percent. Make hot days your light workout.	1. Listen to weather reports noting temperature and wind-chill factor. Unless the equivalent temperature is in the "little-danger" area, avoid outside exercise.
2. Avoid adding to normal salt intake. Do not use salt tablets. Increase consumption of fruits and vegetables.	2. Eat well during cold months: the body needs more calories in cold weather.
3. Avoid lengthy warm-up periods.	3. Warm up carefully until sweating is evident.
4. Wear light-coloured, porous, loose clothing to promote evaporation. Remove special equipment, such as football gear, every hour for 15 minutes.	4. Wear two or three layers of clothing rather than one heavy warm-up suit.
5. Avoid wearing a hat (except for an open visor with brim) because considerable heat loss occurs through the head.	5. Protect the head (warm hat), ears, fingers, toes, nose, and genitals. A hat should cover the ears and face. Fur-lined supporters for men can also prevent frostbite to sensitive parts.
6. Never use rubberized suits, which hold the sweat in and increase fluid and salt/potassium loss.	6. Never use rubberized, airtight suits, which keep the sweat in. When the body cools, the sweat starts to freeze.
7. Remember that wet clothing increases salt and sweat loss, so replace whenever possible.	7. Keep clothing dry, changing wet items as soon as possible.
8. Slowly increase the length of your workout by 5–10 minutes daily for 9 days to acclimatize to the heat.	8. Slowly increase the length of your workout by 5–10 minutes daily for 9 days to acclimatize to the cold.
9. Drink cold water (4.4° C) before (284–560 mL 15 min prior to exercise), during, and after exercise. Hydrate before the workout with two or three glasses of water.	9. Drink cold water freely before, during, and after exercise. Let thirst be your guide.

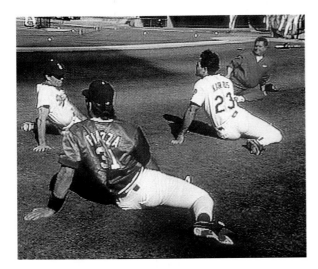

Under the management of Tommy Lasorda, the Dodgers were required to stretch before each practice and each game. The team considerably reduced its injury rate.

running route into the wind for the first half of the route, so that you will be running downwind on the way home when you are likely to be sweating more. In hot weather, plan your route to pass public washrooms or fountains to get water.

Both weather extremes can be dangerous. Heat stroke (when core temperature may rise to 41 degrees Celsius)

symptoms are difficult to reverse unless immediate, rapid cooling takes place. Cessation of sweating, and/or goosebumps on your skin, while exercising in hot weather are early-warning signs of impending heat stroke. Stop exercising immediately, and get water and shade! On the other hand, a 1-degree drop in core temperature will produce pain. Should body temperature drop to 34.4 degrees, shivering ceases and rigidity sets in; at 23.9 degrees, death from heart failure usually occurs.

Properly fitted shoes, appropriate equipment, avoidance of gimmicky exercise devices, and acceptable equipment for contact sports are also important for injury prevention and need special attention. A good-quality shoe is your best protection against injury to the feet, ankles, knees, hips, and lower back.

Use the Recommended Protective Equipment for Your Activity

The use of protective gear can reduce your risk of a serious injury in many activities. Eyeglasses for handball, racquetball, and squash; headgear for bicycling, rollerblading, ice skating, lacrosse, and football; proper wrist, knee, and elbow padding for rollerblading, ice skating, and rugby—all prevent broken bones, concussions, and other serious injuries.

Rollerblading is an example of a relatively new activity in which the use of proper protective equipment

WELLNESS HEROES

Silken Laumann

Silken Laumann, a native of Mississauga, Ontario, has been called "one of Canada's greatest athletes ever." This two-time Olympic medalist and world-class rower has lived through, worked through, and overcome physical tragedy and heartache.

In 1984, Silken's rowing career was blossoming. After winning a bronze medal with her sister Daniele in the 1984 Los Angeles Olympics women's doubles, she took up single sculling. By 1990, she had earned the silver medal at the World Championships, and in 1991 she took the Worlds again and she added a victory in the World Cup.

It was while warming up for a 1992 World Cup race in Germany 10 weeks before the Barcelona Olympics that her life changed forever. In a collision with a German pairs boat, Silken's right leg was sliced open, remaining attached to her body only by remnants of flesh. There was severe damage to her muscles, tendons, and nerves.

After undergoing eight operations and a three-week hospital stay, Silken insisted on being carried from her wheelchair into her racing shell. Though she could not walk, she could row and began training again. Her courage and hard work paid off—amazingly, she was able to compete in the Barcelona Olympics just five weeks later—and won the bronze medal! To Laumann, her Barcelona experience meant "measuring your unique abilities in a set of circumstances that you do not choose. In life, as in sports, we seldom get to choose our own circumstances." She went on to win the silver medal at the 1996 Atlanta Olympic Games, where she concluded her rowing career.

It has been observed that Silken's career exemplified the true spirit of the game: the decorum of courage was more important than winning. Laumann currently resides in Victoria, British Columbia, and continues to influence Canadians as a freelance writer and motivational speaker. ✦

Sources: Adapted from Laura Robinson, *She Shoots, She Scores: Canadian Perspectives on Women and Sport* (Toronto: Thomson Educational Publishing, 1997) pp. 45–50. With permission of the publisher; "Celebrating Women's Achievements," Women in Canadian Sport, National Library of Canada, 2002. Available at www.nlc-bnc.ca/2/12/h12-232-e.html. Accessed March 10, 2003.

greatly reduces injury. The number of people enjoying this form of exercise has increased dramatically in recent years, with over 22 million participants in the United States. Unfortunately, there was a tremendous increase in related injuries serious enough to require emergency care, with an estimated increase of 99 500 from 1993 to 1995 alone. The majority of these involve the wrist (32 percent), lower leg (13 percent), elbow (9 percent), and knee (13 percent). Only 7 percent of those injured were fully outfitted with helmet, wrist guards, elbow pads, and knee pads. Recent data collected by the Canadian Hospitals Injury Reporting and Prevention Program show that the typical injuries from rollerblading include broken wrists, chipped elbows, and bruised knees. The high number of fractures of the upper limbs and other injuries in the upper extremities is predictable, since most inexperienced skaters will attempt to "break" their fall by hyperextending their arms out to the front, side, or back. Contrary to popular belief, the fastest and safest way to stop blading is to drop to both knees. Learning this skill and wearing knee pads are critical injury-prevention techniques in this activity.

*T*ISSUE RESPONSE TO INJURY

The largest organ of the human body is the skin. Much more than some kind of passive envelope, our skin is a stimulus and receptor for touch, pain, pressure, and temperature—that is, a mediator between the body and our environment. Moreover, it is laced with *Langerhans cells* that "catch" bacteria and allergens and work to siphon them to the immune system. Because the skin encases our bodies, it is the first line of defence against any injury-threatening or -producing event. Thus, in physical activities these events result in bruises, blisters, abrasions, punctures, and lacerations (see Table 12.5 on p. 277).

Since all movement in exercise and physical activity takes place around joints, it is important to understand these structures. Joints are classified as fibrous, cartilaginous, or synovial.

Fibrous joints are those where there is no space or *cavity* and bones are held together by fibrous connective tissues such as ligaments. This type of joint is highly resistant and very strong, but has a smaller range of movement. For example, the lower ends of the tibia and the fibula (just in front of the ankle joint) have short, strong ligaments that permit almost no movement.

Cartilaginous joints also have no joint cavity; their articulating bones are tightly connected by cartilage and permit very little free movement. Good examples are the joints between vertebrae in the spine.

Synovial joints have a distinct cavity between the bones, and a sort of sleeve or open-ended *capsule* of ligamentous tissue encases the joint. The capsule serves to connect the bones and protect the contents and integrity of the joint. Along the inner lining of the capsule is the *synovial membrane*, which, among other functions, secretes an egg-white-like fluid to lubricate the joint, provide nourishment to the cartilage on the ends of the articulating bones, and remove debris resulting from wear and tear. The fluid is very viscous at rest, but it becomes less thick as movement increases. In a large synovial joint, such as the knee, there is as much as 3–4 millilitres of this fluid. Other large synovial joints are those of the shoulder, elbow, and hip.

Synovial joints contain one other structural element—*bursae*, self-contained bags of connective tissue lined with their own synovial membrane and filled with synovial fluid. They are also located between skin and bones, tendons and bones, and ligaments and bones. The primary function of bursae is to act as cushions for movement in joints and other areas.

The range and extent of movement is limited not only by the shape and structure of joints but also by *ligaments*. In fact, ligaments' sole function is one of restraint. Muscles perform; ligaments protect against or prevent excessive movement.

Table 12.5 summarizes some of the more common exercise and activity injuries, and some of the prevention and primary forms of treatment. In essence, all exercise and activity injuries—indeed all movement—comes down to the interplay of two forces, gravity and friction. Whether injury occurs during physical activity depends on the magnitude of the forces and on the body tissues involved.

Muscles, bones, even ligaments can, to some extent, adapt or yield to force, but they all have a point of failure or injury. Injury can come from a powerful blow, which is a forceful compression of soft tissue between two hard objects (often bone and the object delivering the blow). Injury can also result from a **chronic** force, as in the "worn running shoe sole" example provided earlier; when the sole is eroded by thousands of steps, and is used by an exerciser several days a week, all those forces are transferred up the leg to the body's tissues.

Then there are the forces of torque (rotary forces) that occur when we add functional or specialized equipment to our bodies. Examples are alpine ski boots and tennis racquets; no matter how well designed, they occasion strong or chronic torque forces.

In general, we can classify exercise and activity injuries by the tissues affected.

Muscles, for example, sustain the **acute** injuries of *contusion* (compressive force) and *strain* (excessive stretch, tear, or rip of muscle fibres, fascia, or tendons).

More-chronic muscle conditions are known as *inflammation* injuries.

Any named injury ending in *itis* is an inflammation of some kind. For example, "tendinitis" is inflammation of a tendon—Achilles tendinitis is a common form. Fasciitis is inflammation of fascia (plantar fasciitis is the most well known form). Inflammation injuries have a gradual onset and generally require long-term treatment. Such injuries are increasing in occupations requiring continuous, repetitive actions. Examples are carpal tunnel syndrome in the wrist, tennis elbow, and repetitive back strain injuries, which last were reported by some two million Canadians aged 12 and older in the 1996–97 National Population Health Survey (Statistics Canada, Catalogue 82-567).

Perhaps the most common and disabling of exercise and activity injuries is *sprain*—a stretching or tearing. (Muscles "strain," joints "sprain.") Sprains are painful, because of ligaments' extensive nerve supply, and very slow to heal, because of their poor blood supply. Ankles, knees, and shoulders seem to be most vulnerable. In sport participation, one of the most common and debilitating ligament injuries is to the anterior cruciate ligament (ACL), one of two that cross to connect the femur (thigh bone) to the tibia (shin bone). Reconstructive surgery is often required for ACL injuries.

Finally, joints can be dislocated, partially or fully (this is especially frequent in the fingers and shoulders). Also, bones can suffer anything from chronic stress fracture (often called "hairline fracture") to complete breakage.

General treatment forms or modalities for primary care of injuries are discussed below, together with prevention and emergency treatment measures. See Figure 12.1 for illustrations of common injuries.

GENERAL TREATMENT MODALITIES

Cryotherapy

The application of cold, or **cryotherapy**, to the skin for 20 minutes or less at a minimum temperature of 10 degrees Celsius causes the constriction of vessels and

---

Chronic Disease or pain of slow onset and long duration.

Acute Disease or pain characterized by sudden onset and a short, severe course.

Cryotherapy The use of cold in the treatment of injury and disease.

Figure 12.1 ✦ Appearance and Signs of Common Exercise and Physical-Activity Injuries

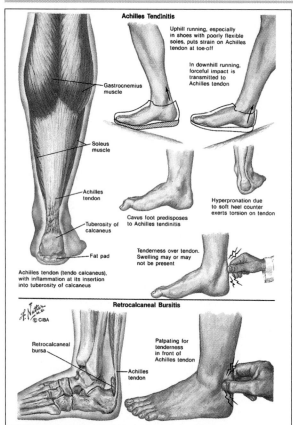

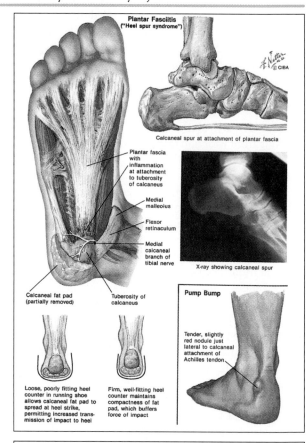

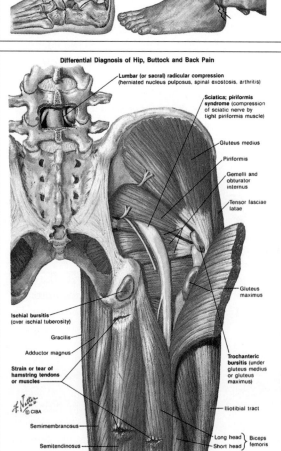

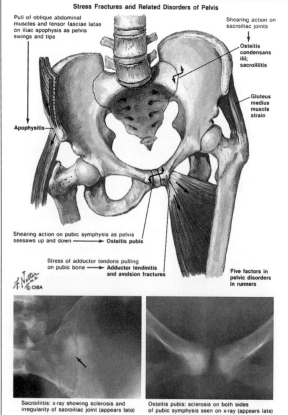

Source: © 1980. Novartis. Reprinted with permission from "Clinical Symposia," Vol. 32/4, illustrated by Frank H. Netter, M.D. All rights reserved.

Table 12.5 ✦ Prevention and Emergency Treatment of Common Exercise and Physical-Activity Injuries

INJURY	GENERAL COMMENTS	PREVENTION AND TREATMENT	NEED FOR A PHYSICIAN
Extremities			
Ankle	Most injuries involve inversion sprains (outer edge of foot turns inward). Ankles are not strong enough for most sports, and are poorly supported by muscles and ligaments that often stretch and tear from high-speed direction changes, cutting, and contact.	Improved support muscle strength offers some protection, along with preventive taping (inversion sprains only). RICE therapy is the preferred treatment. Use crutches for 2 or 3 days if pain is severe.	• If swelling or pain remains for 3 days • If ligament or tendon damage is present • If pain prevents walking • If symptoms of fracture exist
Bruise (charley horse)	A charley horse is nothing more than a thigh contusion from a direct blow to a relaxed thigh muscle (the tissue is compressed against the bone). Bruises to other areas occur in similar fashion.	Prevention involves use of proper equipment in contact sports. RICE therapy is the preferred emergency and home treatment. Replace ice with heat on the third or fourth day.	• If pain and discolouration do not disappear with rest, treatment, and mild exercise • If numbness, weakness, or tingling occurs, or there are signs of vascular compromise, immediate referral is necessary
Elbow (tennis and pitcher's)	The movement causing the condition is a forceful extension of the forearm and a twisting motion (serve in tennis, curve in baseball). The more you play and the older you are, the more likely you are to be afflicted. Pain is present over the outer (lateral epicondyle) or inner (medial epicondyle) elbow and may radiate down the arm. Pain is produced by tears, inflammation, and scar tissue at the attachment of the extensor muscles to the bony prominence of the elbow.	Prevention centres around use of warm-up, correction of poor stroke mechanics, avoiding use of wet tennis balls and heavy, inflexible racquets, and reducing the frequency of curve ball pitches (should be greatly restricted in Little League baseball with growing youngsters).	• If condition remains more than 2 or 3 weeks • If pain makes exercise impossible • If severe swelling is present • If night pain occurs
Fractures	A fracture should be suspected in most injuries where pain and swelling exist over a bone.	Apply ice packs, protect and rest the injured part for 72 hours. In severe cases, splint the bone where the victim lies and transport to emergency room.	• If limb is cold, blue, or numb • If pelvis or thigh are involved • If limb is crooked or deformed • If shock symptoms are present • If rapid, severe swelling occurs
Hamstring strains	The large-muscle group in the back of the upper leg is commonly strained during vigorous exercise. Pain is severe and prohibits further activity. In a few days, discolouration may appear.	Prevention includes proper stretching before exercise, proper diet, improved flexibility, and care in running around wet areas. For treatment use RICE therapy followed by heat application in 3–4 days.	• If severe discolouration occurs • If pain and discomfort remain after 10–15 days of treatment • If numbness, weakness, or tingling occurs, or there are signs of vascular compromise, immediate referral is necessary

(continued)

Table 12.5 ✦ Prevention and Emergency Treatment of Common Exercise and Physical-Activity Injuries *(continued)*

INJURY	GENERAL COMMENTS	PREVENTION AND TREATMENT	NEED FOR A PHYSICIAN
Knee	The knee is a vulnerable joint that depends on ligaments, cartilage, and muscles for support. *Chondromalacia* of the patella, or roughing of the undersurface of the kneecap, is the most common injury; kneecap pain and grating symptoms are evident. A tear of the cartilage is the second most common injury. Pain is evident along the inner or outer part of the knee joint along with swelling. *Ligament* tears are less common but occur from a blow to the leg. Swelling and knee instability result.	Prevention involves flexibility and strength. Exercises should stretch and strengthen the hamstrings, quadriceps, and Achilles tendon. Chondromalacia is treated through use of arch supports or by bulking up the inner part of the heel of the shoe. Aspirin, ibuprofen, or alleve and quadriceps exercises also help. Serious knee injury (cartilage and ligament damage) requires an examination by an orthopedic surgeon. Use of the arthroscope to examine and insert small tools through puncture wounds offers effective treatment and rapid recovery.	• If swelling and pain persist more than 3–5 days • If ligament or cartilage damage is suspected • If chondromalacia is suspected
Shin splints	A shin splint is merely an inflammation of the anterior and posterior tendons of the large bone in the lower leg. It is an overuse syndrome developing in poorly conditioned individuals in the beginning of their training program. Hard surfaces add to the problem.	Avoid hard surfaces, too much mileage, doing too much too soon, using improperly fitted shoes, and running on banked tracks or road shoulders. RICE therapy is recommended for 2–4 days, followed by taping and heat therapy and stretching exercises.	• If condition remains more than 2–3 weeks • If condition recurs after reconvening the exercise routine • If signs or symptoms of a stress fracture occur
Tendinitis	The location of the pain and swelling of the tendon varies in different sports. With considerable running, the Achilles tendon is affected. In those involving repeated movement of the upper arms (swimming, baseball), it is shoulder tendons. When a snapping or rotation of the elbow is involved (tennis/handball), it is the elbow tendons.	For both prevention and treatment, stretch the involved tendon daily and exercise lightly until pain disappears. RICE therapy is helpful in the early stages for three to four days (see *Elbow,* this table). Pain may disappear during a workout, only to return and worsen later.	• If pain and inflammation continue after 2–3 weeks of treatment
Varicose veins	Varicose veins are nothing more than abnormally lengthened, dilated veins. Surrounding muscles support deep veins, whereas superficial veins get little support. In some individuals, vein valves that prevent blood from backing up become defective, enlarged, and lose their elasticity. The condition is uncommon in young people.	Prevention and treatment for those with symptoms or a family history include bed rest and leg elevation, avoiding long periods of standing, use of elastic bandages and support stockings, surgery for severe cases, and removal of intra-abdominal pressure (obesity, tumour, tight girdles).	• If pain is severe enough to make walking difficult • If cosmetic problem is bothersome • If swelling in the calf or foot is present

Table 12.5 ✦ Prevention and Emergency Treatment of Common Exercise and Physical-Activity Injuries *(continued)*

INJURY	GENERAL COMMENTS	PREVENTION AND TREATMENT	NEED FOR A PHYSICIAN
Feet and Hands			
Athlete's foot	Athlete's foot is caused by a fungus and is accompanied by a bacterial infection. Itching, redness, and a rash on the soles, toes, or between the toes is common.	Prevention and treatment are similar; wash between the toes with soap and water, dry thoroughly, use medication containing Tinactin twice daily, and place fungistatic foot powder in shoes and sneakers.	• If treatment does not relieve symptoms in 2–3 weeks
Blisters	Blisters are produced by friction causing the top skin layer to separate from the second layer. Blisters can become severely inflamed or infected unless properly treated. A porous inner sole can be purchased that almost completely eliminates getting blisters on the feet.	Use clean socks, comfortably fitting shoes, and vaseline to reduce friction. Avoid breaking open blisters (skin acts as a sterile bandage). If the blister breaks, trim off all loose skin and apply antibiotic salve. Avoid use of tincture of benzoin and powder that increases friction, because this is more likely to cause blisters than prevent them.	• If inflammation and soreness develop • If redness occurs in the involved limb • If pain or sensitivity occurs under the arms or in the groin area • If blood blister is present
Bunions	Bunions are merely growths on the head of the first or fifth toe that produce inflammation (swelling, redness, pain).	Bunions can be prevented by using properly fitted shoes.	• If symptoms of infection occur
Corns	Hard corns may result from poorly fitted shoes. Inflammation and thickening of soft tissue (top of toes) occur. Soft corns are often caused by excessive foot perspiration and narrow shoes. The corn forms between the fourth and fifth toes in most cases.	Prevention and treatment involves use of properly fitted shoes, soaking feet daily in warm water to soften the area, and protecting the area with a small felt or sponge rubber doughnut. Trim and file corns to reduce pressure.	• If a change of shoes and treatment do not improve the condition
Heel bruise	The most common cause of heel pain is plantar fasciitis—inflammation of the broad band of fibrous tissue that runs from the base of the toes back to the heel and inserts on the inner aspect of the heel. Mild tears and severe bruises are also common.	Prevention involves proper stretching and use of a plastic heel cup. Aspirin should be used to reduce inflammation (two tablets, four times daily); rest is indicated for 5–7 days.	• If pain persists for more than 5–7 days after rest and treatment
Ingrown toenails	The edge of the toenail grows into the soft tissue, producing inflammation and infection.	Prevention and treatment involves proper nail trimming, soaking the toe in hot water two to three times daily, and inserting a small piece of cotton under the nail edge to lift it from the soft tissue.	• If infection occurs

(continued)

Table 12.5 ✦ Prevention and Emergency Treatment of Common Exercise and Physical-Activity Injuries *(continued)*

INJURY	GENERAL COMMENTS	PREVENTION AND TREATMENT	NEED FOR A PHYSICIAN
Stress fracture	A stress fracture is a small crack in a bone's surface, generally a foot, leg, or hand. Unexplained pain may exist over one of the small bones in the hand or foot. X-ray may not reveal small cracks until the bone heals and a callus (scar tissue) forms.	Prevention involves not running too many miles, not increasing mileage too fast, running on soft surfaces, and taking care to progress slowly in a fitness program. Treatment requires rest and proper equipment (especially footwear).	• If unexplained pain exists in the lower back, hip, ankle, wrist, hand, or foot • If night pain occurs • If pain increases with activity
Head and Neck			
Cauliflower ear	A deformed outer ear is common in wrestling, rugby, and football from friction, hard blows, and wrenching in a headlock position. With poor circulation to the ear, fluid is absorbed slowly, and the ear remains swollen, sensitive, and discoloured.	Use protective ear guards, apply vaseline to reduce friction, and apply ice as soon as a sore spot develops. Once a deformed ear develops, only a plastic surgeon can return the ear to normal appearance.	• If symptoms of infection develop • If cosmetic surgery is desired • If swelling is present
Concussion	Any injury to the head producing dizziness or temporary unconsciousness should be considered serious.	Apply ice to the area. Observe the patient for 72 hours for alertness, unequal pupil size (although about one person in four has unequal pupil size all the time), and vomiting. Pressure inside skull may develop in 72 hours.	• If unconsciousness occurred • If bleeding occurs from ears, eyes, or mouth • If there is unequal pupil size, lethargy, fever, vomiting, convulsions, speech difficulty, stiff neck, or limb weakness
Dental injuries	Common in basketball and contact sports from elbow contact.	Chipped tooth—avoid hot and cold drinks. Swelling due to abscess—apply ice pack. Excessive bleeding of socket—place gauze over socket and bite down. Toothache—aspirin and ice packs.	• If tooth is chipped, abscess is present, or bleeding of socket or toothache is present • If tooth is bleeding or knocked out (place in proper solution and see dentist immediately)
Eye (object in eye, contusion from a ball or elbow)	Eye injuries are more common in racquet sports and handball from ball contact, and in contact sports from elbow contact. In racquet sports, the ball may ricochet off the top of the racquet into the eye, or the victim may turn to see where his or her partner is hitting the ball in doubles play.	Protective eye guards should be used in squash, racquetball and handball. Never turn your head in doubles play. Avoid rubbing—you could scratch the cornea. Close both eyes to allow tears to wash away a foreign body. Grasp the lashes of the upper lid and draw out and down over the lower lid. If it feels like an object is in the eye but none can be seen, cornea scrape probably occurred and will heal in 24–48 hours. To remove object, moisten corner of handkerchief and touch object lightly.	• If object is on the eye itself • If object remains after washing • If object could have penetrated the globe of the eye • If blood is visible in eye • If vision is impaired • If pain is present after 48 hours • If pain is present after object has been removed

Table 12.5 ✦ Prevention and Emergency Treatment of Common Exercise and Physical-Activity Injuries *(continued)*

INJURY	GENERAL COMMENTS	PREVENTION AND TREATMENT	NEED FOR A PHYSICIAN
Nasal fracture	The blow may come from the side or front. The side hit causes more deformity. Hemorrhage is profuse (mucous lining is cut), and swelling is immediate.	Prevention involves use of a face guard in football. Bleeding should be controlled immediately (see *Nosebleed*, this table).	• If bleeding continues • If deformity and considerable swelling are present
Extremities			
Neck	Neck injuries are more common in contact sports and require immediate and careful attention. Assume a vertebra is involved, and avoid movement of any kind until a physician or rescue squad arrives.	Neck flexibility exercises should be a part of your warm-up routine. Neck-strengthening exercises are a necessity for contact sport participants.	• If any injury to the neck occurs
Nosebleed	Nosebleed may occur even from mild contact to the nose.	Do not lie down when bleeding starts. Squeeze the nose between the thumb and forefinger just below the hard portion for 5–10 minutes while seated with the head tilted forward. Avoid blowing the nose or placing cold compresses on the bridge of the nose.	• If bleeding occurs frequently and is associated with a cold • If victim has a history of high blood pressure • If emergency treatment fails to stop the bleeding
Torso			
Back	The first 7 vertebrae control the head, neck, and upper back. The next 12 provide attachments for the ribs. The 5 lumbar vertebrae of the lower back support the weight of the upper half of the body. It is this area that plagues millions of people.	Avoid exercise motions that arch the back. Back pain may be caused by muscular and ligamentous sprains, mechanical instability, arthritis, and ruptured discs. Most problems will improve with rest, ice, pain medication, and an exercise program.	• If pain, weakness, or numbness in legs is present • If pain remains after rest and ice therapy • If aching sensation occurs in buttocks or further down the leg
Chest pain	Chest pain provides a heart attack scare to everyone over age 30. Actually, pain could be in the chest wall (muscle, rib, ligament, rib cartilage), the lungs or outside covering, or the pleura, diaphragm, skin, or other organs in the upper part of the diaphragm. Sharp pain that lasts a few seconds, pain at the end of a deep breath or one that worsens with a deep breath, pain on pressing a finger on the spot of discomfort, and painful burning when the stomach is empty are all symptoms that are probably not associated with a heart attack.	Any of the symptoms to the right require immediate hospitalization and physician care.	• If any of the following symptoms are present: mild to intense pain with a feeling of pressure, or squeezing on the chest; pain beneath the breastbone; accompanying pain in the jaw, or down the inner side of either arm; accompanying nausea, sweating, dizziness, or shortness of breath; or pulse irregularity

(continued)

Table 12.5 ✦ Prevention and Emergency Treatment of Common Exercise and Physical-Activity Injuries *(continued)*

INJURY	GENERAL COMMENTS	PREVENTION AND TREATMENT	NEED FOR A PHYSICIAN
Groin strain	The groin muscles (area between the thigh and abdominal region) are easily torn from running, jumping, and twisting. It is a difficult injury to prevent and cure. Pain, weakness, and internal bleeding may occur.	Prevention involves proper stretching prior to exercise. RICE therapy is suggested for treatment.	• If symptoms remain after several days of rest and mild exercise
Hernia	The protrusion of viscera (body organs) through a portion of the abdominal wall is referred to as a hernia. Hernias associated with exercise and sports generally occur in the groin area.	Prevention involves attention to proper form in weight lifting and weight training and care in lifting heavy objects.	• If a protrusion is located that protrudes further with coughing
Hip pointer	A hard blow to the iliac crest or hip produces what is commonly called a hip pointer. The injury is severely handicapping and produces both pain and spasm.	Prevention involves the use of protective hip pads in contact sports. RICE therapy is suggested for treatment.	• If symptoms of a fracture are present
Jock itch	Jock itch is acquired by contact and is associated with bacteria, fungi, moulds, and ringworm.	Prevention and treatment involve practising proper hygiene (showering in warm water, use of antiseptic soap and powder, proper drying); drinking enough water; regularly changing underwear, supporter, and shorts; disinfecting locker benches, mats, and other equipment; and avoiding long periods of sitting in warm, moist areas.	• If condition persists for more than 10 days
Wind knocked out	With a hard blow to the right place, such as a relaxed midsection, breathing is temporarily hampered. Although you will have trouble convincing the victim, breathing will return. The blow has only increased abdominal pressure, produced pain, and interfered with the diaphragmatic cycle reflex due to nerve paralysis or muscle spasm.	The victim should be told to try to breathe slowly through the nose (no easy task for someone who is gasping, dizzy, and 100 percent convinced death is only seconds away). Clothing is loosened at the neck and waist, and ice is applied to the abdomen.	• If breathing is still not normal in 1–2 minutes • If breathing stops (start CPR) • If pain persists in the midsection

Shoulder

Tendinitis	Tendinitis is common in tennis and baseball. Soreness results on the front of the shoulder when elevating the arm from the side.	Ice and aspirin are used. Prevention and treatment involves flexibility and weight-training exercises. Flexibility movements concentrate on back stretching while weight-training choices are lateral lifts and military bench presses.	• If soreness remains for 7–10 days

Table 12.5 ✦ Prevention and Emergency Treatment of Common Exercise and Physical-Activity Injuries *(continued)*

INJURY	GENERAL COMMENTS	PREVENTION AND TREATMENT	NEED FOR A PHYSICIAN
Thorax			
Rib fracture and bruises	Fractures may occur from direct contact or, uncommonly, from muscular contraction. A direct blow may displace the bone and produce jagged edges that cut the tissue of the lungs, producing bleeding or lung collapse.	The type of contact helps reveal rib fracture. Pain when breathing and palpitation are also signs. RICE therapy should be initiated immediately.	• If pain is present when breathing after a direct blow to the thorax • If fracture is suspected • If shortness of breath or difficulty in breathing persists
Miscellaneous Injuries and Illnesses			
Abrasions	Superficial skin layers are scraped off. Injury imposes no serious problem if cleaned properly.	Clean with soap and warm water. Use a bandage if the wound oozes blood. Remove loose skin flaps with sterile scissors if dirty; allow to remain if clean. Check to see if victim has been immunized for tetanus within the last 10 years.	• If all dirt and foreign matter cannot be removed • If infection develops
Common cold	Handshaking with an infected person or breathing in particles after a sneeze are two ways of transmitting a cold virus. Contributing factors may be low resistance, improper nutrition, tension, bacteria entering the respiratory tract, and remaining indoors in winter months, which increases the likelihood of close contact with a contagious person.	A cold will typically last about 7 days. There is no known protection or cure. Antihistamines, decongestants, and cold tablets are of little value. Acetaminophen, combined with rest and plenty of fluids, is sound advice. Exercise only lightly and include 1 or 2 days of rest. No exercise should be attempted if patient has a fever or muscle soreness.	• If fever or sore throat lasts more than a week • If pain is present in one or both ears
Fainting and dizziness	Lack of blood flow to the brain commonly occurs with increasing age and may result in temporary loss of vision or lightheadedness.	Place the victim in a lying position with the feet elevated. If it is not possible to lie down, an alternative position is a sitting posture with the head lowered between the legs.	• If loss of consciousness occurs • If dizziness occurs frequently • If dizziness or fainting occurs with exercise
Frostbite	Frostbite, a destruction of tissue by freezing, is more likely to occur on outer parts of the nose, cheeks, ears, fingers, and toes.	Thaw rapidly in a warm water bath. Avoid rubbing areas with snow. Water should be comfortable to a normal, unfrozen hand (not over 40° C). When a flush reaches the fingers, remove the frostbitten part from the water immediately. For an ear or nose, use cloths soaked in warm water.	• Always see a doctor

(continued)

Table 12.5 ✦ Prevention and Emergency Treatment of Common Exercise and Physical-Activity Injuries *(continued)*

INJURY	GENERAL COMMENTS	PREVENTION AND TREATMENT	NEED FOR A PHYSICIAN
Heat exhaustion/ heat stroke	The body loses heat to the environment and maintains normal temperature by: *Evaporation*—sweat evaporates into the atmosphere. *Radiation*—with body temperature higher than air temperature, heat loss occurs. *Convection*—as body heat loss occurs, air is warmed. This warmed air rises and cooler air moves in to take its place, cooling the body. *Conduction*—heat moves from deeper body organs to skin through blood vessels. The skin acts as a radiation surface for heat loss to the air.	Symptoms of heat exhaustion include nausea, chills, cramps, and rapid pulse. Treatment requires immediate cooling with ice packs to the head, torso, and joints and maintaining proper water and electrolyte balance.	• If rapid improvement is not evident • If multiple cramps occur • If core temperature does not immediately return to normal • If lethargy or confusion is present • If skin is warm and dry
Hypothermia	With extremely cold temperatures and high wind chill, core body temperature may drop below normal levels.	[Prevention involves following the steps outlined in the section "Dress Properly for the Weather" earlier in this chapter.] Treatment calls for warming with blankets, heating pads, replacing wet clothing, and administering warm drinks.	• If core temperature drops below 34.4° C • If lethargy or confusion is present
Infected wounds	Bacterial infection in the bloodstream (septicemia).	Keep area clean, changing the bandage and soaking and cleaning in warm water twice daily. Up to 10–12 days may be needed for normal healing.	• If fever is above 37.8° C • If thick pus and swelling occur the second day
Minor cuts	Minor cuts can develop into serious problems if mistreated or neglected. Avoid use of antiseptics that may destroy tissue and actually retard healing.	Clean the wound with soap and water or hydrogen peroxide, removing all dirt and foreign matter. Use a butterfly bandage or steri-strip to bring the edges of the wound tightly together without trapping the fat or rolling the skin beneath.	• If cut occurs to face or trunk • If deep cut involves tendons, nerves, vessels, or ligaments • If blood is pumping from a wound • If tingling or limb weakness occurs • If cut cannot be pulled together without trapping the fat • If direct pressure fails to stop the bleeding

Table 12.5 ✦ Prevention and Emergency Treatment of Common Exercise and Physical-Activity Injuries *(continued)*

INJURY	GENERAL COMMENTS	PREVENTION AND TREATMENT	NEED FOR A PHYSICIAN
Muscle soreness	You may experience two different types of soreness: general soreness that appears immediately after your exercise session and disappears in 3–4 hours, or localized soreness appearing 8–24 hours after exercise. The older you are, the longer the period between exercise and soreness.	You can help prevent soreness by warming up properly, avoiding bouncing-type stretching or flexibility exercises, and progressing slowly in your program. Doing too much too soon is a common cause. You can expect to have some soreness after your first few workouts, especially if you have been inactive. Don't stop exercising; it will only reoccur later.	• If muscle soreness persists after the second week
Muscle cramps	Muscular cramps commonly occur in three areas: back of lower leg (calf), back of upper leg (hamstring group), and front of upper leg (quadriceps group). Cramps may be related to fatigue, tightness of the muscles, or fluid, salt, and potassium imbalance.	Stretch before you exercise and drink water freely. If cramp occurs, stretch area carefully.	• If multiple cramps occur • If symptoms of heat exhaustion are present

Source: Prepared by Eugene L. Kastleberg, Department of Orthopaedic Surgery, Medical College of Virginia, Virginia Commonwealth University.

reduces the flow of blood to the injured area. When cold is applied for longer than 20 minutes, an intermittent period of **vasodilation** occurs for 4–6 minutes. This prevents tissue damage from too much exposure to cold. At this point, cold is no longer effective. Cold also reduces muscle spasms, swelling, and pain; slows metabolic rate; and increases **collagen** inelasticity and joint stiffness. Cold is somewhat more penetrating than heat, and the effects last longer.

Cold applications should be used immediately after an injury and continued for several days until swelling subsides. Cold can be applied intermittently for 30 minutes (10 minutes on, 10 minutes off, 10 minutes on, per session) every 1½ waking hours in combination with compression, elevation, and rest (see PRICE later in this chapter). *Ice massage* can be used on a small body area by freezing water in a plastic-foam cup to form a cylinder of ice. After removing 1 or 2 inches (2.5–5 cm) of the foam at the top of the cup, the bottom portion of the cup can be used as a handle, and the ice can be rubbed over the skin in overlapping circles for 5–10 minutes until there is a feeling of cold, burning, aching, and numbness in the area. *Ice packs* can be made by placing flaked or crushed ice in a wet towel or self-sealing plastic bag. Unless ice massage is being used, ice should not come in direct contact with the skin.

Thermotherapy

In general, proper **thermotherapy** to an injured area raises skin temperature and increases the amount of blood flow to the area. Heat can also be used to relieve joint stiffness, pain, muscle spasms, and inflammation and to increase the extensibility of collagen tissues. Temperatures should not exceed 46.7 degrees Celsius, and a treatment session should never exceed 30 minutes. Additional cautions in the use of heat include the following:

1. Never apply heat immediately after an injury.
2. Never use heat when there is loss of sensation or decreased arterial circulation.
3. Never apply heat directly to the eyes or genitals or to the abdomen of a pregnant woman.

Vasodilation Increase or opening of the blood vessels.

Collagen The connective-tissue portion of the true skin and of other organs.

Thermotherapy The application of heat.

MYTH AND FACT SHEET

Myth	Fact
1. With injuries to most body parts, you should apply heat.	1. Injuries to soft tissue should be treated initially with PRICE therapy, which requires ice, not heat. Heat should be avoided for 2–3 days until swelling begins to subside. Early use of heat in any form increases swelling, delays healing, and can result in serious tissue changes that may require surgery to correct.
2. You should apply ice directly to your skin for one hour.	2. The maximum amount of time ice should be applied is 20 minutes. Longer periods can actually bring about tissue damage. Ice should not come into contact with the skin unless an ice massage is being used.
3. If you have a heart murmur, you should not exercise.	3. A heart murmur is an abnormal sound caused by turbulent blood flow. The difficulty may be an impaired valve that fails to close completely or valve orifices that are narrowed and slow the flow of blood. A greater-than-normal load is placed on the heart, heart walls may increase in size, and tension increases inside the walls. The heart is less efficient and, in a sense, has to regurgitate blood twice. In what is termed a functional murmur, no structural defect is evident to account for the abnormal sounds. Although you can generally exercise safely with functional murmurs, it is important to consult your physician before starting an exercise program.
4. If you have the wind knocked out of you, you are in danger of dying.	4. The temporary inability to breathe following a blow to a relaxed midsection will slowly subside until natural breathing is restored. Meanwhile, you will gasp for breath; possibly suffer dizziness, nausea, and weakness; and even collapse. A hard blow to the solar plexus increases intra-abdominal pressure, causes pain, and interferes with the diaphragmatic-cycle reflex due to nerve paralysis or muscle spasm. Breathing is only temporarily affected by a blow that momentarily paralyzes the nerve control of the diaphragm. For relief, loosen clothing at the neck and waist, apply ice to the abdomen, and breathe slowly through the nose.
5. A popping or snapping sound in your knee is a sign of serious trouble.	5. The sound generally comes from a tendon flipping over bony fulcrums and may be quite natural in some athletes who simply never really noticed the sound before. "Joint mice," or the presence of some loose cartilage or other tissue, may also produce a clicking sound as the knee flexes and extends. Bone, tendon, ligament, or cartilage damage may not be indicated unless other symptoms are present such as inflammation, swelling, fluid, and knee locking.

4. Never fall asleep while applying heat, and never apply heat over a topical heat ointment.

Heat can be safely applied through the use of moist heat and commercial packs as well as whirlpool and paraffin baths. You can use moist heat at home by soaking a towel in hot water and allowing it to drain for several seconds before applying it to an injured area that is already covered by four to six layers of towelling. The moist towel should not come into direct contact with the skin. In acute cases, cryother-apy is the therapeutic modality of choice (over thermotherapy).

■ Electrotherapy

The use of **electrotherapy** as a form of heat should be performed only by a physician, physical therapist, or licensed athletic trainer. Ultrasound and similar sound-wave treatment modalities should also be administered only by qualified persons.

Diversity Issues

Injury Prevention

During and after adolescence, boys are encouraged to begin strength-training programs that help add muscle mass and improve strength, endurance, and physical appearance. This training also helps boys avoid exercise injuries by strengthening soft tissue and making the body less susceptible to bruises and muscle pulls. Unfortunately, girls are not encouraged at an early age to weight-train, and weight rooms in most public schools in the United States are still male-dominated and not well suited for women. Strength training, particularly with free weights, is still considered a male activity that has not been fully accepted as an appropriate training method for women.

With the advent of aerobics and the increasing number of women frequenting gyms, however, more women are beginning to see the benefits of weight training. Whether they use Nautilus machines or free weights, they are realizing that strengthening their muscles increases overall body strength, increases basal metabolism, and generally improves their appearance. Sometimes, however, women who have never trained with weights tend to overdo it their first time. Lifting too much weight with too many repetitions leads to muscle pulls and soft-tissue injuries, and the associated pain can be very discouraging.

Weight-training injuries for both women and men can be avoided by following a few simple suggestions. The proper lifting techniques described in Chapter 6 for each exercise should be carefully mastered. A first attempt at weight training requires light-to-moderate weights and a relatively high number of repetitions. This approach will slowly prepare the muscles and other soft tissue for heavier weight and fewer repetitions in the future. Training with a partner who acts as a spotter, or protector, is a necessary precaution, particularly when using free weights. A safe, injury-free weight-training program is attainable for all. ✦

Massage

The use of massage to manipulate soft tissue is a helpful adjunct to heat and cold. Stroking, kneading, friction, percussion, and rapid shaking are some of the more common techniques used to increase heat, improve blood flow to the injured area, remove metabolites, overcome edema, improve circulation and the venous return of blood to the heart, and aid relaxation.

Prevention and Emergency Treatment of Common Exercise Injuries and Illnesses

Additional common injuries, illnesses, and problems associated with exercise are discussed in Table 12.5, which serves as a guide for diagnosis, prevention, emergency treatment, and determination of the need for a physician. Almost all of these injuries can be categorized into the four major areas of exercise injuries: sprains, strains, contusions, and fractures. Figure 12.1 illustrates many of these problems. If in doubt, consult a physician immediately or transport the injured person to a hospital emergency room.

PRICE

Emergency home treatment for most muscle, ligament, and tendon strains, and sprains, suspected fractures, bruises, and joint inflammations involves five simple actions known as the PRICE approach:

1. **Prevention/Protection** Prevent the injury by wearing proper equipment and doing a warm-up, or after injury lessen its effects by protecting the injured body part (for example, with crutches).
2. **Rest** To prevent additional damage to injured tissue, stop exercising and immobilize the injured area immediately. If the lower extremities are affected, use crutches to move about.
3. **Ice** To decrease blood flow to the injured area and decrease swelling, apply ice (crushed in a towel or ice pack) directly to the skin immediately for 15–20 minutes. Use cold applications intermittently for 1–72 hours. Do not apply heat.
4. **Compression** To limit swelling and decrease likelihood of hemorrhage and hematoma formation, wrap a towel or bandage firmly around the ice and injured area. Wrap the towel or

Electrotherapy The use of electricity (infrared radiation therapy, shortwave and microwave diathermics, and ultrasound therapy) in the treatment of disease or injury.

BEHAVIOURAL CHANGE AND MOTIVATIONAL STRATEGIES

There are many things that might interfere with the use of some practices known to prevent exercise-related injuries. Here are some of these barriers (roadblocks) and strategies for overcoming them.

Roadblock	Behavioural Change Strategy
Although you are aware of the value of proper warm-up before exercise, you never seem to do it. It seems so natural to change into your workout clothing and immediately start the 4.8-kilometre jog or the tennis match. Yet you have noticed a tightness in the calf muscles after exercise for a week or so now.	Most people are impatient and want to get right into exercise without wasting time. This mindset is difficult to overcome. One approach may be to avoid viewing warm-up as a separate component of your program. Continue what you are doing but divide the jog into three continuous segments: (1) Begin jogging immediately but very slowly for the first kilometre, progressing from a 0.4-kilometre walk to a slow jog; (2) stop and stretch for at least five minutes, emphasizing calf and Achilles tendon exercises (see Chapter 7); and (3) complete the remaining 13.8 kilometres of your jog. Other forms of exercise can also be planned that permit considerably less effort in the initial 5–10 minutes to build in a warm-up period.
You are totally exhausted at the end of your workout and feel nauseated, uncomfortable, and sore.	Most individuals develop the habit of saving the most vigorous part of their workout routine for the final 5–10 minutes, before stopping and standing around to talk or sitting down to relax. Failure to use a cool-down period produces the roadblock symptoms. You can avoid this problem by adding one more segment to the 4.8-kilometre jog. Segment 3 should involve the most vigorous portion of the workout for about 3.0 kilometres or 10–20 minutes followed by a fourth segment involving a 0.8-kilometre slow jog or walk and a brief stretching period to taper off at the end of your workout.
List roadblocks interfering with your approach to exercise injury prevention. 1. _____ 2. _____ 3. _____	Now, cite the behavioural change strategies that can help you overcome the roadblocks you listed. If you need to, refer back to Chapter 3 for behavioural change and motivational strategies. 1. _____ 2. _____ 3. _____

bandage only to hold the ice, not so tightly as to restrict circulation.

5. **Elevation** To help drain excess fluid through gravity, improve the venous return of blood to the heart, and reduce internal bleeding and swelling, raise the injured area above heart level.

Home treatment should begin as soon as possible. The procedure should be: (1) evaluate the injured area; (2) apply ice for 20 minutes; (3) compress the ice firmly against the injury; (4) replace the ice pack with a compress wrap and pad; (5) rest the injured area; (6) reapply ice within 1–1½ hours; (7) remove the wrap and elevate the area before you go to bed; and (8) begin ice therapy immediately on rising in the morning. On the fourth or fifth day, discontinue cold treatments and begin to apply moist heat or dry heat or use a whirlpool twice daily for 15–20 minutes. Depending on the severity of the injury and amount of swelling and pain, mild exercise can resume in four or five days.

A great deal of misinformation is circulated on home emergency treatment. Remember that incorrect treatment can worsen the injury or actually produce serious side-effects that may require surgery later.

Shock

Many injuries, such as fractures, concussions, profuse bleeding, heart attack, back and neck damage, and severe joint trauma, can produce shock. *Shock* is one of the body's strongest natural reactions to disease and injury. It slows blood flow, which acts as a natural tourniquet and reduces pain with serious injury. All three types of shock can kill: *traumatic* (injury or loss of blood), *septic* (infection-induced), and *cardiogenic* (from a heart attack). Shock is much easier to prevent than to treat.

With the above injuries and illnesses, always assume that shock is present; splint any broken bones; handle the victim with care; stop any bleeding; and keep the victim warm at all times.

USE OF MEDICATION IN THE TREATMENT OF EXERCISE-RELATED INJURIES

Numerous prescription and nonprescription (over-the-counter) drugs are available to combat infection, treat fungi, control pain and bleeding, and reduce inflammation. It is wise, however, to consult your physician before using any medication. It is also important to update your medicine cabinet to make certain you are stocking the basics for common illnesses and injuries. Take a moment to analyze your home pharmacy by completing Lab Activity 12.2: Evaluating Your Home Medicine Cabinet at the end of this chapter. Then compare your findings to the recommended home pharmacy in Table 12.6.

Infection can often be prevented by including at least one antiseptic and one wound protectant in your home medicine kit. Your physician may also prescribe an antibiotic—either a topical dressing or a systemic medication.

Pain may be controlled through the skin by applying a topical anesthetic to inhibit pain sensations through quick evaporation and cooling or by *counterirritating* the skin so you are no longer aware of the pain. Liniments, analgesic balms, heat, and cold are examples of **counterirritants**, which actually trick the brain into ignoring soreness. Pain signals reach the brain along two types of nerve fibres—C fibres, which are not covered by a fatty material called myelin, and myelinated fibres, which have the fatty covering. The C fibres transmit dull, aching-type pain and soreness whereas the myelinated fibres transmit sharper pain. The

> **Counterirritants** Medication, heat, cold, electricity, and so forth used to eliminate pain and inflammation.

Table 12.6 ✦ Your Home Pharmacy

MEDICAL CONCERN	MEDICATION
Allergy	**Antihistamines**
Cold and coughs	Cold tablets, cough drops
Constipation	**Milk of magnesia**
Diarrhea	Antidiarrheal, paregoric, immodium
Eye irritations	Eye drops
Exercise injury problems (inflammation)	See your physician; enteric or coated **aspirin,** NSAID medication
Exercise injury problems (pain)	**Acetaminophen, aspirin,** use of heat and cold
Pain and fever (children)	Children's aspirin, acetaminophen, liquid acetaminophen, enteric or coated aspirin, rectal suppositories
Fungus	**Antifungal preparations**
Sunburn (preventive)	**Sunblock** (a minimum 15 SPF is recommended; 30 SPF would be safer)
Sprains	**Elastic bandages**
Stomach, upset	Antacid (nonabsorbable)
Wounds (general)	**Adhesive tape, bandages, sodium bicarbonate (soaking agent)**
Wounds (antiseptics)	**Ethyl alcohol (60–90%),** isopropyl alcohol
Wounds (protectant)	Topical antibiotics

Note: Items in bold print are basic requirements; other preparations are also useful and should be considered.

brain can only process so many pain signals at once. When the two types of nerve fibres are activated simultaneously, the myelinated fibres override the C fibres and you perceive only the sharper pain and sensations of heat, cold, and pressure, not the dull ache.

Some central nervous system drugs such as acetaminophen (Tylenol) and aspirin also reduce pain by acting on the nerves that carry the pain impulse to the brain.

Inflammation to soft tissue can be reduced through the use of one of several drugs. Aspirin is effective for conditions such as tendinitis, bursitis, chondromalacia, and tendosynovitis. Some enzymes can help treat swollen joints, reduce inflammation, edema, pain, swelling, and redness. NSAIDs (nonsteroidal anti-inflammatory drugs) are also quite effective in eliminating inflammation. A physician's prescription and guidance is needed,

however, because side-effects may occur and dangers exist with long-term use.

NUTRITION AND HEALING

Individuals who do not eat correctly and have poor nutritional status do not heal as rapidly as normal. Although the recommended nutrient intakes (RNIs) (see Chapter 8) for protein and for some vitamins and minerals increase during periods of recovery from illness and injury, a sufficient safety margin exists in the RNI to promote normal healing and recovery, provided you are consuming adequate fluids and calories.

SUMMARY

Protecting Your Body from Injury and Illness

Many exercise-related injuries are preventable. You can significantly reduce your risk of injury and illness by using a preconditioning period before beginning your exercise program, warming up and cooling down properly, analyzing your medical history, progressing slowly in the early stages of your program, monitoring body signals, dressing properly for the activity, and mastering proper form.

Tissue Response to Injury

The healing process is unique to each individual. Factors such as age, nutrition, treatment, and type and severity of the injury play a major role. In the acute stage immediately following an injury, the body attempts to keep things localized to prevent further damage and aid the healing process that will occur over the next five or six weeks. Complete regeneration and repair, however, may require up to a year.

General Treatment Modalities

The immediate and continued use of cold applications over the first several days after a soft-tissue injury should be followed by heat therapy during the repair, regeneration, and remodelling stages of healing. Numerous techniques to apply heat and cold can be safely used.

Prevention and Emergency Treatment of Common Exercise Injuries and Illnesses

Proper home emergency treatment for a soft-tissue injury to an extremity requires the use of PRICE. Certain symptoms suggest the need for immediate care by a physician. If you are in doubt, take the injured person to an emergency room or physician as soon as possible.

Some injuries involving fractures, concussions, bleeding, heart attack, and severe joint trauma can produce shock. Because shock is considerably easier to prevent than it is to treat, precautions should be taken with all patients when dealing with these types of injuries.

Use of Medication in the Treatment of Exercise-Related Injuries

Your medicine cabinet should contain the basic items necessary for the emergency treatment of common exercise injuries. Over-the-counter medications to treat inflammations, fungi, pain, fever, wounds, and basic problems such as allergies, colds, constipation, diarrhea, and eye irritations should be readily available.

Nutrition and Healing

Sound nutrition is important during recovery from both injury and illness. Nutritional needs increase somewhat during the recovery period, and it is important to continue to eat well, avoid skipping meals, drink plenty of water and other fluids, and consider the use of a multiple vitamin and mineral supplement.

STUDY QUESTIONS

1. What is the difference between warm-up and stretching? How do you know when you are warmed up? How do you "cool down"? Provide examples in your answers.

2. Define and give one example for each of these terms: sprains, strains, contusions, fractures. Using these categories, go through Table 12.5 and recategorize the injury forms under these four headings.

3. Describe cryotherapy. How long should it be applied?

4. Explain the concept of PRICE and how you would use this important procedure in exercise injury treatment.

5. How would you treat frostbite? Shock? Hypothermia?

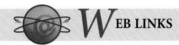

WEB LINKS

St. John Ambulance, Canada; information on CPR training
www.sja.ca

Canadian Academy of Sports Medicine
www.casm-acms.org/

Canadian Physical Medicine and Rehabilitation Services
www.canadianwellness.com/physical/physical.asp

Sports Medicine—classifications
http://sportsmedicine.about.com/

eSportmed.com
www.esportmed.com/store/showtas.cfm?tas=Z136

Running Injuries
www.clark.net/pub/pribut/spsport.html

Sport and Exercise Injury Prevention
www.amateur-sports.com/injuries.htm

Sports Injury Care and Specific Injuries
www.cramersportsmed.com/injury.htm

REFERENCES

NATA News. "American Heart Association Issues Nation's First Guidelines for Identifying Athletes at Risk of Sudden Cardiac Death" (November 1996).

Lab Activity 12.1

Evaluating Your Potential for Foot and Leg Injuries

INSTRUCTIONS: *Injuries to the feet and legs are common in most sports activities. If you continue the same activity long enough, overuse injuries are almost certain. There are also certain aspects in the makeup of the lower extremities that may require some adjustment to prevent injury. To evaluate your potential for lower extremity injury, examine yourself carefully in the following areas:*

1. **Length of both legs below the ankle:** Stand erect, with your ankles together, and ask a helper to measure the distance from the floor to a spot marked with a magic marker at the bony protrusion of your ankle.

2. **Length of both legs above the ankle:** Sit in a chair with your feet on the floor, heels together, and toes pointed. If a carpenter's level placed on both knees is uneven, your problem is above the ankle.

3. **Morton's toe:** Stand erect without shoes or socks and determine whether your second toe is longer than your big toe.

4. **Excessive pronation:** Examine your running or athletic shoes for excessive wear on the outside back of the shoe heel.

Results

1. Does the length of your legs differ by more than 1.6 millimetres?

2. Is the problem below the ankle or from the ankle to the knee?

3. Is your second toe longer than your big toe?

4. Are your shoes wearing unevenly?

5. Are you experiencing pain in your lower back, hip, knees, ankles, or feet during or following exercise?

If you answered Yes to any of the questions, consult an orthopedic physician for advice on how to prevent a future injury.

Lab Activity 12.2

Evaluating Your Home Medicine Cabinet

INSTRUCTIONS: *It is very important to analyze your medicine cabinet at least once a year and discard outdated prescriptions and other medicine. Replace used items, discard unnecessary items, place dangerous medicine out of the reach of children, and purchase newly needed products. Because you are beginning a new exercise program, some new items may be needed to prepare you for the treatment of common injuries. Complete the three steps below to evaluate and update your medicine cabinet.*

1. Prepare a list of all items in your home medicine cabinet and complete the form below.

Item	Date	Purpose	Effectiveness
_____	____	_____	_____
_____	____	_____	_____
_____	____	_____	_____
_____	____	_____	_____
_____	____	_____	_____
_____	____	_____	_____
_____	____	_____	_____
_____	____	_____	_____
_____	____	_____	_____
_____	____	_____	_____
_____	____	_____	_____

2. List all unneeded and outdated items that can be discarded.

_____ _____
_____ _____
_____ _____
_____ _____
_____ _____

(continued)

3. Study Table 12.6 to make certain your cabinet contains the bare necessities for treatment of common exercise injuries and ailments. List the items you are missing and may want to consider purchasing.

———————————————   ———————————————

———————————————   ———————————————

———————————————   ———————————————

———————————————   ———————————————

———————————————   ———————————————

13

Preventing Heart Disease, Cancer, and Other Diseases

CHAPTER OBJECTIVES

By the end of this chapter, you should be able to:

1. Cite the prevalence and describe the causes of heart disease.
2. Cite the prevalence and describe the causes of cancer.
3. Describe how to prevent or postpone the development of heart disease.
4. Describe how to prevent cancer.
5. Discuss the role of physical fitness in preventing heart disease, cancer, and other diseases.

WHEN FRANK WAS young, he assumed he was invulnerable. He knew intellectually that he would someday die; sooner or later, everyone does. But that was not a reality Frank had internalized. In fact, he acted as though he were impervious to the effects of his health decisions. He smoked cigarettes, rarely exercised, took on too much work thereby "stressing himself out," did not eat well by often choosing fatty meals at fast-food restaurants, and spent prolonged periods lounging in the sun.

Frank eventually paid the price for his health-related choices. By the time he reached his fiftieth year, he had a cough diagnosed as lung cancer and had blocked arteries that threatened a heart attack. Although he had yet to develop skin cancer, his doctor warned him that cancer was possible unless he altered his exposure to the sun's harsh rays. Contributing to his heart condition was the amount of stress to which he subjected himself, the cigarettes he smoked, and his lack of regular exercise. Contributing to the threat of his developing cancer elsewhere than in the lungs was his ingestion of foods high in fat. Frank's early years may have been carefree, but his later adult life was fraught with discomfort and fear. He realized he would not live as long as he might have.

Unfortunately, Frank's situation, extreme though it may sound, is not all that unusual. Too many people have experienced the death of a loved one from either heart disease, cancer, or some other disease. If you have not experienced any of these illnesses yourself, you certainly know others who have—parents, grandparents, relatives, friends. This is not surprising because heart disease and cancer alone account for 55 percent of all deaths that occur in Canada each year. Throw in stroke, which is also a developmental disease associated with an unhealthy lifestyle, and you have accounted for over 60 percent of the deaths that occur in this country every year.

In this chapter, we will define heart disease, cancer, and other serious and potentially fatal diseases and conditions and discuss what causes them. More importantly, we will describe how to prevent their occurrence or at least how to delay their arrival. Much of that latter discussion pertains to lifestyle decisions that include physical fitness and wellness considerations.

*H*EART DISEASE

One of the authors of this book once moved into a new house and experienced a most frustrating situation. Every few weeks the faucets had to be dismantled to

---

Coronary heart disease (CHD) A condition in which the heart is supplied with insufficient blood due to clogging of coronary arteries.

Occluded Clogged arteries that no longer allow the normal amount of blood to pass through them are said to be occluded.

Plaque A collection of blood fats and other substances that combine to clog blood vessels.

Atherosclerosis A condition in which plaque has formed and blocks the passage of blood through a blood vessel.

Angina pectoris Chest pain caused by restricted blood flow to the heart.

Lipoproteins A substance consisting of lipids and proteins that travels through the blood system transporting triglycerides and cholesterol.

Triglyceride A fatty substance in lipoproteins.

Low-density lipoproteins (LDLs) Fatty particles in the blood that carry cholesterol to cells throughout the body.

High-density lipoproteins (HDLs) Fatty particles in the blood that pick up unused cholesterol and transport it for processing and elimination from the body.

---

clean out the debris. (The builder said this was to be expected in a new house, that lead and material from inside the pipes accumulates and clogs the faucets.) Every few weeks the screens in the taps got clogged and had to be taken out and cleaned.

The situation with the faucets is analogous to that of the body's fluid system, which includes the heart, the blood, and the blood vessels. As the faucets carry water to where it is needed, so the blood vessels carry blood to where it is needed. As the pumping station somewhere in town pumps the water, so the heart pumps the blood. And as pipes can become clogged with debris, so can your blood vessels.

■ How the Heart Functions

The heart's main function is to pump blood containing oxygen and nutrients to the various parts of the body. The heart also receives blood filled with waste products (such as carbon dioxide) that it pumps into the lungs for elimination through breathing. If blood vessels become obstructed or if they rupture, thereby interfering with the passage of oxygenated blood, the part of the body deprived of blood can die. And if the heart's blood supply itself is blocked, it, too, can die. That is what happens when a heart attack occurs. Because the arteries supplying the heart are called the coronary arteries, any problem with them is called either **coronary heart disease (CHD)** or coronary artery disease.

■ Coronary Heart Disease (CHD)

Some people are born with heart disease. They may have a heart chamber missing or malformed, a valve between the chambers of the heart not opening or closing adequately, or a weak heart that is unable to pump with enough power to distribute enough blood throughout the body. Others may have blood vessels that do not work normally because they are malformed. Still others may have heart disease because they have had rheumatic fever (which affects the heart valves), or they may experience an irregular heartbeat known as an *arrythmia*.

The most prevalent form of heart disease, however, is CHD. The coronary arteries can become **occluded** when blood fats and other substances collect on their inside walls, thereby narrowing the opening through which blood can flow (see Figure 13.1). This collection of blood fats and other substances can also break loose and travel through the arteries until it gets caught and blocks the flow of blood at that point. That is called a *thrombosis*. The clogging material is called **plaque**, and the condition is known as **atherosclerosis**. Plaque consists of fatty substances, cholesterol, cellular waste products, calcium, and the clotting material *fibrin*. If blood flow is restricted, a person can become fatigued easily

Figure 13.1 ✦ Coronary Artery Blockage

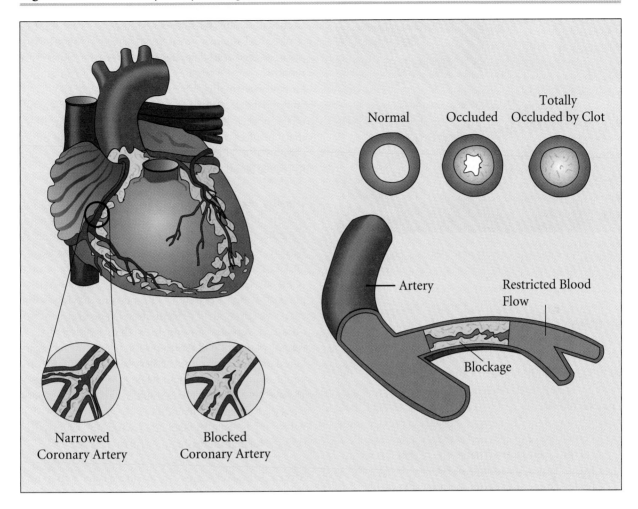

and may feel **angina pectoris** when active. If the coronary arteries are so narrowed or blocked that little, if any, blood can pass through, the part of the heart deprived of oxygenated blood can die. And if that part is important or involves a large enough section of the heart, the person to whom this happens can die.

Fat and Cholesterol

Lipoproteins consist of **triglycerides**, a blood protein (to make the fat soluble in the portion of the blood that is water), and cholesterol. Although some people are suspicious of the role of triglycerides in causing CHD, researchers have found no clear-cut association between the two. The real culprit in CHD is the cholesterol found in the foods we eat, and that is manufactured by the liver. When we eat foods high in saturated fats, the liver is stimulated to manufacture cholesterol. Add that to the cholesterol in the foods of animal origin that we eat, and the amount in our blood can be excessive.

Low-Density and High-Density Lipoproteins (LDLs and HDLs)

There are several different kinds of lipoproteins, of which **low-density lipoproteins (LDLs)** and **high-density lipoproteins (HDLs)** have the most significance for CHD. LDLs are produced in the liver and released into the bloodstream where they carry cholesterol to cells throughout the body. Cholesterol helps form cell membranes and the covering that protects nerve fibres; aids in the formation of vitamin D and the sex hormones androgen, estrogen, and progesterone; and helps produce bile salts that aid in digestion of fats. When LDLs carry more cholesterol than the body requires, however, they can build up on the artery walls.

HDLs are also produced by the liver and released into the bloodstream. Although they also carry cholesterol, HDLs pick up unused cholesterol and return it to the liver where it is used to produce bile salts. In addition, it is thought that HDLs provide a protective layer to help prevent a buildup of substances on artery walls.

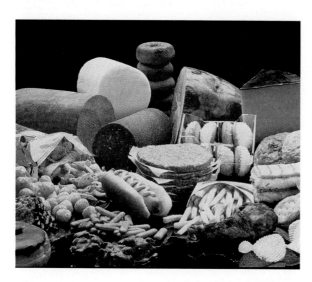

The average Canadian eats too much fat and cholesterol, substances that contribute to both heart disease and cancer.

When LDL is elevated and HDL is too sparse, there is a likelihood that arteries will be clogged and CHD will be promoted. It is recommended that HDL (the *good* cholesterol) levels exceed 9 millimoles per litre (mmol/L) of blood for adult men and women and that LDL (the *bad* cholesterol) levels remain less than 3 mmol/L. A total cholesterol/HDL ratio of 5 to 1 (20 percent of total cholesterol being of the HDL variety) begins to provide some protection from CHD. Physical activity can increase HDL levels in the bloodstream. That is one reason it is recommended as a way of preventing CHD.

To determine if the composition of your blood is healthful, complete Lab Activity 13.1: Is Your Blood in Tune? at the end of this chapter.

◼ Other Risk Factors for Heart Disease

You already know that the foods we eat and the cholesterol our bodies produce are two reasons blood vessels can become clogged. There are also other causes of clogged coronary arteries and the development of heart disease.

Hypertension High blood pressure, or hypertension, is an independent risk factor for cardiovascular disease and can increase the risk by two- or threefold (Berenson et al., 1998). Twenty-five percent of Canadian men and 18 percent of Canadian women have high blood pressure. **Hypertension** is systolic blood pressure in excess of 140 millimetres Hg or diastolic blood pressure in excess of 90 millimetres Hg. **Systolic blood pressure** refers to the force of the blood against the arterial blood-vessel walls when the left ventricle contracts and blood is pumped out of the heart. **Diastolic blood pressure** represents the force of the blood against the arterial walls when the heart is

relaxed. High blood pressure forces the heart to work harder than normal and places the arteries under strain. Eventually, hypertension contributes to heart attacks, strokes, and atherosclerosis. In 90 percent of high-blood-pressure *essential hypertension* cases, the causes are unknown. In the remaining 10 percent, it is caused by a kidney abnormality, a tumour of the adrenal gland, or a congenital defect of the aorta (the main artery leading out of the heart). Regular physical activity and a healthier diet are often recommended for people whose blood pressure is too high. In some cases, medication is needed to reduce blood pressure to healthier levels.

Obesity or Overweight The National Population Health Survey (1996–97) found that 48 percent of Canadian adults are considered overweight. Of these, 19 percent were categorized as having some excess weight and 29 percent as obese. These values have remained relatively constant since the 1994–95 survey when 49 percent were overweight (19 percent having some excess weight and 30 percent obese). The prevalence of obesity is greater among men than women. Excess weight places added strain on the heart and increases blood pressure and blood cholesterol. For these reasons, people who gain more than 9 kilograms after the age of 18 have been found to have doubled their risk of experiencing a heart attack. In addition, obesity is linked to diabetes and is usually associated with lack of physical activity, further increasing the risk of heart attack.

Stress Excessive stress also increases a person's chances of contracting heart disease. That is because stress results in an increase in cholesterol in the blood, an increase in heart rate, higher blood pressure, and other effects detrimental to normal heart functioning. Stress results in the release of hormones called *catecholamines*, which prepare the body to respond physically—the fight-or-flight response discussed in an earlier chapter. The heart beats faster, blood pressure increases, and blood-glucose and cholesterol levels increase. If stress occurs often, these detrimental effects become chronic and can lead to CHD.

Two researchers (Friedman and Rosenman, 1974) have even found a coronary-prone personality type. They call it the Type A behaviour pattern, characterized by being focused on time (hurried and time-pressured), competitive, aggressive, hostile, and polyphasic (doing two or more things at a time). The opposite, Type B behaviour pattern, seems to protect people from developing CHD (see Chapter 10). More recent research indicates that hostility is the major ingredient in the Type A behaviour pattern. That is, people who are easily angered and who are often hostile are the most susceptible to CHD. Stress also too frequently interferes with

MYTH AND FACT SHEET

Myth	Fact
1. If CHD runs in your family, there is not much you can do to prevent getting it.	1. CHD is related to a number of factors of which heredity is but one. Other risk factors include smoking, lack of exercise, fatty diets, obesity, and high blood pressure. You can do much to eliminate or diminish the effects of these risk factors.
2. All cholesterol is bad.	2. The cholesterol that accumulates on the walls of the arteries, LDL, is bad for you. HDLs, however, help to carry blood fats out of the body and therefore are helpful.
3. You can recognize if your blood pressure is high, but there is little you can do to lower it.	3. High blood pressure occurs without any noticeable symptoms, but with a healthier diet and regular physical activity, blood pressure can be lowered, even without medication.
4. Everything causes cancer.	4. This is simply not true. Although cancer can result from toxins, carcinogens in cigarette smoke, chemicals, and viruses, saying that everything causes cancer is merely an excuse for ignoring specific causes.
5. Cancer affects all groups of people to the same extent.	5. More black men and women than white men and women die of cancer. White men and women contract skin cancer to a much greater extent than black men and women.

people engaging in regular exercise. They become so concerned with managing the source of the stress—whether that be their classes, jobs, finances, or home lives—that they allow too little time, if any, for physical activity.

Sedentary Lifestyle We have just discussed the effect of stress on physical activity. In addition, a sedentary lifestyle does not allow for the production of sufficient HDLs, strengthen the heart muscle, or help control mild hypertension. To make matters worse, inactivity is associated with being overweight and obesity, two other risk factors for CHD. And inactivity deprives you of an outlet for the release of built-up stress by-products (for example, cholesterol). Research indicates that sedentary individuals have a 1.2–2-fold increased risk of premature death. With nearly 60 percent of Canadian adults not being physically active, our population remains at high risk for heart disease (Heart & Stroke Foundation of Canada, 1999).

Smoking Tobacco The National Population Health Survey (1996–97) revealed that 29 percent of Canadian adults (15 years and over) smoke cigarettes either daily or occasionally. Although a steady decline in smoking rates occurred from 1977 to 1986, the smoking rates since 1991 have remained constant (National Population Health Survey, Statistics Canada, 1996–97). Research has linked smoking with various diseases such as cancer, emphysema, and heart disease. When a person smokes, the blood vessels constrict thereby causing increased blood pressure. In addition, the heart speeds up in response to nicotine, a central nervous system stimulant. Furthermore, cigarettes contain substances that can damage the inside walls of the arteries. Once arteries

Hypertension High blood pressure; usually greater than 140 systolic blood pressure and/or greater than 90 diastolic blood pressure.

Systolic blood pressure The force of the blood against the arterial blood-vessel walls when the left ventricle contracts and blood is pumped out of the heart.

Diastolic blood pressure The force of the blood against the arterial walls when the heart is relaxed.

DIVERSITY ISSUES

Smoking Rates

Since 1999, the federal government has been using data from the Canadian Tobacco Use Monitoring Survey (CTUMS) to track tobacco use in this country. The latest results from the first half of 2002 for CTUMS confirms that smoking rates in Canada are declining. Here are some of the statistics from wave 1, 2002:

- In 2002, approximately 21 percent of the population over age 15 were daily or occasional smokers. This is down from 25 percent in 1999. Men have a slightly higher rate (23 percent) than women (20 percent).

- Rates for youth aged 15–19 are also down: 22 percent in this category smoke, down from 28 percent in 1999. Interestingly, in this age category, more females (24 percent) smoke than males (20 percent).

- The young adult category (ages 20–24) contains the highest percentage of smokers—31 percent—although this too is down, from 35 percent in 1999. For this group, the numbers for men and women are about even.

Although these CTUMS results are definitely heartening, smoking is still the leading cause of preventable death in Canada, responsible for more than five times the number of deaths caused by car accidents, murder, suicide, and alcohol abuse—combined. Given these statistics, it's certain that the federal government will continue to monitor and try to reduce tobacco use in the Canadian population ✦

Sources: Adapted from Canadian Tobacco Use Monitoring Survey (CTUMS), Summary of Results for Wave 1 (February to June) of 2002. Available at **www.hc-sc.gc.ca/hecs-sesc/ tobacco/research/ctums/2002/summary.html**. Accessed March 10, 2002; Health Canada, News Release. Smoking Rates Continue to Drop. June 28, 2002. Available at **www.hc-sc.gc.ca/english/ media/releases/2002/2002_52.htm**. Accessed March 10, 2002. Adapted and reproduced with the permission of the Minister of Public Works and Government Services Canada, 2003. *Health Canada assumes no responsibility for any errors or omissions which may have occurred in the adaptation of its material.*

Family History Not all risk factors are amenable to change. Heredity, for example, is not. Some people are born with a predisposition to heart disease. However, that predisposition only means there is the *potential* to develop CHD—your lifestyle will influence whether and when you do. Some people prefer to use a family history of heart disease as an excuse for behaving in ways that are unhealthy for the heart. That is unfortunate because they might be able to delay or even prevent CHD if they change their behaviour.

Seventy-five percent of Canadian adults have at least one of the major heart disease risk factors (hypertension, elevated blood cholesterol, regular smoking, and sedentary lifestyle). Diseases of the heart are the most expensive diseases for Canadians, accounting for $18 billion each year. To determine your risk of acquiring CHD, complete Lab Activity 13.2: RISKO: A Heart Health Appraisal at the end of this chapter.

How to Prevent Coronary Heart Disease (CHD)

It is possible to manage many of the risk factors for CHD. Hypertension can be controlled by some combination of diet, exercise, and medication. Being overweight or obese can be controlled by diet and exercise. Stress can be managed by a change in lifestyle and some form of regular relaxation. Sedentary lifestyles can be remedied by participation in an exercise program. Smoking can be stopped by joining a smoking-cessation program or quitting cold turkey. And periodic medical screenings can be useful to analyze blood lipids and evaluate the functioning of the heart. The good news is that you have a great deal of influence over whether you develop CHD. If you are serious about preventing CHD, you can do so.

The Role of Physical Activity

Physical activity is one of the most important components of a CHD-prevention program. That is because it is either directly or indirectly related to so many of the risk factors. Physical activity exercises the heart muscle, encourages the production of HDLs, and aids in the control and prevention of mild hypertension. It enhances cardiorespiratory endurance and increases stroke volume of the heart (the amount of blood pumped out of the heart with each contraction). It also is an excellent stress-management technique because it uses the stress by-products that prepare the body to respond physically to a stressor. And physical activity can help you maintain desirable weight and the proper amount of lean-body mass.

have been damaged, it is easier for cholesterol and other substances to adhere to and accumulate in them. All of this, coupled with carbon dioxide from cigarette smoke replacing oxygen in the bloodstream, means the heart is overworking and heart disease is more likely.

These effects are somewhat direct and obvious, but there are less direct and less obvious CHD-related benefits of physical activity as well. Engaging in regular exercise will tone your body, provide you with confidence in your ability to perform physically, and make you feel better about yourself. In short, it will improve your self-esteem. The result will be less stress, fewer catecholamines produced, and therefore less potential damage to your heart.

Physical activity also encourages smoking cessation. Smoking is incompatible with aerobic activity because carbon monoxide replaces oxygen in the bloodstream. Furthermore, doing one good thing for your health, such as becoming physically fit, encourages other healthy lifestyle adjustments.

It is for these and other reasons that an effective CHD-prevention program includes a physical-activity component. As prestigious an organization as the Heart and Stroke Foundation of Canada recognizes the importance of physical activity in preventing CHD. The Foundation, in its position statement on physical activity, recommends that regular physical activity, when properly undertaken, can be effective in preventing and limiting the disabling effects of heart disease and stroke. Its specific recommendations are that people of all ages be active on a daily basis, and that they incorporate fitness-enhancing activity into their normal routine. Also, schools should ensure that quality daily physical and health education is provided. The Foundation stresses that physical activity is a vital component in maintaining good health as well as in cardiac and stroke rehabilitation.

CANCER

Cancer is a disease involving abnormal cell growth. Cells grow wildly, divide rapidly, and assume irregular shapes; thus, tumours develop, and invade nearby normal tissue. The abnormal cells can spread to other parts of the body via the bloodstream and lymphatic system in a process called **metastasis**. Disability and/or death can ensue (see Table 13.1).

Cancer is the leading cause of death in Canada. In 2001, an estimated 134 100 new cases of cancer were diagnosed and 68 600 deaths were attributed to cancer (Cancer Bureau, CCDPC, Health Canada, 2001). This represents a 3.8 percent increase in the number of new diagnoses and a 9.4 percent increase in the number of deaths due to cancer since 1997.

Lung cancer is by far the leading cause of death from cancer in both men and women, but that need not

be the case. If everyone who now smokes cigarettes quit, the incidence of lung cancer would decline dramatically. The 2001 Canadian Cancer Statistics indicate the importance of women receiving breast cancer screenings and of men undergoing prostate exams, given that these are the second leading causes of cancer death among women and men, at 5500 and 4300, respectively.

Cancer is really more than one disease. Some cancers are caused by chemicals, others by environmental pollutants, some by radiation from the sun, and still others by viruses. As we have already discussed, cancers also occur in different parts of the body. Even the treatment for different cancers can vary. In some cases, surgery is necessary to remove the cancerous tissue. Sometimes, radiation or chemotherapy is required. Often, a combination of these three treatments is used.

◾ Causes of Cancer

Cancer develops from a number of different causes. By far the leading cause of cancer is the use of tobacco. An estimated 75 percent of all lung cancer cases are thought to be caused by smoking cigarettes. Smoking a pipe or cigar or chewing tobacco can cause cancer of the mouth and its parts. The use of tobacco products is associated with cancer of the larynx, pharynx, esophagus, pancreas, and bladder.

High-fat diets are associated with cancer of the colon, rectum, prostate, stomach, and breast. Conversely, diets low in fat, but high in fruits and vegetables, seem to offer protection against certain cancers.

Repeated exposure to the sun is also a cause of skin cancer. It is the radiation from the sun that is the culprit here. Particularly vulnerable are people with fair skin who burn easily.

Excessive use of alcohol exposes one to the risk of oral cancer and cancers of the larynx, throat, esophagus, and liver, especially when accompanied by the use of smokeless tobacco.

Other causes of cancers include occupational hazards (exposure to toxins or chemicals or other **carcinogens**), viruses, obesity, environmental pollutants (such as those contained in automobile exhaust), and hereditary and genetic factors.

Metastasis The process in which cancerous cells from one part of the body travel to other parts of the body.

Carcinogens Agents (toxins, chemicals, and so forth) that can cause cancer.

Table 13.1 ✦ Estimated New Cases and Deaths for Cancer Sites by Gender, 2001

SITE	NEW CASES (1999 ESTIMATE)			DEATHS (1999 ESTIMATE)			DEATHS/CASES RATIO (1999 ESTIMATE)		
	Total	M	F	Total	M	F	Total	M	F
All Cancers	**134 100**	**68 600**	**65 400**	**65 300**	**34 600**	**30 700**	**0.49**	**0.50**	**0.47**
Lung	21 200	12 100	9200	18 000	10 700	7400	0.85	0.89	0.80
Breast	19 500	19 500	—	5500	—	5500	0.28	—	0.28
Prostate[1]	17 800	17 800	—	4300	4300	—	0.24	0.24	—
Colorectal	17 200	9300	7900	6400	3400	3000	0.37	0.37	0.38
Non-Hodgkin's Lymphoma	6200	3400	2800	2700	1400	1250	0.44	0.42	0.45
Bladder	4700	3500	1250	1500	1050	460	0.32	0.30	0.37
Kidney	3900	2400	1500	1450	890	550	0.37	0.37	0.36
Melanoma	3800	1950	1800	820	490	330	0.22	0.25	0.18
Leukemia	3500	2000	1500	2100	1200	940	0.61	0.61	0.62
Body of Uterus	3500	—	3500	670	—	670	0.19	—	0.19
Pancreas	3100	1500	1650	3100	1500	1650	1.00	0.99	1.01[2]
Oral	3100	2100	980	1050	730	320	0.34	0.34	0.33
Stomach	2800	1750	1000	1950	1200	770	0.70	0.67	0.76
Ovary	2500	—	2500	1500	—	1500	0.60	—	0.60
Brain	2400	1300	1050	1550	880	670	0.66	0.67	0.64
Thyroid	1900	510	1400	160	50	110	0.09	0.10	0.08
Multiple Myeloma	1700	960	760	1250	670	590	0.73	0.70	0.77
Cervix	1450	—	1450	420	—	420	0.29	—	0.29
Esophagus	1350	930	420	1450	1050	400	1.09[2]	1.15[2]	0.95
Larynx	1250	1000	240	520	430	90	0.42	0.42	0.38
Hodgkin's Disease	810	430	380	120	70	55	0.15	0.16	0.14
Testis	790	790	—	35	35	—	0.05	0.05	—
All Other Sites	9500	4900	4600	8700	4600	4100	0.91	0.93	0.89

— = not applicable

[1] The number of new prostate cases was estimated on the basis of data years 1980–1989.

[2] The high ratio (in excess of 1.0) for cancers of esophagus and pancreas may result from incomplete registration of this cancer before death.

Note: Incidence figures exclude an estimated 70 000 new cases of non-melanoma skin cancer (ICD-9 173). Total of rounded numbers may not equal rounded total number.

Source: Cancer Bureau, CCDPC, Health Canada National Cancer Institute of Canada: Canadian Cancer Statistics 2001, Toronto, Canada, 2001.

To determine how susceptible you are to contracting cancer, complete Lab Activity 13.3: Determining Your Risk of Getting Cancer at the end of this chapter.

■ Cancer Prevention

Although not all cancers can be prevented, the Canadian Cancer Society states that 60–70 percent of cancers in Canada could be prevented if Canadians adopted healthier lifestyles. If people gave up smoking, ate diets consisting of less fat and more vegetables and fruits, limited the amount of alcohol they ingested, and protected themselves from exposure to the sun, the decrease in the incidence of cancer would be significant. Here are some things you can do to decrease your chances of contracting cancer or, if you do contract it, to detect it early:

1. Abstain from using tobacco in any form, including the smokeless variety.

2. Eliminate or reduce your consumption of alcohol; drink only in moderation.

3. Avoid contact with known carcinogens whenever possible.

4. Decrease your exposure to the sun; avoid sunbathing for long periods of time; and use a sunscreen with the appropriate sun protection factor (SPF) for your skin type anytime you plan to be in the sun.

5. Follow a dietary plan that increases your consumption of vitamins A and C, cruciferous vegetables (for example, cauliflower and broccoli), and fibre. Reduce your consumption of artificial sweeteners, heat-charred food, nitrite-cured or smoked foods, fats, and calories.

6. Maintain recommended body weight and fat.

7. Memorize the seven warning signs of cancer (see Table 13.2) and be alert to these changes if they occur in your body.

8. Obtain cancer screenings as recommended (see Table 13.3) to identify early signs of cancer.

9. Learn how to do breast (females) and testicular (males) self-examinations and do them regularly.

10. Check for changes in your skin that might indicate skin cancer.

11. Report any family history of cancer to your doctor and have that history noted on your medical records.

Table 13.4 summarizes the things you can do to prevent your developing cancer.

■ Physical Activity and Cancer Prevention

Physical activity has been found to help prevent the onset of cancer. The exact reason for this is unclear, although several theories have been proposed. For example, some researchers attribute the decreased incidence of cancer among people who are physically active to their being

Table 13.2 ✦ The Seven Warning Signs of Cancer

Report any of the following signs of cancer to your doctor:

Change in bowel or bladder habits

A sore that does not heal

Unusual bleeding or discharge

Thickening or lump in breast or elsewhere

Indigestion or difficulty in swallowing

Obvious change in wart or mole

Nagging cough or hoarseness

Source: American Cancer Society, *Cancer Facts & Figures—1993* (New York: American Cancer Society, 1993), p. 12. Used by permission. © American Cancer Society, Inc.

WELLNESS HEROES

Terry Fox

Terry Fox was diagnosed with osteogenic sarcoma (bone cancer) in his right leg in 1977. His leg was amputated about 15 centimetres above his knee. While in hospital, Terry was so overcome by the suffering of cancer patients that he decided to run across Canada to raise funds for cancer research. His journey was called The Marathon of Hope.

Terry's Marathon of Hope took place in 1980. His additional objective was to raise the awareness of all Canadians of the critical need to find a cure for cancer. Terry's fierce determination resulted in his running about 43 kilometres every day for 143 days.

Before reaching his goal he was overcome by a return of his cancer and died in June 1981; however, by February 1, 1981, Terry's hope of raising one dollar from every Canadian was realized—the Marathon's fund totalled $24.17 million. And to date, over $300 million has been raised worldwide. All funds support innovative cancer research and are distributed by the National Cancer Institute of Canada. This event is the largest one-day fundraiser for cancer research in the world.

The success of the annual Terry Fox Run is made possible by the dedication and hard work of thousands of volunteers who organize over 6,600 run sites in Canada. Across the country over 1.5 million participants walk, jog, and bike to raise funds in the name of Terry Fox. One national and nine provincial Terry Fox Run offices, with 21 full-time employees, support this magnificent work in Canada.

In 2001, there were an estimated 242 000 participants from more than 50 countries as disparate as United Arab Emirates, South Africa, Mexico, India, and Ghana, and over $6.25 million was raised by them. In total, over $20 million was raised worldwide that year. It is a fitting tribute to a man who knew that cancer has no nationality. ✦

Sources: Adapted from http://www.terryfoxrun.org/english/foundation/history/; "the Terry Fox Run Around the World," The Terry Fox Foundation. Available at http://www.terryfoxrun.org. © Copyright 2003, The Terry Fox Foundation.

Table 13.3 ✦ Canadian Cancer Society's Guidelines for Early Detection and Screening for Cancer

Although healthcare agencies mostly agree with the following guidelines, your family doctor will recommend appropriate tests to monitor your health, based on your medical history and your lifestyle. Screening tests do not exist for every type of cancer and when they do, they are not always 100 percent accurate. There is no single test for all types of cancers. Visit your doctor or dentist if you notice a change in your normal state of health.

TEST OR PROCEDURE	SEX	AGE	GUIDELINES FOR EARLY DETECTION AND SCREENING
Mammography	Female	50–69 High risk	Every two years if you are aged 50–69. Women under 50 or over 69 should check with their doctor. Combine with clinical breast examination and BSE. Individualized plan of surveillance as outlined by your doctor. High-risk groups include: first-degree relative (mother, daughter, sister) with breast cancer, family history of cancer.
Clinical breast examination	Female	All women	By a doctor or trained health professional at least every two years. Combine with mammography and BSE.
Breast self examination	Female	Adult women— particularly after age 40	Regular BSE is not as effective as mammography or clinical breast examination in finding breast cancer, but breast self examination helps you learn what is normal for your breast and to notice any changes. Report changes to your doctor. Combine with mamography and clinical breast examination.
Pap test/ Pelvic examination	Female		Pap test once you become sexually active at any age, and even if you don't have sex anymore. Pap testing is performed every 1–3 years depending on the screening guidelines in each province.
Skin examination	Female/male	All ages	Regular skin examination and report any changes to your doctor.
Fecal Occult Blood Test (FOBT)	Female/male	Age 50 and over High risk	At least every two years to detect colorectal cancer. Positive tests should be followed up with a colonoscopy or double contrast barium enema. People at high risk of colorectal cancer should discuss an individualized plan of surveillance with their doctor. High-risk groups include: those with inflammatory bowel disease, other bowel disorders, previous colorectal cancer, benign polyps, and a strong family history of colorectal cancer.
Digital rectal examination (DRE)	Female/male	50 and over	Every year. Digital rectal examination can be helpful to detect cancers of both the rectum and prostate.
PSA test (Prostate Specific Antigen)	Male	50 and over High risk	Men over 50 should discuss the benefits and risks of early detection using PSA and DRE with their doctor. Men at high risk of prostate cancer—such as men of African ancestry, and those with a strong family history of prostate cancer—may wish to discuss the need for testing at a younger age.
Testicular self-examination (TSE)	Male	15 and over	Monthly testicular self-examination is an early detection measure. Report any changes to your doctor.

Source: 2002 Canadian Cancer Society. All rights reserved.

leaner. Excess fat is associated with cancer of the colon, prostate, endometrium, and breast. Whether physical activity has a direct effect on cancer or an indirect effect by reducing body fat is unknown.

The National Cancer Institute in the United States also reports that men who exert the energy equivalent of walking 10 or more miles (16.1 or more kilometres) per week have half the risk of developing colon cancer

Table 13.4 ✦ How to Prevent Cancer

Research continues to show that up to 70% of cancers can be prevented. Take the following steps to reduce your risk of developing cancer.

1. **Be a non-smoker and avoid second-hand smoke.**

   Smoking causes about 30 percent of all cancer deaths in Canada. Lung cancer is the leading cause of cancer death for men and women in Canada. Smoking also increases your risk of developing cancers of the mouth, throat, larynx, cervix, pancreas, esophagus, colon, rectum, kidney, and bladder.

   Nonsmokers exposed to secondhand smoke are also at higher risk of getting cancer and other lung diseases. Health Canada estimates that more than 300 nonsmokers die from lung cancer each year because of secondhand smoke.

   If you are a smoker, quit. If you are a nonsmoker, avoid secondhand smoke.

2. **Eat 5–10 servings of vegetables and fruit a day. Choose high fibre, lower fat foods. If you drink alcohol, limit your intake to 1–2 drinks a day.**

   Research suggests as much as one-third of all cancers may be related to what we eat and drink. Eat 5 to 10 servings of vegetables and fruit a day. Eat plenty of whole-grain fibres. Keep your dietary fat intake low and if you drink, limit your alcohol consumption to 1 to 2 drinks per day. For a healthy diet, balance your daily meals with foods from the four food groups described in *Canada's Food Guide to Healthy Eating*.

3. **Be physically active on a regular basis: this will also help you maintain a healthy body weight.**

   Most people know that regular exercise is necessary to remain healthy. Studies strongly suggest that exercise reduces your risk of colon cancer. Also, the evidence of a link between physical activity and preventing breast cancer is convincing.

4. **Protect yourself and your family from the sun.**

   Reduce sun exposure between 11 a.m. and 4 p.m. Check your skin regularly and report any changes to your doctor.

   This year, tens of thousands of Canadians will develop skin cancer because of overexposure to UV (ultraviolet light). Skin cancer is the most frequently diagnosed cancer in Canada.

   Reduce sun exposure between 11 a.m. and 4 p.m. Seek shade or create your own. Keep babies under one year old out of direct sun. Tanning parlours and sunlamps are not safe.

   When you are in the sun, always remember: SLIP, SLAP, SLOP.

   - SLIP on clothing to cover your arms and legs.
   - SLAP on a wide-brimmed hat.
   - SLOP on sunscreen (SPF 15 or higher).

5. **Follow cancer screening guidelines.**

   For women, discuss mammography, Pap tests, and breast exams with a health professional.

   For men, discuss testicular exams and prostate screening with a health professional.

   Both men and women should also discuss screening for colon and rectal cancers.

   Even people with healthy lifestyles can develop cancer. One way to detect cancer early is to have regular screening tests. These tests can often find cancer when it is still at an early stage. The earlier the cancer is found, the more successful the treatment is likely to be.

6. **Visit your doctor or dentist if you notice any change in your normal state of health.**

   Know your body and report any changes to your doctor or dentist as soon as possible (for example, sores that do not heal, a cough that goes on for more than two weeks or a change in bowel habits). Health care professionals are trained to spot the early warning signs of cancer and other diseases.

7. **Follow health and safety instructions at home and at work when using, storing, and disposing of hazardous materials.**

   At home and at work, take care to follow safety instructions when using, storing, and disposing of household pesticides or any other chemicals.

   Health Canada and Environment Canada have guidelines for handling cancer-causing substances. By following these guidelines, you can protect yourself against the risk posed by these materials. These guidelines are printed on the packaging and posted in workplaces.

Source: Canadian Cancer Society. All rights reserved.

DIVERSITY ISSUES

Environmental Tobacco Smoke and Children

A small child held by someone who is smoking will breathe in more cancer-causing chemicals than the smoker. Every day young children are forced to breathe secondhand smoke at home, at school, in restaurants, in public places, in cars, and on buses. Half of all Canadian children have at least one parent who smokes.

Environmental tobacco smoke (ETS), or second-hand smoke, is the most common and harmful form of indoor air pollution. It is made up of *mainstream smoke* and *sidestream smoke.* Mainstream smoke is what smokers breathe into their lungs and then out into the air. Sidestream smoke comes from the burning end of the cigarette between puffs.

Secondhand smoke has up to 4000 chemicals in it, more than 50 of which are known to cause cancer in humans. In fact, three cancer-causing chemicals found in secondhand smoke are so dangerous that the North American air quality rules used by most governments say no one should ever be exposed to them. Sidestream smoke has more tar, nicotine, carbon monoxide, and other chemicals that cause cancer than the mainstream smoke from filtered cigarettes. When a cigarette burns, about 85 percent of the smoke that goes into the air is sidestream smoke.

Secondhand smoke has serious effects on children's health. Children of parents who smoke cough and wheeze more, have more ear infections, go to the hospital more often with bronchitis and pneumonia, and have reduced lung function. Children with asthma have more asthma attacks due to secondhand smoke, and their attacks tend to be more severe. Children whose parents smoke 10 or more cigarettes a day have a greater chance of becoming asthmatic. There is a possible link between a mother's smoking and an infant's risk of dying from sudden infant death syndrome (SIDS).

Secondhand smoke also affects the unborn child of a mother who smokes or is exposed to second-hand smoke. Nicotine can be measured in the blood of a pregnant woman exposed to secondhand smoke. Nicotine speeds up the heartbeat of the fetus, slows down the growth of babies' lungs and air passages, and can also cause miscarriages and stillbirths. Carbon monoxide from secondhand smoke can cut down the unborn baby's oxygen supply by 25 percent, and this has an effect on the baby's growth.

There are many things you can do to protect your children and yourself. Make your home and car smoke-free areas. Find out about the smoking policy in your child's as well as your own school; if they are not smoke-free, work with school officials to clean the air. Urge your local or provincial government to pass laws that ban smoking in public places, schools, restaurants, public transportation, and workplaces. Tobacco legislation is considered the most efficacious method of reducing ETS exposure. ✦

Source: Adapted from "Growing Up in Smoke," off *Canadian Cancer Society* Web page, accessed March 30, 1999 **www.cancer. ca/info/pubs/growsme1.htm.** This material reprinted with the permission of the Canadian Cancer Society (**www.cancer.ca**)

of less active men. One theory explaining this finding is that exercise increases the rate of transit of food through the digestive tract. If there are carcinogens in the fecal stream, the faster they proceed through the system, the less chance there is that they will attach themselves to mucosa lining the tract and develop into cancer.

There is also evidence that women who exercise regularly are less prone to develop cancer of the breast or of the reproductive system. One theory relates a lower rate of these cancers and exercise to the amount of body fat. Fat is needed to make estrogen. This theory hypothesizes that excess fat increases the risk of these cancers because it leads to too much estrogen being produced.

These findings pertain to moderate amounts of exercise. That does not mean that intense exercise is also protective. In fact, some researchers believe that intense exercise is actually detrimental because it suppresses the immune system, resulting in the body being less able to ward off carcinogens. The discovery by researchers that prostate cancer is more common among male athletes lends credence to this theory.

■ Early Detection and Diagnosis of Cancer

Many cancers are highly curable if they are detected early. For example, both breast and testicular cancer detected in their earliest stages are well over 90 percent curable. The later the cancer is detected, the less positive is the prognosis. That is why it is so important to detect cancer as early as possible. Obtaining regular medical checkups is one way of assuring that cancers are found in their earliest stages. Medical screenings recommended are listed in Table 13.3. Another method of early detection is by performing regular self-examinations. Two of the most frequently recommended self-examinations are of the breast for women and of the testicles for men. Figures 13.2 and 13.3 show you how to perform these self-examinations.

Figure 13.2 ✦ Breast Self-Examination

While mammography and clinical breast examination are the most reliable methods of finding breast cancer, regular breast self-examination (BSE) helps you to learn what is normal for your own breasts and to recognize when something may be wrong.

What to look for when doing breast self-examination (BSE)

You are looking for changes in your breasts. First, you need to learn what is normal for your breasts. It may be normal for your breasts to feel a bit lumpy. You should check for any place in your breast that feels thicker or harder than the rest of your breast.

Use a mirror

Always begin checking your breasts by standing in front of a mirror. Leave your arms by your side. Look at your breasts. Slowly turn from side to side. Are there any changes in size and shape from the last time you looked? Check for rashes or puckery skin. Look for any discharge from your nipples.

Arms up

Lift your arms above your head while still looking in the mirror. Put your hands behind your ears. Look at your breasts and under your arms. Lower your hands to your nose. Squeeze your palms together. Are there any changes?

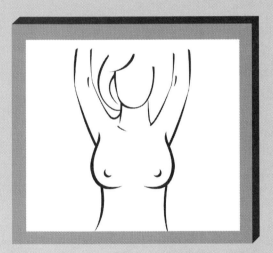
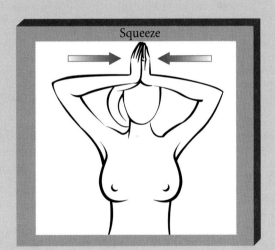

Keep standing

Complete the following steps for both breasts. Use the opposite hand for each breast. Start just below your collarbone. Cover all of your breast, even the nipples. Hold the fingers of your hand together. Keep your fingers stiff and your hand flat. Use the pads of your fingers, not the tips.

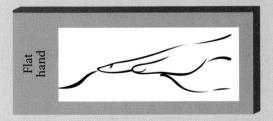
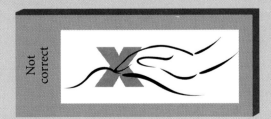

Bend your wrist to go over the curves of your breast. Keep constant contact and pressure with your skin. Make small circles covering the entire breast using one of the methods pictured on the next page.

(continued)

Figure 13.2 ✦ Breast Self-Examination *(continued)*

Grid method

Make small circles in straight lines starting just below your collarbone. Cover the area outlined by the box. Make small circles all the way across your breast. Go slowly. Now move your fingers down. Repeat the small circles back and forth across your breast.

Keep moving down until you are below your breast. You may need to make many circles to check your whole breast. Make sure you check your nipple. Hold fingers stiff. Bend your wrist to go under your arm. Complete these steps for both your breasts.

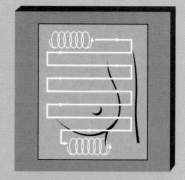

Circular method

Make small circles starting at the outside edge of your breast. Cover the area outlined by the circle. Make the small circles all the way around your breast. Go slowly. Now move your fingers in toward your nipple. Go around the breast again. The circle will be smaller this time.

Keep moving in toward your nipple. You may need to make many circles to check your whole breast. Make sure you check your nipple. Hold fingers stiff. Bend your wrist to go under your arm. Complete these steps for both your breasts. After you cover the whole area of your breast, check under your arm and up to your collarbone too. Relax your arm by your side. Slide your hand under that arm. Make small circles like you did over your breast.

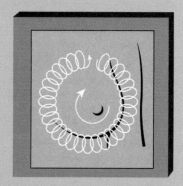

Lie down

Lie on your back on a firm surface. Put one hand behind your head. Hold the fingers of your other hand together. Check both breasts again, using the pads of your fingers and bending your wrist to cover the curves of your breasts.

Large breasts

If your breasts are large, they may fold over on your chest. This fold may feel like a firm ridge. Do not panic. This ridge is normal for large breasts. Lift them up to check all parts for changes.

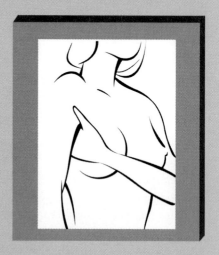

What to do if you find a change

Most of the time, the changes women find in their breasts are not cancer. If you do find a change in your breasts, call your doctor or clinic that day. Visit your doctor as soon as you can. Your doctor will be able to do tests to tell you what the change in your breast means. The sooner you have these tests the better.

A visit to your doctor will give you peace of mind if your lump is not cancer. And it may save your life if you need medical treatment.

Want to learn more?

If you want to learn more about checking your breasts:

• Ask your doctor or a trained health professional.
• Call the Cancer Information Service at 1-(888)-939-3333.

Source: Canadian Cancer Society, 2003 (**www.cancer.ca**)

Figure 13.3 ✦ Testicular Self-Examination *(continued)*

Follow the instructions in the diagram carefully and examine your testes immediately after your next hot bath or shower. Heat causes the testicles to descend and the scrotal skin to relax, making it easier to find unusual lumps.

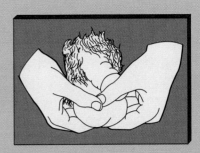

Examine each testicle by placing the index and middle fingers of both hands on the underside of the testicle and the thumbs on the top. Gently roll the testicle between your thumb and fingers, feeling for small lumps.

Changes or anything abnormal will appear at the front or side of your testicle. Did you find any unusual lumps? Are there any unusual signs of any kind? Are there any markings or lumps at any site?

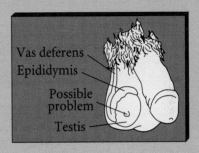

Vas deferens
Epididymis
Possible problem
Testis

Keep in mind that not all lumps are a sign of testicular cancer. Unusual lumps at any location, however, should be checked by a physician. Early detection greatly increases your chances of a complete cure. Repeat the examination every month and record your findings.

SEXUALLY TRANSMITTED DISEASES

Certain diseases can interfere with sexual activities. These used to be called venereal diseases (VD), named for Venus, the Roman goddess of love. Today, they are known less euphemistically as **sexually transmitted diseases (STDs)**. Although more than 20 organisms are linked to STDs, we discuss only the most prevalent STDs.

■ Gonorrhea

Popularly known as "the clap," "the drip," and many equally descriptive names, **gonorrhea** is caused by the *Neisseria gonorrhoeae* bacterium. In 2001, gonorrhea was the second most frequently reported STD in Canada. The incidence of the disease, however, which peaked at 56 336 cases in 1981, has decreased steadily with fewer than 6360 cases in 2001 Centre for Infectious Disease Prevention and Control, Health Canada, 2002).

Gonorrhea is transmitted by intercourse and by oral–genital and anal–genital contact. Because the bacteria need the warmth and moisture provided by the mucous membranes of the vagina, mouth, or anus, it is unlikely (though not impossible) that a person could acquire gonorrhea from using someone else's towel or from sitting on a public toilet seat unless the bacteria have just been deposited there and the area is warm and moist. A male exposed to the bacterium through sexual intercourse has about a 20 percent chance of developing gonorrhea, whereas a female likewise exposed has about an 80 percent chance of contracting gonorrhea. The difference is due to the vaginal environment, which is - conducive to the growth of the bacteria.

Effects of Gonorrhea Gonorrhea affects the urogenital tract in both sexes: the urethra in males and the urethra, vagina, and cervix in females. However, the symptoms are somewhat different in men and women. The early symptoms in men are a milky, bad-smelling discharge from the penis, feelings of urgently having to urinate,

Sexually transmitted diseases (STDs) Bacterial, viral, and parasitic diseases that are transmitted through sexual contact, which usually affect the genital area and may cause serious disease complications throughout the body.

Gonorrhea An STD that is caused by a bacterium. Although the disease can be treated with antibiotics, if left untreated it can lead to serious complications, including bladder and kidney disease and diseases of the pelvic and genital areas.

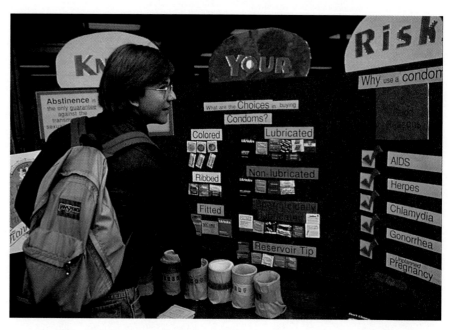

Sexually transmitted diseases are always a risk, but that risk can be minimized with safer-sex techniques such as using a condom.

and a burning sensation when doing so. If untreated, the infection can cause swelling of the testicles and damage the prostate gland, resulting ultimately in sterility. Additional complications may include kidney and bladder damage.

Whereas infected men are usually aware something is wrong with them, women may not notice the early signs of gonorrhea. One reason for this is that the symptoms are similar to those in common vaginal infections: a slight burning sensation in the genital area and a mild discharge from the vagina. Women may also be asymptomatic. An estimated 80 percent of women who have gonorrhea are unaware of it until the disease has become more severe. If left untreated, gonorrhea invades the uterus, fallopian tubes, and ovaries. Pelvic infection may result, causing sterility or requiring surgical removal of infected pelvic organs. An additional concern in women is that gonorrhea can be passed from an infected mother to her infant as it passes through the vaginal canal during delivery, often resulting in blindness. To prevent this from occurring, the eyes of newborns are routinely treated with antibiotic drops.

Treatment of Gonorrhea Diagnosis of gonorrhea is not as simple as it is for some of the other STDs. It requires laboratory examination of a sample taken from the infected area with a cotton swab or growing the bacteria under laboratory conditions. The disease usually responds to penicillin treatment or, if the patient is allergic to penicillin, to tetracycline drugs. However, there is a growing concern about penicillin-resistant strains of gonorrhea, and researchers are attempting to develop other drugs that will effectively eradicate the disease.

Those treated for gonorrhea are advised to return for a follow-up examination in about ten days to be certain that the medication has been effective and that the infection has not recurred. During treatment, abstinence from sexual intercourse and other sexual activities that may transmit the bacteria is advised.

■ Syphilis

Known in the past as the "great pox" or the "great impostor" because people thought it resembled smallpox, **syphilis** now is often referred to as just "the syph." Syphilis is caused by the *Treponema pallidum*, a corkscrewlike organism that resembles bacteria and that is part of a group of such organisms called *spirochetes*. In 2001, 281 cases of syphilis were reported in Canada, which marked a 60 percent increase over the number reported in 2000 (Centre for Infectious Disease Prevention and Control, Health Canada, 2002).

Because *Treponema pallidum* can survive only in the warmth and moisture provided by the mucous membranes of the human body, it quickly dies outside the body. For this reason, syphilis cannot usually be contracted from a toilet seat (unless the spirochete has recently been deposited there just prior to someone else with an open sore sitting on the seat, the chances of which are extremely remote). Syphilis is transmitted during sexual intercourse, oral–genital or anal–genital contact, or by kissing a person who has a syphilitic sore in the mouth. These activities provide the spirochete with a route of entrance to the body.

Effects of Syphilis The disease progresses through four stages. In stage 1 (primary stage), a painless sore, called a **chancre** (pronounced shanker), appears three to four weeks after the spirochete enters the body. The chancre looks like a pimple or wart and appears where the spirochete entered the body, often on the lips or the vaginal wall. The chancre may go unnoticed in women or be ignored in men because it is painless and disappears in a few weeks without treatment.

Stage 2 (secondary stage) occurs about six weeks after contact. Symptoms may include a rash over the entire body, welts around the genitals, low-grade fever, headache, hair loss, and sore throat. These symptoms also disappear without treatment. However, if the symptoms are noticeable, most victims see a doctor at this time. Thus, it is uncommon for cases of syphilis in North America to progress to the third stage.

Stage 3 (latency stage) begins about two years after contact (up to five years in some people). After a year, the victim cannot transmit the disease to anyone else. The only exception is that a pregnant woman can transmit the disease to her fetus through the placental wall. Latency may last 40 or more years. During this time, the organism infects and irreparably damages the heart, brain, and other organs. By stage 4 (tertiary stage), the disease may lead to heart failure, blindness, other organ damage, and finally death.

Treatment of Syphilis Syphilis can be detected by means of a simple blood test. Because it is such a dangerous disease and can be transmitted to unborn babies, a blood test for syphilis is done on pregnant women during the prenatal period. Syphilis generally responds well to penicillin or, in some cases, to other antibiotics. Because no immunity develops to the disease, prompt diagnosis and treatment after any possible exposure are essential.

When syphilis is passed from the mother to the fetus prior to birth, it is known as congenital syphilis. Until the sixteenth week of pregnancy, the fetus is protected from spirochetes by a membrane called Langhan's layer. However, after the sixteenth week, spirochetes can pass through the placental barrier and enter the fetus's bloodstream, causing birth defects, physical abnormalities, and mental retardation.

Once syphilis is contracted, the individual should refrain from all sexual activity that can transmit the spirochete. Treatment should also consist of follow-up examinations to determine whether antibiotics have been effective in eliminating the spirochete. As with gonorrhea and the other STDs, because the disease-causing organism needs a route of entry into the body, the use of a condom can help prevent the spread of syphilis.

Genital Herpes

There are two types of *herpes simplex* viruses. Type 1 causes cold sores in the mouth, and type 2 causes **genital herpes**. However, there is growing evidence that they are more related than previously thought. Genital herpes is one of the most prevalent STDs in the world.

Effects of Herpes Approximately 2–10 days after the virus enters the body, some symptoms such as sores and swollen glands (around the groin), flulike symptoms (fever, muscle aches), and pain in the genital area during urination or intercourse may occur. Other symptoms may include fatigue, swelling of the legs, and watery eyes. The disease progresses through four stages:

1. **Prodromal stage** An itching, or tingling sensation (**prodrome**) develops near the site where the virus invaded the body, with the skin turning red and becoming sensitive; prodrome is also an early symptom of a recurrent infection or outbreak.

2. **Blister stage** A sore or cluster of sores appears; fever, swollen glands, and other symptoms may occur; after 2–10 days, the sores break open (on future outbreaks, fever and swollen glands usually do not occur).

3. **Healing stage** Sores shrink; scabs form; pain, swollen glands, and fever subside (scabs fall off by the end of the second week).

4. **Inactive stage** The virus retreats to nearby nerve cells; stress and poor health may cause the virus to re-emerge.

Syphilis A serious STD caused by a spirochete; untreated syphilis has very serious complications and is eventually fatal. Treatment includes the use of antibiotics, but some strains of syphilis are resistant to treatment.

Chancre A painless sore on the penis, mouth, or anus or in the vagina where the spirochete that causes syphilis has entered the body.

Genital herpes An STD caused by the herpes simplex, type 2 virus. The disease is incurable. Carefully treated, it is not a serious disease, but its spread to the rest of the body can result in serious complications. It has been linked to the onset of cervical cancer.

Prodrome A system of an approaching disease.

Because the virus remains dormant in the nerve cells, recurrences can be experienced. However, these are not as frequent as most people believe. Although some people may experience future outbreaks several times monthly, others may encounter them only rarely. Approximately one-third of those with the disease never have a recurrence, and another third have outbreaks only rarely. Furthermore, recurrences of herpes are usually shorter and less painful than the initial outbreak.

Herpes has potentially more harmful effects on women than on men. Women who have herpes genitalis are eight times more likely to develop cervical cancer than noninfected women. In addition, a herpes-infected pregnant woman has a one-in-four chance of transmitting the infection to her infant during delivery, and the risks to the infant include death. Consequently, the recommended course of action for pregnant women with herpes is to deliver by cesarean section (incision through the abdomen and uterus to remove the fetus rather than delivery through the vaginal canal).

Treatment of Herpes Herpes is treated with the drug Acyclovir, which can relieve some symptoms and suppress recurrences of the disease. To prevent passing the virus to others, individuals with herpes should refrain from sex from the onset of the prodrome until sores have completely healed and should use a condom during other times.

Chlamydia

Caused by a viruslike bacterium called *Chlamydia trachomatis,* **chlamydia** has been the most common STD since 1991. Some estimate that chlamydia is up to ten times more prevalent than gonorrhea and may be present in as many as 4 percent of all pregnant women. Up to 10 percent of university students may also be infected. In 2001, 47 622 cases of genital chlamydia were reported in Canada (Centre for Infectious Disease Prevention and Control, Health Canada, 2002).

Effects of Chlamydia In women, chlamydia can cause infections in the vagina and pelvic inflammatory disease, which can lead to infertility. Symptoms include vaginal discharge, itching and burning of the vulva, and some discomfort when urinating. However, as many as 70 percent of female chlamydia infections go undetected until more serious problems develop. As with other STDs, chlamydia can create problems during birth deliveries if the pregnant woman is infected. Conjunctivitis, an inflammation of the eye, can be contracted by the newborn during delivery, and blindness can result. These conditions can be prevented with ointments containing tetracycline or erythromycin applied to the newborn's eyes.

In men, chlamydia can cause inflammation of the urinary and reproductive tracts and, in extreme circumstances, sterility. Symptoms include a mild burning sensation when urinating, followed by a thin, watery, clear discharge. Left untreated, it can also lead to swelling of the testicles.

Treatment of Chlamydia Chlamydia can be easily detected with a simple culture test that can be performed by university health services. Once detected, it can be treated effectively with a week-long administration of the antibiotic tetracycline. As with other treatments consisting of antibiotics, it is important to finish the entire dosage of the tetracycline; otherwise, the infection may recur and be more resistant to the drug than before.

Genital Warts

The result of a viral infection (*human papilloma virus,* or HPV), **genital warts** occur on most areas of the genitals and anus. In females, the warts typically appear in the lower area of the vagina. In males, they appear on the glans, foreskin (if not circumcised), and shaft of the penis and may appear in the anal area in some homosexual men. The incubation period for HPV is approximately three months after contact with an infected person. University health centres report that genital warts are quite prevalent among students.

Effects of Genital Warts Researchers have found that several strains of HPV are associated with the development of cervical cancer. This revelation has led to a more urgent need for prevention of what was previously thought to be a relatively benign STD.

Some lesions are moist and some are dry. The moist lesions are the ones that respond well to treatment. Large warts should be biopsied for cancerous cell growth.

Diagnosis is made by the appearance of the warts. In the moist areas of the body, they tend to be white, pink, or white to grey. In the dry areas, they are usually yellow and yellow-grey.

Treatment of Genital Warts The usual treatment is administration of the drug podophyllin, an irritant that causes the outer skin in the area containing the virus to slough off. Thus, the drug does not kill the virus, but merely removes the infected tissue. Podophyllin is applied by the health practitioner to each lesion, allowed to dry, and then washed off four hours later by the patient. Sometimes, an antibiotic ointment is prescribed as well to treat infection at the site and to help keep the wart moist. The podophyllin is usually applied once a week for five or six weeks or for the time it takes to control the infection. However, genital warts often recur after the first bout, even if treated. Recurrences can be experienced for several months or years until immunity develops. In some cases, warts are removed by laser surgery, electrosurgery, freezing with liquid hydrogen, or surgical incision.

Pelvic Inflammatory Disease

With the exception of AIDS, **pelvic inflammatory disease (PID)** is the most dangerous and the most difficult to diagnose of all the STDs affecting women. That is because its symptoms may not be obvious until damage has already occurred. Left untreated, PID can result in infertility and even death.

Effects of Pelvic Inflammatory Disease Symptoms of PID include abdominal pain or tenderness, pain during intercourse, increased menstrual cramps, profuse bleeding during menstruation, irregular menstrual cycles, vaginal bleeding at times other than when menstruating, lower-back pain, nausea, loss of appetite, vomiting, vaginal discharge, burning sensation during urination, chills, and fever. Unless PID is promptly diagnosed and treated, scar tissue forms inside the fallopian tubes. This scar tissue can result in infertility by partially or totally blocking the tubes, preventing the egg from entering the uterus or the sperm from fertilizing the egg. Scar tissue also increases the risk of a tubal pregnancy (in which the fertilized egg becomes implanted inside the fallopian tube rather than the uterus).

Treatment of Pelvic Inflammatory Disease Diagnosis of PID is based on medical and sexual history, a pelvic examination, and laboratory tests. Treatment is by administration of an antibiotic and is usually effective. However, any structural damage done to pelvic organs may be irreversible or, at the least, require more extensive medical treatment.

HIV Infection and AIDS

Acquired immunodeficiency syndrome (AIDS) is a condition caused by infection with the **human immunodeficiency virus (HIV)**. It is called a syndrome because it consists of a number of conditions resulting from a decreased ability of the body's immunological system to ward off infections and other threats to health. Among the syndrome's manifestations are pneumonia, cancer, and other opportunistic infections (infections resulting from lowered resistance of a weakened immune system). HIV is transmitted through bodily fluids, predominantly blood, semen, and vaginal secretions. It can also be transmitted from an infected pregnant woman to her fetus. In order to infect someone, HIV must have a route of entry into

the body. The most common ways HIV is transmitted are through sex and the use of intravenous drugs. Sexual intercourse, oral–genital sex, or anal intercourse in which bodily fluids are exchanged are particularly risky activities. Intravenous drug use, in which a needle is shared, may result in HIV being directly deposited into the bloodstream.

Prevalence of HIV Infection and AIDS The number of people infected with HIV and the number of people with AIDS keeps increasing, so any figures given here may soon be outdated. As of the end of 2001, the World Health Organization estimated that there were approximately 40 million people globally living with HIV.

In Canada, about a dozen people become infected every day with HIV. The current estimate is 49 800. This represents 4190 new cases of HIV diagnosed in Canada in 1999, and a 24 percent increase in infections from 1996 to 1999 (Centre for Infectious Disease Prevention and Control, Health Canada, 2001).

Canada's first case of AIDS was reported in 1982. During the next decade, most HIV infections occurred among men who had sex with men (MSM), injecting drug users (IDU), and among those who received infected blood and blood products.

Since then, local, provincial, and federal groups and agencies have succeeded in reducing the rate of infection in the gay and bisexual male population; stringent blood-screening standards now ensure that we are safe from infection through the blood supply. At the

Chlamydia A common STD caused by a viruslike bacterium; can lead to sterility, inflammation in the reproductive and urinary tracts, and pelvic inflammatory disease. Treated with antibiotics.

Genital warts An STD of the genital and perineal areas of both men and women caused by a virus; linked to an increased incidence of cancer.

Pelvic inflammatory disease (PID) An extremely serious STD for women. PID can lead to infertility, tubal pregnancy, and structural damage to pelvic organs.

Acquired immunodeficiency syndrome (AIDS) An STD that weakens the human immune system, leading to serious opportunistic diseases; fatal in the long run.

Human immunodeficiency virus (HIV) Virus transmitted primarily through sexual contact and intravenous drug use that weakens the immune system and often develops into full-blown AIDS.

same time, improved treatments have increased the life expectancy of some Canadians infected with HIV.

The news about HIV/AIDS in Canada, however, is not all good. HIV infection rates for MSM are lower than in the past, but other Canadians—particularly those marginalized by socioeconomic factors—are becoming infected at increasing rates. HIV infection is increasing rapidly among people living in poverty (especially women and Aboriginal peoples) and prison inmates, and injection drug users now account for almost half of all newly reported HIV cases. MSM still account for the majority of persons living with HIV/AIDS (Health Canada Web page).

Especially worrisome are the number of young people, many in their teens, now living with HIV/AIDS and the number of Canadians who are not aware of their HIV status. Of course, many more of our fellow citizens are infected with HIV but have not yet developed AIDS.

Effects of HIV Infection Once in the body, HIV invades the cells of the immune system, resulting in its becoming less and less effective over time. Increasing incapacity results, with death being inevitable. Symptoms include loss of appetite, weight loss, fever, night sweats, skin rash, diarrhea, tiredness, lack of resistance to infection, and swollen lymph glands. Among the common conditions of full-blown AIDS, which usually develops some eight to ten years after HIV infection, are Kaposi's sarcoma (a form of cancer of the blood vessels that can be evidenced by purple skin lesions), other cancers, pneumonia, and brain dementia.

Treatment of HIV Infection Rather than testing for the presence of the virus itself, HIV infection is diagnosed with a blood test (called ELISA—enzyme-linked immunosorbent assay) that identifies the presence of antibodies that develop in response to HIV. If the test is positive for these antibodies, another, more sophisticated test (Western blot) is administered to confirm this result. However, it may take anywhere from three to eight months for enough of these antibodies to develop to be identifiable through the AIDS test. Consequently, someone may test negative even though he or she is infected. Further, this person may still transmit the virus to other people.

Although HIV infection is incurable and almost inevitably leads to death, some medications appear to delay debilitating symptoms. The most well-known of

these drugs is AZT (azidothymidine). Recent studies have found that a combination of AZT with other drugs is most effective in prolonging symptom-free living among people infected with HIV.

Ways of preventing HIV infection include abstaining from high-risk sexual activities, using a condom with the spermicide nonoxynol-9 if sexually active, limiting the number of sexual partners, maintaining a monogamous relationship with someone who is HIV-free, and refraining from the use of intravenous drugs. For pregnant women who are HIV-infected, the administration of AZT can dramatically decrease the risk of their babies being born infected. Therefore, if they have participated in high-risk behaviours (or even if they have not), they might want to have an AIDS test to determine whether AZT is warranted.

OTHER DISEASES AND CONDITIONS

Prevention of several other diseases and conditions has also been associated with exercise, including diabetes, obesity, and hypertension.

Diabetes

Diabetes is a disease of the pancreas in which an insufficient amount of **insulin** is produced to make use of sugars and other carbohydrates in a normal way. The result is increased blood-glucose levels, which can lead to a number of other states of ill health. The seventh leading cause of death in Canada, diabetes contributes to the development of heart disease, stroke, kidney failure, and blindness. Symptoms of diabetes include frequent urination and thirst, extreme hunger, rapid weight loss, blurred vision or a sudden change in visual acuity, overtiredness, and drowsiness. Among the more than 1.5 million diabetics in Canada, some need to take insulin into their bodies to help regulate the amount of glucose in their blood. Others, however, can control insulin insufficiency (sometimes called *glucose intolerance*) by diet and exercise. Exercise uses up the excess blood glucose, and diet can limit the amount of sugar and carbohydrates ingested in the first place.

Obesity

The relationship between leanness and colon and other cancers, and between body fat, production of estrogen, and subsequent breast cancer, was mentioned earlier in this chapter. Obesity, 20 percent or more above recommended weight, is also related to CHD, stroke, hypertension, diabetes, and other conditions. Exercise helps

---

Insulin A hormone produced in the pancreas that aids in the digestion of sugars and other carbohydrates.

BEHAVIOURAL CHANGE AND MOTIVATIONAL STRATEGIES

Many things might interfere with your behaving in ways to prevent CHD and cancer. Here are some barriers (roadblocks) and strategies for overcoming them.

Roadblock	Behavioural Change Strategy
Friends or relatives may smoke cigarettes. That means that you may be tempted to do so yourself. Even though we like to think we act independently, other people's behaviours influence us, particularly if we like and respect those people. Furthermore, you do not even have to smoke to be subjected to the harmful effects of tobacco products. All you need do is inhale sidestream smoke, which can affect your susceptibility to CHD and cancer.	Two behavioural change strategies appropriate here are contracting and social support. Find a friend or relative who would like to give up smoking. This will not be difficult. Smokers often try to quit; the problem is that they are usually unsuccessful. Draw up a contract for each of you to smoke less gradually over a period of weeks (gradual programming). Use the contract format described in Chapter 3. If you do not presently smoke, make your contract address your not starting to smoke and the other person's contract specific to gradually reducing the number of cigarettes smoked per week. Each of you then signs the other's contract as a witness. The support you can provide each other, and the pressure of a contract that will periodically be evaluated, can be just the motivation needed to counteract the influence of other smoking friends and relatives.
You may find exercise uncomfortable. Your muscles may ache, your clothes and body may get sweaty, and you may not enjoy the activity itself. With this attitude, you cannot be expected to maintain an exercise program even if you are motivated to begin one. After all, most people do not want to feel uncomfortable and will choose not to be so.	Use goal-setting strategies to establish realistic and achievable fitness goals. If you are experiencing aches and pains, you are overtraining or exercising inappropriately. As has been pointed out, the old maxim "No pain, no gain" has long been discarded by fitness experts. You should feel good after a workout. You can also use selective awareness. Focus on the benefits of the exercise: how it will burn up calories, make you look and feel better, help you be healthier, make the clothes you bought when you weighed less fit once again, and so forth. If you focus on the benefits rather than on the temporary discomfort caused by perspiration, you will be more likely to maintain your exercise program.
You may enjoy eating foods high in saturated fats. Many of us grew up on french fries and hot dogs or hamburgers. They taste good, are easy to prepare, and are relatively inexpensive. Unfortunately, they also put us at risk for both CHD and certain cancers.	Use reminder systems to encourage the buying and eating of healthier foods. Put notes on your refrigerator and pantry to remind you to refrain from eating certain foods when you are looking for a snack. And place a picture of a clogged artery at the top of your shopping list to remind you not to buy unhealthy foods. You can also use covert modelling. Find a friend who eats well, who looks good, and whose behaviour you would like to follow. Then observe what this friend eats. After obtaining a good picture of how this friend selects and prepares foods, model your behaviour on him or her. Eat and prepare similar foods—at least those that you enjoy eating and that are also low in fat and other unhealthy food ingredients.
List roadblocks interfering with your working at preventing CHD and cancer. 1. _____ 2. _____ 3. _____	Now cite behavioural change strategies that can help you overcome the roadblocks you just listed. If you need to, refer back to Chapter 3 for behavioural change and motivational strategies. 1. _____ 2. _____ 3. _____

reduce body fat, tone muscles, and decrease body weight. When that occurs, the heart has to pump less forcefully because blood vessels are not occluded, the blood has to travel less distance, and blood glucose is reduced because it is being used for muscular contractions during physical activity. For these reasons, obesity is best treated by diet control in conjunction with an exercise program.

◼ Hypertension

When blood vessels are partially blocked, the heart has to work harder to pump blood through them. This increased tension of the blood against the walls of the blood vessels is called *hypertension*, or high blood pressure. Blood pressure is measured as diastolic and systolic blood pressure. The recommended blood pressure reading is 120 systolic/80 diastolic. Usually, readings above 140 systolic and/or 90 diastolic are considered high.

Because high blood pressure creates stress on the walls of the arteries, it can result in the rupture of these blood vessels. When that happens in the brain, a stroke occurs. In addition, high blood pressure can create small tears on the walls of the coronary arteries, making it easier for plaque to attach and accumulate and CHD to develop.

In many cases, hypertensives need medication for the remainder of their lives. In many other cases, however, exercise and diet can help control hypertension. Exercise uses blood fats that otherwise might accumulate on the walls of blood vessels. Exercise also helps the heart become stronger so it can pump blood as required. In addition, physical activity contracts muscles around blood ve ssels so blood is more efficiently transported through the circulatory system.

Summary

◼ Coronary Heart Disease (CHD)

CHD is the second leading cause of death in Canada. It involves a blockage of blood to the heart, depriving it of necessary oxygen and nutrients without which a heart attack can occur and part of the heart muscle can die. Death can even be the result.

Coronary arteries can be occluded by an accumulation of blood fats and other substances on their walls. This clogging material is known as *plaque*, and the resulting condition as *atherosclerosis*. The fatty particles that can collect on the walls of the arteries are called *lipoproteins*. Lipoproteins consist of triglycerides, a blood protein, and cholesterol.

HDLs and LDLs are produced in the liver and released into the bloodstream where they carry cholesterol that is needed by the body. Excess cholesterol carried by LDLs can accumulate on the artery walls, eventually clogging coronary arteries and causing heart disease. HDLs carry excess cholesterol back to the liver and possibly provide a protective layer of grease to help prevent a buildup of substances on the walls of the arteries. When LDL is elevated and HDL is too sparse, there is a likelihood that arteries will be clogged and CHD will be promoted.

Risk factors for CHD include diets high in fats, hypertension, obesity and overweight, stress, sedentary lifestyle, the use of tobacco, and a family history of CHD.

Physical activity is an excellent means of preventing CHD because it relates to several risk factors. It exercises the heart muscle, encourages the production of HDL, aids in the control of mild hypertension, develops cardiorespiratory endurance, reduces catecholamines produced in response to stress, helps maintain desirable weight, and discourages cigarette smoking.

◼ Cancer

Cancer is a disease involving abnormal cell growth. These cells can spread to other parts of the body by metastasis. Cancer is the leading cause of death in Canada. As many as 80 percent of cancer cases, however, could be prevented with a change in lifestyle.

Cancer can be caused by chemicals, environmental pollutants, radiation from the sun, or viruses. The greatest cause of cancer, however, is the use of tobacco. An estimated 75 percent of all lung cancer cases are thought to be caused by cigarette smoking, and the use of tobacco is associated with cancer of the larynx, pharynx, esophagus, pancreas, and bladder.

The number of cancer cases could be dramatically reduced if people ate diets low in fats and high in fruits and vegetables (in particular, cruciferous vegetables), refrained from tobacco use, eliminated or reduced their consumption of alcohol, and decreased their exposure to the sun.

Moderate physical activity seems to protect people from developing cancer. This is particularly true for cancer of the colon, prostate, endometrium, and breast. Theories about why this relationship exists point to exercise leading to lower body fat, less production of estrogen, and increased rate of transit of food through the digestive tract.

The earlier cancer is detected, the more effective is the treatment. To identify the presence of cancer early, obtain regular medical screenings and perform regular self-examinations (such as breast and testicular self-examinations).

Sexually Transmitted Diseases

Sexually transmitted diseases are diseases primarily contracted through sexual activity. Examples of STDs are gonorrhea, syphilis, genital herpes, chlamydia, genital warts, pelvic inflammatory disease, and HIV infection and AIDS.

Gonorrhea is caused by the *Neisseria gonorrhoeae* bacterium and is treated with penicillin. Early symptoms may include painful urination, a milky, smelly discharge, and an urgent need to urinate. Women are often asymptomatic but may experience a slight burning sensation in the genital area and a mild vaginal discharge.

Syphilis is caused by a corkscrew-like organism called *Treponema pallidum* and is treated with penicillin. In stage 1, a painless sore (chancre) appears in the infected area. In stage 2, symptoms may include a body rash, welts, fever, headache, hair loss, and a sore throat. Stage 3 is a latency period that may last up to 40 years or more. In stage 4, syphilis may lead to heart failure, blindness, other organ damage, and finally death.

Genital herpes is caused by the *herpes simplex* virus and is treated with the drug Acyclovir (although this treatment only diminishes the severity and frequency of outbreaks, as genital herpes is presently incurable). Early symptoms may include sore and swollen glands, flulike symptoms, and pain in the genital area during urination or sexual intercourse. Genital herpes progresses through four stages: prodromal, blister, healing, and inactive. The virus remains dormant in the nerve cells with periodic recurrences possible.

Chlamydia, the most prevalent STD, is caused by the *Chlamydia trachomatis* bacterium and is treated with the antibiotic tetracycline. Symptoms include vaginal discharge, itching and burning of the vulva, and some discomfort when urinating. However, as many as 70 percent of female chlamydia infections go undetected until more serious problems develop.

Genital warts are caused by the *human papilloma virus* (HPV) and are treated with the drug podophyllin (sometimes an antibiotic ointment is prescribed as well). However, warts tend to recur. They can sometimes be removed through laser surgery, electrosurgery, freezing with liquid hydrogen, or surgical incision.

Pelvic inflammatory disease (PID), which can cause infertility and even death if left untreated, is treated by administration of an antibiotic. Symptoms include abdominal pain or tenderness, pain during intercourse, increased menstrual cramps, profuse bleeding during menstruation, irregular menstrual cycles, vaginal bleeding at times other than when menstruating, lower-back pain, nausea, loss of appetite, vomiting, vaginal discharge, burning sensation during urination, chills, and fever.

Acquired immunodeficiency syndrome (AIDS) is caused by the human immunodeficiency virus (HIV) and is presently incurable. HIV is transmitted through bodily fluids (blood, semen, vaginal secretions) most commonly encountered through sex or the use of intravenous drugs. HIV infection is treated with the drug azidothymidine (AZT) and a combination of other drugs that seem to prolong symptom-free living. Methods of prevention include abstaining from sex, using a latex condom with the spermicide nonoxynol-9, limiting the number of sexual partners, maintaining a monogamous relationship with an HIV-free partner, and refraining from the use of intravenous drugs.

Other Diseases and Conditions

Exercise can also be effective in preventing or responding to other diseases, including diabetes, obesity, and hypertension. Exercise uses up blood glucose and other blood fats, expends calories, and makes the heart and circulatory system operate more efficiently. As a result, exercise and diet are mainstays in the treatment and prevention of these conditions.

STUDY QUESTIONS

1. What are the main causes of heart disease, and which are preventable?

2. What are the main causes of cancer?

3. What are the warning signs of cancer?

4. What is the suspected connection between physical activity and cancer prevention?

5. What is the most common type of STD in Canada, and what are its symptoms and treatment?

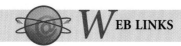

WEB LINKS

Canadian Cancer Statistics 2001
www.hc-sc.gc.ca/hpb/lcdc/bc/stats.html

Canadian Cancer Society
www.cancer.ca

Health Canada
www.hc-sc.gc.ca/english/

Canadian Fitness and Lifestyle Research Institute
www.cflri.ca

Heart and Stroke Foundation of Canada
www.hsf.ca

World Health Organization
www.who.int/home-page/

REFERENCES

Friedman, Meyer, and Ray H. Rosenman. *Type A Behaviour and Your Heart.* Greenwich, CT: Fawcett, 1974.

Berenson, G.S., S. Srinivasan, W. Bao, et al. "Association Between Multiple Cardiovascular Risk Factors and Atherosclerosis in Children and Young Adults." *New England Journal of Medicine* 338 (1998): 1650–1656.

Centre for Infectious Disease Prevention and Control, Health Canada. *National HIV Prevalence and Incidence Estimates for 1999: No Evidence of Decline in Overall Incidence.* Bureau of HIV/AIDS, STD and TB Update Series, Health Canada Population and Public Health Branch, May, 2001.

Division of Sexual Health Promotion and STD Prevention and Control, Centre for Infectious Disease Prevention and Control, Health Canada. 2002. *Reported Cases and Rates of Notifiable STD from January 1 to December 31, 2001, and January 1 to December 31, 2000.*

Heart and Stroke Foundation of Canada. *The Changing Face of Heart Disease and Stroke in Canada 2000.*

Heart and Stroke Foundation of Canada. *General Information—Incidence of Cardiovascular Disease (2002).*

National Cancer Institute of Canada. *Canadian Cancer Statistics 2001.* Toronto, Canada, 2001.

Statistics Canada, catalogues 91-002, vol. 7, no. 3; 91-512; 91-213. Canadians and smoking: An update. Health and Welfare Canada, 1991. General Social Survey, Statistics Canada, 1991. Survey on Smoking in Canada, Cycle 3, 1994. National Population Health Survey, Statistics Canada, 1996/97.

World Health Organization (2001). AIDS epidemic update, December 2001. **www.unaids.org/epdemic_update/report?dec01/index.html**

Lab Activity 13.1

Is Your Blood in Tune?

INSTRUCTIONS: *The composition of your blood is very important when it comes to preventing CHD. You can easily have your physician check your blood-fat levels. Sometimes, this is done with a simple finger prick, but to be as accurate as possible, it should be done by having blood drawn from a vein after you have fasted for about 12 hours. Record the results of that assessment below by checking the appropriate rating.*

_____ Total cholesterol is below 5.2 mmol/L: No further evaluation necessary, recheck in 5 years.

_____ Total cholesterol is 5.2–6.2 mmol/L (borderline high cholesterol): Evaluate risk factors to see what lifestyle changes you can make (diet, exercise, and so forth). If your physician says you are not in the high-risk category for CHD, active treatment is not necessary, but recheck in 1–8 weeks.

_____ Total cholesterol is above 6.2 mmol/L (high cholesterol): Analyze and measure HDL, LDL, and triglycerides.

Once the above is completed, answer the following questions:

Yes	No		
_____	_____	**1.**	Is your total cholesterol no more than $4.5 \times$ HDL cholesterol?
_____	_____	**2.**	Is your cholesterol-to-HDL ratio at least 5 to 1?
_____	_____	**3.**	Is your HDL reading above 0.90 mmol/L?
_____	_____	**4.**	Is your LDL cholesterol less than 6.2 mmol/L?

If the answers to these questions are Yes, your lipid profile is good. Regardless of how your lipid profile turned out, list the important changes you can make to lower your total cholesterol and increase your HDL cholesterol over the next 12 months.

1. _____

2. _____

3. _____

4. _____

5. _____

Lab Activity 13.2

RISKO: A Heart Health Appraisal

INSTRUCTIONS: *Complete the following activity to assess your general risk for developing coronary heart disease.*

✦ Understanding Heart Disease

Estimates are that almost 80 000 Canadians die of coronary heart disease every year. In the United States, it's the single leading cause of death—as well as in many other countries.

Scientists have identified certain factors linked with an increased risk of developing coronary heart disease. Some of these factors are unavoidable, like increasing age, being male or having a family history of heart disease. However, many other risk factors can be changed to lower the risk of heart disease. High blood pressure, high blood cholesterol, cigarette smoking, and physical inactivity are the four major modifiable risk factors; obesity is a contributing risk factor. Diabetes also strongly influences the risk of heart disease.

RISKO is a way for you to evaluate your risk of coronary heart disease on the basis of your risk factors. RISKO scores are based on blood pressure, cholesterol, smoking, and weight. (Physical inactivity is also an important risk factor, but it was not part of the statistical base from which RISKO was derived.)

✦ Men

1. Systolic Blood Pressure

If you *are not* taking anti-hypertensive medications and your systolic blood pressure is:

                                                                                  Score

124 or less	0 points	Between 175 and 184	12 points
Between 125 and 134	2 points	Between 185 and 194	14 points
Between 135 and 144	4 points	Between 195 and 204	16 points
Between 145 and 154	6 points	Between 205 and 214	18 points
Between 155 and 164	8 points	Between 215 and 224	20 points
Between 165 and 174	10 points		_____

(continued)

Lab Activity 13.2 *(continued)*
RISKO: A Heart Health Appraisal

If you *are* taking anti-hypertensive medications and your systolic blood pressure is:

Score

120 or less	0 points	Between 164 and 175	12 points
Between 121 and 127	2 points	Between 176 and 190	14 points
Between 128 and 135	4 points	Between 191 and 204	16 points
Between 136 and 143	6 points	Between 205 and 214	18 points
Between 144 and 153	8 points	Between 215 and 224	20 points
Between 154 and 163	10 points		

_____

2. Blood Cholesterol

Locate the number of points for your total and HDL cholesterol in the table below.

	HDL							
Total	25	30	35	40	50	60	70	80
140	4	2	0	0	0	0	0	0
160	5	3	2	0	0	0	0	0
180	6	4	3	1	0	0	0	0
200	7	5	4	3	0	0	0	0
220	7	6	5	4	1	0	0	0
240	8	7	5	4	2	0	0	0
260	8	7	6	5	3	1	0	0
280	9	8	7	6	4	2	0	0
300	9	8	7	6	4	3	1	0
340	9	9	8	7	6	4	2	1
400	10	9	9	8	7	5	4	3

_____

3. Cigarette Smoking

If you:

Do not smoke	0 points
Smoke less than a pack a day	2 points
Smoke a pack a day	5 points
Smoke two or more packs a day	9 points

_____

4. Weight

Locate your weight category in the table below. If you are in:

Weight category A	0 points
Weight category B	1 point
Weight category C	2 points

FT	IN	A	B	C
5	1	Up to 162	163–250	251+
5	2	Up to 167	168–257	258+
5	3	Up to 172	173–264	265+
5	4	Up to 176	177–272	273+
5	5	Up to 181	182–279	280+
5	6	Up to 185	186–286	287+
5	7	Up to 190	191–293	294+
5	8	Up to 195	196–300	301+
5	9	Up to 199	200–307	308+
5	10	Up to 204	205–315	316+
5	11	Up to 209	210–322	323+
6	0	Up to 213	214–329	330+
6	1	Up to 218	219–336	337+
6	2	Up to 223	224–343	344+
6	3	Up to 227	228–350	351+
6	4	Up to 232	233–368	359+
6	5	Up to 238	239–365	366+
6	6	Up to 241	242–372	373+

Total Score _____

✦ **Women**

1. Systolic Blood Pressure

If you *are not* taking anti-hypertensive medications and your systolic blood pressure is:

Score

125 or less	0 points	Between 172 and 183	10 points
Between 126 and 136	2 points	Between 184 and 194	12 points
Between 137 and 148	4 points	Between 195 and 206	14 points
Between 149 and 160	6 points	Between 207 and 218	16 points
Between 161 and 171	8 points		

_____

If you *are* taking anti-hypertensive medications and your systolic blood pressure is:

117 or less	0 points	Between 145 and 154	10 points
Between 118 and 123	2 points	Between 155 and 168	12 points
Between 124 and 129	4 points	Between 169 and 206	14 points
Between 130 and 136	6 points	Between 207 and 218	16 points
Between 137 and 144	8 points		

_____

(continued)

Lab Activity 13.2 *(continued)*
RISKO: A Heart Health Appraisal

2. Blood Cholesterol

Locate the number of points for your total and HDL cholesterol in the table below.

				HDL				
TOTAL	25	30	35	40	50	60	70	80
140	2	1	0	0	0	0	0	0
160	3	2	1	0	0	0	0	0
180	4	3	2	1	0	0	0	0
200	4	3	2	2	0	0	0	0
220	5	4	3	2	1	0	0	0
240	5	4	3	3	1	0	0	0
260	5	4	4	3	2	1	0	0
280	5	5	4	4	2	1	0	0
300	6	5	4	4	3	2	1	0
340	6	5	5	4	3	2	1	0
400	6	6	5	5	4	3	2	2

_____

3. Cigarette Smoking

If you:

Do not smoke	0 points
Smoke less than a pack a day	2 points
Smoke a pack a day	5 points
Smoke two or more packs a day	9 points

_____

4. Weight

Locate your weight category in the table below. If you are in:

Weight category A   0 points

Weight category B   1 point

Weight category C   2 points

Weight category D   3 points

FT	IN	A	B	C	D
4	8	Up to 139	140–161	162–184	185+
4	9	Up to 140	141–162	163–185	186+
4	10	Up to 141	142–163	164–187	188+
4	11	Up to 143	144–166	167–190	191+
5	0	Up to 145	146–168	169–193	194+
5	1	Up to 147	148–171	172–196	197+
5	2	Up to 149	150–173	174–198	199+
5	3	Up to 152	153–176	177–201	202+
5	4	Up to 154	155–178	179–204	205+
5	5	Up to 157	158–182	183–209	210+
5	6	Up to 160	161–186	187–213	214+

FT	IN	A	B	C	D
5	7	Up to 165	166–191	192–219	220+
5	8	Up to 169	170–196	197–225	226+
5	9	Up to 173	174–201	202–231	232+
5	10	Up to 178	179–206	207–238	239+
5	11	Up to 182	183–212	213–242	243+
6	0	Up to 187	188–217	218–248	249+
6	1	Up to 191	192–222	223–254	255+

_____

Total Score _____

✦ What Your Score Means

Note: If you're diabetic, you have a greater risk of heart disease. Add 7 points to your total score.

0–2	You have a low risk of heart disease for a person of your age and sex.
3–4	You have a low-to-moderate risk of heart disease for a person of your age and sex. That's good, but there's room for improvement.
5–7	You have a moderate-to-high risk of heart disease for a person of your age and sex. There's considerable room for improvement in some areas.
8–15	You have a high risk of developing heart disease for a person of your age and sex. There's lots of room for improvement in all areas.
16 and over	You have a very high risk of developing heart disease for a person of your age and sex. You should act now to reduce all your risk factors.

✦ Some Words of Caution

1. RISKO is a way for adults who don't have signs of heart disease now to measure their risk. If you already have heart disease, it's very important to work with your doctor to reduce your risk.

2. RISKO is not a substitute for a thorough physical examination and assessment by your doctor. It's intended to help you learn more about the factors that influence the risk of heart disease, and thus to reduce your risk.

3. If you have a family history of heart disease, your risk of heart disease will be higher than your RISKO score shows. If you have a high RISKO score and a family history of heart disease, taking action now to reduce your risk is even more important.

4. If you're a woman under 45 years old or a man under 35 years old, your real risk of heart disease is probably lower than your RISKO score.

5. If you're overweight, have high blood pressure or high blood cholesterol, or smoke cigarettes, your long-term risk of heart disease is higher even if your risk of heart disease in the next several years is low. To reduce your risk, you should eliminate or control these risk factors.

(continued)

Lab Activity 13.2 *(continued)*
RISKO: A Heart Health Appraisal

✦ **How to Reduce Your Risk**

1. **Quit smoking for good.** Many programs are available to help.

2. **Have your blood pressure checked regularly.** If your blood pressure is less than 130/85 millimetres Hg, have it rechecked in two years. If it's between 130–139/85–89, have it rechecked in a year. If your blood pressure is 140/90 or higher, you have high blood pressure and should follow your doctor's advice. If blood pressure medication is prescribed for you, remember to take it.

3. **Stay physically active.** Physical inactivity, besides being a risk factor for heart disease, contributes to other risk factors including obesity, high blood pressure, and a low level of HDL cholesterol. To condition your heart, try to get 30–60 minutes of exercise three or four times a week.

   Activities that are especially beneficial when performed regularly include:
   a. Brisk walking, hiking, stair-climbing, aerobic exercise, and calisthenics
   b. Jogging, running, bicycling, rowing, and swimming
   c. Tennis, racquetball, soccer, basketball, and touch football

   Even low-intensity activities, when performed daily, can have some long-term health benefits. Such activities include:
   a. Walking for pleasure, gardening, and yard work
   b. Housework, dancing, and prescribed home exercise

4. **Lose weight if necessary.** For many people, losing weight is one of the most effective ways to improve their blood pressure and cholesterol levels.

5. **Reduce high blood cholesterol through your diet.** If you're overweight or eat lots of foods high in saturated fats and cholesterol (whole milk, cheese, eggs, butter, fatty foods, fried foods), make changes in your diet. Look for *The American Heart Association Cookbook* at your local bookstore; it can help you.

6. **Visit or write your local Canadian Heart and Stroke Foundation for more information and copies of free pamphlets.** Some subjects covered include reducing your risk of heart attack and stroke, controlling high blood pressure, eating to keep your heart healthy, how to stop smoking, and exercising for good health. *For more information, contact your local Canadian Heart and Stroke Foundation (www.heartandstroke.ca).*

Source: RISKO, A Heart Health Appraisal, 1994. Copyright American Heart Association. Reproduced with permission.

Lab Activity 13.3

Determining Your Risk of Getting Cancer

INSTRUCTIONS: *Select the response that best describes you for each item and record the point value for each response selected in the space provided. Total your points for each section separately.*

Lung Cancer

1. Sex
   a. Male (2)
   b. Female (1)

   1. ____1____

2. Age
   a. 39 or less (1)
   b. 40–49 (2)
   c. 50–59 (5)
   d. 60+ (7)

   2. ____1____

3. Smoker (8)
   Nonsmoker (1)

   3. ____1____

4. Type of smoking
   a. Current cigarettes or little cigars (10)
   b. Pipe and/or cigar but not cigarettes (3)
   c. Ex-cigarette smoker (2)
   d. Nonsmoker (1)

   4. ____1____

5. Number of cigarettes smoked per day
   a. 0 (1)
   b. Less than ½ pack per day (5)
   c. ½–1 pack (9)
   d. 1–2 packs (15)
   e. More than 2 packs (20)

   5. ____1____

6. Type of cigarettes
   a. High tar/nicotine (10)[a]
   b. Medium tar/nicotine (9)
   c. Low tar/nicotine (7)
   d. Nonsmoker (1)

   6. ____1____

[a]High T/N=More than 20 mg tar and 1.3 mg nicotine.
   Medium T/N=16–19 mg tar and 1.1–1.2 mg nicotine.
   Low T/N=15 mg or less tar and 1.0 mg or less nicotine.

(continued)

Lab Activity 13.3 *(continued)*
Determining Your Risk of Getting Cancer

7. Duration of smoking
   a. Never smoked (1)
   b. Ex-smoker (3)
   c. Up to 15 years (5)
   d. 15–25 years (10)
   e. More than 25 years (20)

   7. ___1___

8. Type of industrial work
   a. Mining (3)
   b. Asbestos (7)
   c. Uranium and radioactive products (5)

   8. _____

   Lung Total ___7___

Colon/Rectal Cancer

1. Age
   a. 39 or less (10)
   b. 40–59 (20)
   c. 60 and over (50)

   1. ___10___

2. Has anyone in your immediate family ever had:
   a. Colon cancer (20)
   b. One or more polyps of the colon (10)
   c. Neither (1)

   2. ___1___

3. Have you ever had:
   a. Colon cancer (100)
   b. One or more polyps of the colon (40)
   c. Ulcerative colitis (20)
   d. Cancer of the breast or uterus (10)
   e. None (1)

   3. ___1___

4. Bleeding from the rectum (other than obvious hemorrhoids or piles)
   a. Yes (75)
   b. No (1)

   4. ___1___

   Colon/Rectal Total ___13___

Skin Cancer

1. Frequent work or play in the sun
   a. Yes (10)
   b. No (1)

   1. ___10___

2. Work in mines, around coal tars, or around radioactivity
   a. Yes (10)
   b. No (1)

   2. ___1___

3. Complexion—fair or light skin   3. ___1___
    a. Yes (10)
    b. No (1)
                                        Skin Total ___12___

Women Only—Breast Cancer

   1. Age Group   1. ___10___
      a. 20–34 (10)
      b. 35–49 (40)
      c. 50 and over (90)

   2. Race/ethnicity   2. ___25___
      a. Oriental (5)
      b. African-American (20)
      c. White (25)
      d. Mexican-American (10)

   3. Family history   3. ___10___
      a. Mother, sister, aunt, or grandmother
        with breast cancer (30)
      b. None (10)

   4. Your history   4. ___10___
      a. Previous lumps or cysts (25)
      b. No breast disease (10)
      c. Previous breast cancer (100)

   5. Maternity   5. ___20___
      a. First pregnancy before 25 (10)
      b. First pregnancy after 25 (15)
      c. No pregnancies (20)
                                    Breast Total ___75___

Women Only—Cervical Cancer[b]

   1. Age group   1. ___10___
      a. Less than 25 (10)
      b. 25–39 (20)
      c. 40–54 (30)
      d. 55 and over (30)

   2. Race/ethnicity   2. ___10___
      a. Oriental (10)
      b. Puerto Rican (20)
      c. African-American (20)
      d. White (10)
      e. Mexican-American (20)

[b]Lower portion of uterus. These questions do not apply to women who have had total hysterectomies.

(continued)

Lab Activity 13.3 *(continued)*
Determining Your Risk of Getting Cancer

3. Number of pregnancies   3. _10_
   a. 0 (10)
   b. 1–3 (20)
   c. 4 and over (30)

4. Viral infections   4. _1_
   a. Herpes and other viral infections or ulcer
      formations on the vagina (10)
   b. Never (1)

5. Age at first intercourse   5. _5_
   a. Before 15 (40)
   b. 15–19 (30)
   c. 20–24 (20)
   d. 25 and over (10)
   e. Never (5)

6. Bleeding between periods or after intercourse   6. _1_
   a. Yes (40)
   b. No (1)

                                              Cervical Total _37_

Women Only—Endometrial Cancer[c]

1. Age group   1. _5_
   a. 39 or less (5)
   b. 40–49 (20)
   c. 50 and over (60)

2. Race/ethnicity   2. _20_
   a. Oriental (10)
   b. African-American (10)
   c. White (20)
   d. Mexican-American (10)

3. Births   3. _15_
   a. None (15)
   b. 1–4 (7)
   c. 5 or more (5)

4. Weight   4. _50_
   a. 50 or more pounds overweight (50)
   b. 20–49 pounds overweight (15)
   c. Underweight for height (10)
   d. Normal (10)

[c]Body of uterus. These questions do not apply to women who have had total hysterectomies.

5. Diabetes
  a. Yes (3)
  b. No (1)

5. ____|____

6. Estrogen hormone intake
  a. Yes, regularly (15)
  b. Yes, occasionally (12)
  c. None (10)

6. ___10___

7. Abnormal uterine bleeding
  a. Yes (40)
  b. No (1)

7. ____|____

8. Hypertension
  a. Yes (3)
  b. No (1)

8. ____|____

Endometrial Total ___105___

✦ Analysis of Results

Lung

1. Men have a higher risk of lung cancer than women equating them for type, amount, and duration of smoking. Since more women are smoking cigarettes for a longer duration than previously, their incidence of *lung and upper respiratory tract (mouth, tongue, and larynx)* cancer is increasing.
2. The occurrence of lung and *upper respiratory tract* cancer increases with age.
3. Cigarette smokers have up to 20 times or even greater risk than nonsmokers. However, the rates of ex-smokers who have not smoked for ten years approach those of non-smokers.
4. Pipe and cigar smokers are at a higher risk for lung cancer than nonsmokers. Cigarette smokers are at a much higher risk than nonsmokers or pipe and cigar smokers. *All forms of tobacco, including chewing, markedly increase the user's risk of developing cancer of the mouth.*
5. Male smokers of less than one-half pack per day have five times higher lung cancer rates than nonsmokers. Male smokers of one to two packs per day have 15 times higher lung cancer rates than nonsmokers. Smokers of more than two packs per day are 20 times more likely to develop lung cancer than nonsmokers.
6. Smokers of low-tar/low-nicotine cigarettes have slightly lower lung cancer rates.
7. The frequency of lung and *upper respiratory tract* cancer increases with the duration of smoking.
8. Exposures to materials used in these industries have been demonstrated to be associated with lung cancer. Smokers who work in these industries may have greatly increased risks. Exposures to materials in other industries may also carry a higher risk.

(continued)

Lab Activity 13.3 *(continued)*
Determining Your Risk of Getting Cancer

If your lung total is:

24 or less	You have a low risk for lung cancer.
24–49	You may be a light smoker and would have a good chance of kicking the habit.
50–74	As a moderate smoker, your risks of lung and upper respiratory tract cancer are increased. If you stop smoking now, these risks will decrease.
75 and over	As a heavy cigarette smoker, your chances of getting lung and upper respiratory tract cancer are greatly increased. Your best bet is to stop smoking now—for the health of it. See your doctor if you have a nagging cough, hoarseness, persistent pain or sore in the mouth or throat.

Colon/Rectal

1. Colon cancer occurs more frequently after the age of 50.
2. Colon cancer is more common in families with a previous history of this disease.
3. Polyps and bowel diseases are associated with colon cancer.
4. Rectal bleeding may be a sign of colorectal cancer.

If your colon total is:

29 or less	You are at a low risk for colorectal cancer.
30–69	This is a moderate-risk category. Testing by your physician may be indicated.
70 and over	This is a high-risk category. You should see your physician for the following tests: digital rectal exam, guaiac slide test, and proctoscopic exam.

Skin

1. Excessive ultraviolet causes cancer of the skin. Protect yourself with a sunscreen medication.
2. These materials can cause cancer of the skin.
3. Light complexions need more protection than others.

Numerical risks for skin cancer are difficult to state. For instance, a person with a dark complexion can work longer in the sun and be less likely to develop cancer than a light complected person. Furthermore, a person wearing a long-sleeve shirt and wide-brimmed hat may work in the sun and be less at risk than a person in the sun for only a short period who wears a bathing suit. The risk goes up greatly with age.

The key here is that if you answer Yes to any question, you need to protect your skin from the sun or any other toxic material. Changes in moles, warts, or skin sores are very important and need to be seen by your doctor.

Breast

If your breast total is:

Under 100 — Low-risk women should practise monthly breast self-examination and have their breasts examined by a doctor as part of a cancer-related checkup.

100–199 — Moderate-risk women should practise monthly breast self-examinations and have their breasts examined by a doctor as part of a cancer-related checkup. Periodic breast X-rays should be included as your doctor may advise.

200 or higher — High-risk women should practise monthly breast self-examinations and have the above examinations more often. See your doctor for the recommended (frequency of breast physical examinations or X-ray) examinations related to you.

Cervical

1. The highest occurrence is in the 40-and-over age group. The numbers represent the relative rates of cancer for different age groups. A 45-year-old woman has a risk three times higher than a 20-year-old.
2. Puerto Ricans, blacks, and Mexican-Americans have higher rates of cervical cancer.
3. Women who have delivered more children have a higher occurrence.
4. Viral infections of the cervix and vagina are associated with cervical cancer.
5. Women with earlier intercourse and with more sexual partners are at a higher risk.
6. Irregular bleeding may be a sign of uterine cancer.

If your cervical total is:

40–69 — This is a low-risk group. Ask your doctor for a Pap test. You will be advised how often you should be tested after your first test.

70–99 — In this moderate-risk group, more frequent Pap tests may be required.

100 or more — You are in a high-risk group and should have a Pap test (and pelvic exam) as advised by your doctor.

Endometrial

1. Endometrial cancer is seen in older age groups. The numbers by the age groups represent relative rates of endometrial cancer at different ages. A 50-year-old woman has a risk 12 times higher than a 35-year-old woman.
2. Caucasians have a higher occurrence.
3. The fewer children one has delivered, the greater the risk of endometrial cancer.
4. Women who are overweight are at greater risk.
5. Cancer of the endometrium is associated with diabetes.
6. Cancer of the endometrium may be associated with prolonged continuous estrogen hormone intake. This occurs in only a small number of women. You should consult your physician before starting or stopping any estrogen medication.
7. Women who do not have cyclic regular menstrual periods are at greater risk.
8. Cancer of the endometrium is associated with high blood pressure.

(continued)

Lab Activity 13.3 *(continued)*
Determining Your Risk of Getting Cancer

If your endometrial total is:

45–59	You are at very low risk for developing endometrial cancer.
60–99	Your risks are slightly higher. Report any abnormal bleeding immediately to your doctor. Tissue sampling at menopause is recommended.
100 and over	Your risks are much greater. See your doctor for tests as appropriate.

Source: American Cancer Society, *Cancer Facts & Figures—1993* (New York: American Cancer Society, 1993), p. 12. Used by permission. © American Cancer Society, Inc.

Women and Physical Fitness

CHAPTER OBJECTIVES

By the end of this chapter, you should be able to:

1. Define and contrast terms such as essential versus storage fat and fast-twitch versus slow-twitch muscle fibres.

2. Identify sex differences in physiological performance.

3. Identify risk factors for osteoporosis.

4. Evaluate your daily intake of calcium and iron.

5. Detail the role of iron supplementation in iron-deficiency anemia versus sports anemia.

6. Evaluate the safety and benefits of exercise during pregnancy and lactation.

WHEN LIZA WAS A senior in high school 25 years ago, she had an interest in cross-country running but was discouraged from exercising by those who feared exercise was hazardous to women's health. In fact, her school had very few facilities for women and had no competitive teams for women's sports. Today, Liza jogs 50 kilometres per week and often competes in road races. She rides in long-distance bicycle races and has begun training for her first ultramarathon at age 43. This mother of four maintains a very active lifestyle and is in excellent physical condition. At her last class reunion, she was given the "Best Preserved" award for both men and women from her senior class. When asked her secret, Liza responded that she began a walking program in college and simply never stopped!

The Canadian Association for the Advancement of Women in Sport (CAAWS) is dedicated to ensuring that girls and women have access to the complete range of opportunities and choices and have equity as participants in all sports and physical activities. Women are capable of adapting to strenuous training programs and have large maximal aerobic capacities. Although there are some sex differences in performance, women can improve cardiorespiratory endurance, decrease body-fat percentage, increase muscle endurance and strength, and improve performance. In fact, women of all ages can benefit from physical conditioning programs.

Such a large number of women are successfully participating in endurance exercise programs that it is evident that sex should not be a deterrent to women participating in aerobic sports. The large number of national and international female athletes who have set world records in every sport in which men commonly compete has shown that women have the ability to tolerate the physiological demands of strenuous endurance exercise.

We also know that there are many health benefits to be derived from participating in physical-conditioning programs. Active women tend to be leaner, to have a more positive blood-lipid profile, to respond more favourably to mental stress, to have less high blood pressure, to be less prone to cardiorespiratory and metabolic diseases, and even to be less susceptible to cancer than sedentary women. Also, exercisers are less prone to developing crippling diseases such as osteoporosis in adult years than nonexercisers.

In this chapter, we will explore sex differences in physiological performance and discuss the potential benefits women can derive from participating in physical-conditioning programs. We will then explore special considerations for women such as osteoporosis, iron-deficiency anemia, sports anemia, menstrual disorders, pregnancy, lactation, and exercise. We want to emphasize that additional benefits, such as the improved self-esteem and sense of self-satisfaction most people derive from participation in physical-conditioning programs, are certainly not sex-specific. If you have not been involved in an exercise program, get started today.

PHYSIOLOGICAL DIFFERENCES BETWEEN WOMEN AND MEN RELATED TO ATHLETIC PERFORMANCE AND PHYSICAL FITNESS

Four major categories of sex differences in athletic performance and physical fitness will be considered in this section. These include differences in the energy systems

Adenosine triphosphate (ADP) A substrate present in muscle tissue that combines with phosphate to form ATP for muscle contractions.

Creatine phosphate (CP) A substrate present in muscle tissue that is broken down into its components (creatine and phosphate) in order to provide phosphates for the production of ATP.

Stroke volume The amount of blood pumped per beat of the heart; usually expressed in units of millilitres per beat.

for both anaerobic power and maximal aerobic power, body composition, and muscular strength. On average, women weigh less and are shorter than men, but they have more fat tissue and less muscle mass. This remains true even when female athletes are matched against male athletes for any sport. Some of the differences in performance can thus be explained by the difference in physical stature.

Anaerobic Power

As mentioned earlier, the major energy systems in the body are the anaerobic and aerobic metabolism systems. Almost no research has been conducted on the anaerobic capability of female athletes. Therefore, we can only discuss potential differences in performance between males and females.

The energy that is released when food is broken down in the body is not directly used by the muscles to do work. Instead, it is used to manufacture a substance called **adenosine triphosphate (ATP)**, the primary energy molecule of the body. It is either stored in small amounts in the muscles or manufactured through the process of metabolism. Only when energy is liberated from the breakdown of ATP can the cells of the body perform work.

The immediate energy system is composed of ATP and **creatine phosphate (CP)** stored in the muscles. Research has shown that the muscular concentrations of ATP and PC are similar in women and men. Women tend to have a smaller total muscle mass due to differences in physical stature, and so their total amount of ATP and PC is less than that of the average male. For this reason, their total anaerobic capacity is less than that of the average male.

The lactic acid system is a second source of energy for anaerobic activities. It provides energy for high-intensity activities lasting from 30 seconds to two or three minutes in duration. Research has shown that women tend to have lower levels of lactic acid in their blood after maximal exercise than men do. This implies that the capacity of this system is lower in women than it is in men. A probable explanation for this difference is that women have a smaller total muscle mass than men.

When the capacities of the ATP, PC, and lactic acid systems are evaluated, women have less anaerobic capacity than men. The effect on performance is that women have less power and less explosive capability than men. This partially explains the difference in world-record performances for most weight-lifting and track and field events, such as sprint races or the shot put.

Maximal Aerobic Power

The aerobic metabolism energy system is used primarily in activities lasting longer than three minutes and is the major energy source for daily activities and endurance

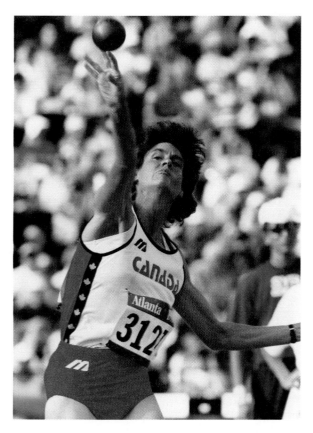

Due to differences in the ATP, PC, and lactic acid systems in men and women, women have less power and less explosive capability than men.

Table 14.1 ✦ Sex Differences in Maximal Oxygen Consumption (mL O_2/kg/min) (50th percentile)

AGE	MALES	FEMALES
20–29	48.0	35.7
30–39	42.2	33.1
40–49	37.5	29.4
50–59	33.6	25.0
60+	30.1	22.0

Source: Based on Health/Fitness Assessment Tutorial, University of Massachusetts, "Percentile Scores for Maximal Oxygen Uptake." Available at **http://omega.cc.umb.edu/ ~umexcsci/tables.html#table2**. Accessed March 11, 2003.

exercise. As with the anaerobic energy systems, the maximal aerobic power, or maximal oxygen consumption (VO_2max), of females is also lower than that of males. Before puberty, there is no difference in VO_2max between girls and boys. Most researchers estimate that the VO_2max of women is 15–25 percent lower than that of adult males past 20 years of age. Table 14.1 shows sex differences in VO_2max. As you can see, from age 20, men have consistently higher VO_2max values than women. It is also clear that there is a consistent decline in VO_2max, or maximal aerobic power, every decade past the age of 20 for both women and men. For both sexes, there is a 25 percent decline in VO_2max in the 40-plus years of life after age 20. This decrease in aerobic power is reflected in lesser endurance times among adult athletes.

There are numerous causes of the lower VO_2max in women as compared to men. Because VO_2max is a product of oxygen delivery to the muscles times the amount of oxygen extracted from the blood by the muscles, several major systems are involved. The cardiorespiratory system is responsible for the amount of oxygen delivered to the muscles. In particular, the cardiac output determines the amount of oxygen delivered to the muscles. The maximal **stroke volume** is lower in women than in

men because women have smaller hearts than men. Also, as can be seen in Table 14.2, the maximal heart rate is lower in women than in men regardless of age. Thus, the overall output of the heart is lower in women than in men because of a lower number of beats and a smaller amount of blood pumped by the heart with each beat.

Another factor affecting sex differences in the amount of oxygen delivered to the muscles is the difference in blood volume and in amount of hemoglobin in the blood. Women tend to have lower total blood volume than men. Hemoglobin is responsible for carrying oxygen in the bloodstream to the muscles. Women also have lower concentrations of hemoglobin in the blood than men. Because the total amount of blood and its oxygen-carrying capacity are both lower in women, the maximal aerobic capacity of women is lower than that of men.

In terms of the amount of oxygen removed from the blood to be used by the muscles, women also have less capacity because they have small muscle masses. If

Table 14.2 ✦ Sex Differences in Resting and Maximal Heart Rate (50th percentile)(in beats/min)

AGE	RESTING		MAXIMAL	
	Males	*Females*	*Males*	*Females*
20–29	64	67	192	188
30–39	63	68	188	183
40–49	64	68	181	175
50–59	63	68	171	169
Over 60	63	65	159	151

Source: Data from J. H. Wilmore, M. Pollock, and S. M. Fox, *Health and Fitness Through Physical Activity* (New York: Wiley, 1978).

you compare the amount of oxygen used per unit of muscle, there is very little difference between women and men. But when the total amount of oxygen used by muscles is compared, women have less capacity. For this reason, it is important to learn different ways of expressing the VO_2max when examining sex differences.

The VO_2max is highest in women who participate in endurance sports. Table 14.3 shows body composition and VO_2max data for female athletes of varying ages. As can be seen, women who participate in cross-country skiing have the highest measured VO_2max. The next-highest values occur in women engaging in activities such as the triathlon, track and field, cycling, and cross-country running. Sports with a very low aerobic capacity, such as golf, have the lowest VO_2max values. It is also interesting to note that some of the highest recorded VO_2max values have been for women older than 30.

■ Body Composition

The average adult female is 7.6–10 centimetres shorter and 11.3–13.5 kilograms lighter and has 4.5–6.8 kilograms more fat tissue than the typical adult male. Even for athletes, these differences are usually present. The average sex differences in body-fat percentage are shown in Table 14.4. In every age category, women have a higher percentage of body fat than men. For both sexes, the body fat percentage increases as they get older.

The reason for a higher percentage of body fat in women as compared to men is based on the types of fat

Table 14.3 ✦ Body Composition and Maximal VO_2 Data for Female Athletes of Varying Ages

ATHLETIC GROUP OR SPORT	AGE	HEIGHT (cm)	WEIGHT (kg)	RELATIVE FAT (%)	MAXIMAL VO₂ (mL/kg/min)
Basketball	19.1	169.1	62.6	20.8	42.9
Bicycling	—	167.7	61.3	15.4	57.4
Dancing, ballet	15.0	161.1	48.4	16.4	48.9
General	21.2	162.7	51.2	20.5	41.5
Golf	33.3	168.9	61.8	24.0	34.2
Gymnastics	15.2	161.1	50.4	13.1	45.2
	19.4	163.0	57.9	23.8	36.3
Pentathlon	21.5	175.4	65.4	11.0	45.9
Racquetball	23.0	173.0	68.0	14.0	—
Skating, figure	16.5	158.8	48.6	12.5	48.9
Skiing, alpine	19.5	165.1	58.8	20.6	52.7
Cross-country	20.2	163.4	55.9	15.7	61.5
	24.3	163.0	59.1	21.8	68.2
Swimming	19.4	168.0	63.8	26.3	37.6
Distance	—	166.3	60.9	17.1	43.2
Tennis	39.0	163.3	55.7	20.3	44.2
Track and field	19.9	161.3	52.9	19.2	57.5
	32.4	169.4	57.2	15.2	59.1
	43.8	161.5	53.8	18.3	43.4
Sprint	20.1	164.9	56.7	19.3	—
Cross-country	15.6	163.3	50.9	15.4	50.8
Discus	21.1	168.1	71.0	25.0	—
Jumpers/hurdlers	20.3	165.9	59.0	20.7	—
Shot put	21.5	167.6	78.1	28.0	—
Triathlon	—	—	—	12.6	58.7
Volleyball	19.9	172.2	64.1	21.3	43.5
Weight lifting					
Bodybuilders	27.0	160.8	53.8	13.2	—

Source: From Jack H. Wilmore and David L. Costill, *Training for Sport and Activity: The Physiological Basis of the Conditioning Process,* 3rd ed. © 1988 Wm. C. Brown Publishers Communications, Inc., Dubuque, IA. All rights reserved. Reprinted by permission.

in the body. **Essential fat** is stored in the muscles, heart, lungs, liver, spleen, intestines, kidneys, and bone marrow. **Storage fat** includes fat tissue that protects the internal organs and **subcutaneous fat**. The higher body-fat level of women compared to men is determined primarily by a higher percentage of sex-specific essential fat in women. Women need a minimum of 12 percent body fat to maintain their essential body-fat stores and conduct all the necessary functions for normal body metabolism, while men only need 3 percent body fat. When women reduce their body-fat stores below 12 percent, menstrual disorders and hormone irregularities are likely to occur.

This higher level of body fat, coupled with a decrease in muscle mass, adversely affects physiological performance in females. Endurance activities are affected the most. In general, any activity that demands that body weight be supported will be most adversely affected by a high amount of body fat and a lesser amount of muscle mass. This is one reason women tend to have poorer performances in distance-running events.

Let's take another look at Table 14.3. The wide range of body-fat percentages shown illustrates the diversity among women who participate in different sports. Women who participate in some anaerobic sports have lower body-fat percentages than women who participate in aerobic sports. Thus, the energy system used is not the primary criterion for estimating body-fat percentage among female athletes. Female athletes tend to manipulate their body-fat percentage in order to improve performance. The optimal percentage of body fat for the particular sport and the aesthetic value of having a low body-fat percentage are important determinants for maintaining a particular body-fat percentage for female athletes.

▇ Muscular Strength

In general, women's muscular strength is about 70 percent that of men. Part of the explanation for this

Table 14.4 ✦ Sex Differences in Fat Percentage (fiftieth percentile)

AGE	MALES	FEMALES
20–29	21.6	25.0
30–39	22.4	24.8
40–49	23.4	26.1
50–59	24.1	29.3
Over 60	23.1	28.3

Source: Data from J.H. Wilmore, M. Pollock, and S. M. Fox, *Health and Fitness Through Physical Activity* (New York: Wiley, 1978).

phenomenon is that different types of muscle fibres are used in different types of sports—specifically, **slow-twitch (ST)** and **fast-twitch (FT) fibres**.

Both women and men who participate in endurance sports have a higher percentage of ST fibres. Women and men who participate in anaerobic sports have a higher percentage of FT fibres. Actually, there is no difference between men and women in terms of who has the largest percentage of ST fibres. The sex difference appears in the *size* of the muscle fibres, not the percentage. Female athletes who participate in endurance sports have 66 and 71 percent of the male FT and ST fibre areas, respectively. This smaller total muscle mass in women accounts for the difference in total muscle strength.

Have you ever wondered why women in a weight-training class do not experience the same degree of muscular **hypertrophy** as men even though they use the same training program? Both women and men will increase in strength with a weight-training program. In fact, the actual percentage increase in strength may be higher for women than for men. Yet women seldom experience the muscular bulkiness seen in men following intense weight-training programs. The primary reason for this is that muscular hypertrophy is controlled by the male sex hormone testosterone. The level of testosterone in the blood is about ten times higher in men than in women. Because women have lower levels of testosterone, they will experience less muscular development, even though they will gain strength from participating in a weight-training program.

You must also remember that because women have a smaller total muscle mass than men, they will also have less muscle hypertrophy than men. Finally, because women have more subcutaneous body fat than men, much of the muscular hypertrophy they experience is masked beneath the layers of fat. As women lose more

Essential fat The amount of fat required for normal physiological functioning.

Storage fat Fat that is stored in the adipose tissue.

Subcutaneous fat The layer of adipose tissue directly beneath the skin.

Slow-twitch (ST) fibres The type of muscle fibres used in endurance sports; equipped metabolically to meet the demands of aerobic activities of long duration.

Fast-twitch (FT) fibres The type of muscle fibres used in anaerobic, power sports; metabolically equipped to meet the demands of short-duration, high-intensity activities.

Hypertrophy An increase in size.

MYTH AND FACT SHEET

Myth	Fact
1. Walking does not provide cardio-protective benefits to women.	1. A recent study involving 84 000 nurses, ages 40–65, who had no evidence of heart disease upon initiation of the study in 1986, refutes this statement. The study reported that the women who used a brisk (at least 4.8 km/h) or very brisk (at least 6.4 km/h) striding pace had a 54 percent lower risk of coronary heart disease. Nevertheless, walking at *any* pace was cardio-protective. The nurses who walked at a slower pace still had a 32 percent reduction in coronary heart disease compared to those who did not walk at all.
2. Contact sports such as hockey and soccer are more dangerous for women than they are for men.	2. No research has shown that women are more physiologically vulnerable to injury than their male counterparts who are involved in sports. In fact, a Health Canada study of Canadian youth revealed that although gender differences were very small for injuries occurring in other venues, males at all age levels were more likely than their female counterparts to experience a sport-related injury.
3. People expend very few calories while working around the house.	3. According to a recent report, during a 15-minute period, a 69.8-kilogram person expends 96 calories scrubbing floors, 79 calories washing windows or mopping, 44 calories vacuuming or dusting, 40 calories washing dishes or ironing, and 35 calories making beds. Painting expends 310 calories an hour; scraping paint, 260; and raking leaves, 220. Engaging in such activities on a regular basis can help you maintain a healthful weight, regardless of age or sex.
4. Symptoms of overtraining are typically only psychological in nature.	4. Psychological symptoms of overtraining include poor concentration and feelings of disorientation. You may become irritable, anxious, or depressed. You may also fail to sleep well. Physical symptoms such as chronic soreness and weakness typically occur. Overtraining also can lead to chronic colds and infections.

body fat, they will see greater muscle definition, but they need not worry about becoming too "masculine" as a result of participating in a weight-training program.

Girls and young women are not prohibited from participating in any type of physical activity simply because of their sex (see Table 14.5). Using the guidelines in the table, women can benefit from participating in endurance and anaerobic training programs just as much as men.

SPECIAL CONSIDERATIONS FOR WOMEN: OSTEOPOROSIS

A crippling disease common to older people in general, and to older women in particular, is osteoporosis. With

this disease, the bones become porous and fragile and break with very little exertion. An estimated 1.4 million Canadians are affected by this degenerative disease. There are over 21 000 osteoporosis-related hip fractures in Canada annually.

Furthermore, at least one-third of all women age 65 or older will suffer a fracture of the spine at some point in their lives. Such fractures can be difficult to treat because the break is usually not clean. The bone literally explodes into countless fragments that cannot be reassembled. If an artificial joint-replacement operation is not possible, the person may be confined to a wheelchair for years.

Although osteoporosis progresses faster in women than in men, this crippling disease constitutes a primary health concern for most older adults. The causes of osteoporosis are multiple and somewhat confusing, as

Table 14.5 ✦ "On the Move" Top 10 Success Factors

The Canadian International Working Group on Women and Sport (2002) designed a program called "On the Move," a national initiative to help increase the physical activity of Canadian girls and young women aged 9–18. The organization has summarized 10 factors that will help to increase females' participation in physical activity programs:

1. Fun: It is important to make physical activity a fun and positive experience; there should be no tryouts or skill/fitness-oriented prerequisites.
2. A Mix of Physical and Social Activities: A multi-activity approach that offers experiences outside the traditional realm of sport makes participation in a physical activity program more appealing. Offering facility-dependent choices and including some less physical options from time-to-time keep the program interesting.
3. Input into Program Design: What works for one age group or community may not work with another; ask participants what they find fun, enjoyable, challenging and basically, what they want to do.
4. Girls and Young Women Only: Research and On the Move experiences support the concept of female-only programming. This provides females the opportunity to participate in physical activities in their own way.
5. A Safe and Supportive Environment: A secure environment is crucial, especially for those females with low participation rates due to lack of skills, lack of positive experiences with physical activity and sport and therefore, lack of self-confidence with respect to their participation. Stress that mistakes are okay, that they are accepted for who they are, that female bodies come in all shapes and sizes, and that they are supported by program facilitators.
6. Peer Age Groupings: Group females according to their peer levels and make sure the age range is suitable to support challenges but not to overwhelm the younger girls. Offer older participants volunteer opportunities to serve as program leaders and role models for the younger ones.
7. Basic Skill Learning: Instructing participants on the basic skills allows them to develop their skills and leads to greater confidence while participating in a variety of physical activities. Focus on fun rather than competition and performing perfectly.
8. Role Model Leader: Leaders should be female, enthusiastic, positive, encouraging, and accepting. They should be well trained and capable of responding to the diversity of issues that face participants.
9. Food: Incorporate healthy food into the program launch event and include snacks at program sessions. Take advantage of these opportunities to talk about nutrition, healthy eating, self-esteem, and body image.
10. Choice of Clothing and Music: Because girls and young women are sometimes self-conscious about their bodies and can suffer from a negative body image, let them choose their own clothing. As their comfort level increases, they will begin to dress more suitably for fuller physical participation. Music adds to creating an appealing environment and reduces tension levels.

will be explained later. Though we strongly recommend that men and women meet the recommended nutrient intake (RNI) for daily calcium intake, it is not yet clear whether adequate calcium intakes can prevent osteoporosis or merely help to slow it down. In any case, there are two major types of osteoporosis.

Type I Osteoporosis

The interior of any long bone is **trabecular bone**. When dietary calcium intake is high, calcium is redeposited in the trabecular bone. Thus, trabecular bone is very metabolically active, and the amount of calcium deposited in this type of bone is partially dependent on the levels of certain hormones in the bloodstream and certain vitamins and minerals in the diet.

Type I osteoporosis typically is characterized by losses of trabecular bone and is associated with low estrogen levels accompanying menopause or surgical removal of the ovaries. Type I is also identified by the kind of bone breaks that occur. With Type I osteoporosis, the bones may become so fragile that even an individual's own body weight can overburden the spine, causing the vertebrae to disintegrate and crush down. When such breaks occur, major nerves may also become pinched and cause excruciating pain in the individual. Trabecular bone loss usually begins in the third decade of life. Six times as many women as men experience Type I osteoporosis after age 65.

Trabecular bone The interior of the bone, which looks like a dense, lacy crystal network and makes up part of the body's calcium bank.

Type II Osteoporosis

Cortical bone can lose its calcium deposits, but usually at a much slower rate than trabecular bone can. Cortical bone losses usually begin at age 40. In Type II osteoporosis, both cortical and trabecular bone loses its calcium deposits, but at a much slower pace. As the person ages, the vertebrae may slowly begin to compress into wedge shapes, usually painlessly, and cause the hunchback posture common in older adults. This type of osteoporosis occurs twice as often in women as in men but is seen in both sexes after age 70.

Developing Peak Bone Mass

Peak bone mass is developed up to age 24. Between the ages of 25 and 30, peak bone mass is usually maintained. However, after approximately age 30, bone loss begins to occur. Although this process cannot be reversed, the rate of bone loss can often be retarded. It is important to be aware that your bones are strongest and most dense in your late teenage and early adult years, because right now you can reduce your likelihood of developing osteoporosis. Once the decline in bone mineralization begins, men typically experience a lifetime bone-density loss of 20–30 percent. Women have a more accelerated bone-mineral loss, resulting in 50 percent or more lifetime bone-density losses.

As has already been described, the type of osteoporosis you may be at risk of developing depends on the type of bone affected and the rate at which that bone is lost. Other risk factors, however, may help you determine whether you may be predisposed to developing this disease.

Risk Factors

Your predisposition to developing osteoporosis depends on both environmental and hereditary factors. The single strongest predictor is age, followed by sex. Additional risk factors include nutritional status, body weight, cigarette smoking, hormonal health, physical inactivity, and alcohol consumption. The effects of many of these risk factors are additive, but we do not know the relative con-

tribution of each risk factor. We recommend that you eliminate as many risk factors as possible.

Age Bones lose their density as you get older because you produce less bone-building equipment and more bone-dismantling equipment. Thus, you should try to obtain enough calcium during young adulthood that when the bone-dismantling process begins, you have optimal bone density. If you build strong bones up to the age of 24, your skeleton will remain stronger throughout your life. To promote maximal calcium stores in the bones, experts recommend an RNI of 1200 milligrams per day for young adults and 800 milligrams per day for men and women past the age of 24. One cup (227 mL) of either whole or 1 percent milk contains approximately 300 milligrams of calcium. Thus, women need to drink 3–4 cups of milk per day in order to meet the RNI. One cup of plain yogurt contains approximately 415 milligrams of calcium. Thus, only three cups of yogurt are needed to meet the RNI.

Sex and Hormones Both men and women lose bone density as they get older, but women tend to lose much greater amounts than men do and are therefore more susceptible to bone breakage. After menopause, women are especially susceptible to developing osteoporosis because the ovaries decrease their estrogen output. However, premenopausal women whose ovaries are removed are also at very high risk because their bodies do not produce estrogen. Research has shown that young women who are long-distance runners for years are prone to athletic **amenorrhea**. Many of these women can only have a period following estrogen administration. If they fail to obtain estrogen-replacement therapy, however, these young women become very susceptible to osteoporosis.

Obviously, men do not usually produce large amounts of the estrogen hormone. Thus, lack of estrogen cannot be used to explain the increased incidence of osteoporosis in older men. Researchers have found that men tend to suffer more fractures when their testes have been removed or when the testes begin to lose their functional capability, as often occurs as a part of the aging process. It seems feasible to assume that both female and male sex hormones contribute significantly to osteoporosis.

Being Underweight and Physical Inactivity Osteoporosis occurs much more frequently in women who are underweight. Thus, while obesity is linked very strongly to all types of cardiorespiratory disease, osteoporosis is equally strongly linked to women who are too stringent in maintaining their body weight.

Cortical bone A very dense, ivorylike bone that forms an outer shell that protects and encompasses trabecular bone; it also composes the shafts of all long bones in the body.

Amenorrhea Absence of the menstrual cycle.

For years, researchers have known that when you are confined to bed rest, your bones lose density, just as the muscles atrophy. The strong relationship between muscle strength and bone density is important because if you want to maintain strong bones, you need to engage in weight-bearing activities. This will be discussed in more detail later in this section.

Cigarette Smoking Smokers have a higher incidence of fractures than nonsmokers. One reason for this may be that smokers tend to weigh less than nonsmokers. Also, women who smoke tend to experience menopause at an earlier age than nonsmokers do.

Alcohol Consumption Alcoholics have long been known to have less bone density than nonalcoholics. Even men who are alcoholics tend to have more bone fractures than nonalcoholic males do. The possible link may be that alcohol causes the body to lose more fluid, and so more calcium is lost in the urine. Thus, calcium is leached out of the bones to maintain the blood level of calcium. Also, alcoholics tend to have poor nutritional habits and typically avoid foods known to be rich sources of calcium. Alcohol also tends to affect the ovaries of women, upsetting the normal hormonal balance that is necessary to maintain healthy levels of calcium in the bones.

Evidence Supporting Risk Factors Strong evidence suggests that obesity, African ancestry, estrogen use, and high peak bone mass are related to decreased susceptibility to osteoporosis. Factors such as being of northern European descent, older age, surgical removal of ovaries before menopause, and extensive bed rest also increase susceptibility to osteoporosis (see Table 14.6). Moderate evidence suggests that heavy exercisers (with the exception of underweight amenorrheic females) have a lower incidence of osteoporosis, while smokers and heavy drinkers are at greater risk. More research is needed to ascertain the impact of factors such as Asian ancestry, number of live births, diabetes mellitus, and caffeine consumption.

◼ Prevention of Osteoporosis

As the previous discussion suggests, several factors are related to the delay or prevention of osteoporosis, especially exercise and calcium nutrition.

Exercise As was mentioned earlier in this textbook, much research has been conducted on the impact of exercise on the development of bone density. You may

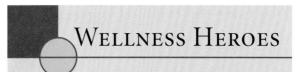

WELLNESS HEROES

CAAWS

The Canadian Association for the Advancement of Women in Sport (CAAWS), recognized as the leading sport and physical organization for girls and women in Canada, has the mission of ensuring that girls and women have access to a complete range of opportunities and choices and have equity as participants and leaders in sport and physical activity. This national not-for-profit organization works in partnership with Sport Canada and Canada's sport and active-living communities to achieve gender equity in the sport community. CAAWS operates with a strong base of volunteers and a small team of effective and efficient staff.

CAAWS provides expert advice, positive solutions, and support to the sport and active-living communities. Innovative and responsive attitudes ensure that CAAWS adapts quickly to change. Policies, plans, and actions are based upon these attitudes and are supported by a solid foundation of research and information.

CAAWS provides an opportunity for people to contribute in a variety of enjoyable and productive ways to girls and women in sport and physical activity. The organization's strategy for change is based on strong and vibrant partnerships. CAAWS' movement for gender equity is not a negative process to disenfranchise men; rather, it is viewed as a long-overdue process to bring women to an equitable level.

CAAWS was created in 1981 in response to the growing recognition that change could only take place when women began to speak about the issues. A year earlier, Sport Canada's Women's Program had been launched to deal with various inequities. Today, CAAWS has positioned itself as an agent of change, using cooperation, collaboration, and consultation to bring gender equity for girls and women to the sport community. Since April 1998, the CAAWS Web site has provided information to well over one million visitors. ✦

Source: Adapted from "Who We Are," off *Canadian Association for the Advancement of Women in Sport (CAAWS)* Web page, accessed January 8, 2003 **www.caaws.ca.**

Table 14.6 ✦ Risk Factors for Osteoporosis

FACTORS THAT INCREASE RISK	FACTORS THAT DECREASE RISK
Northern European ancestry	African ancestry
Female sex	High dietary calcium intake
Low dietary calcium intake	High peak bone mass by age 24
Older age	Heavy chronic exercise history
Postmenopausal status for women	Obesity
Surgical removal of ovaries before menopause	Estrogen use
Surgical removal of testes	
Extensive bed rest	
Increased alcohol consumption	
Cigarette smoking	
Being underweight	

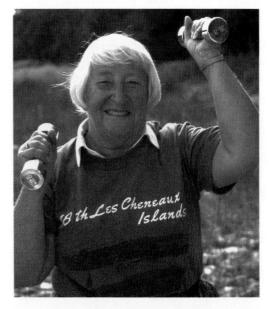

Many types of exercise help to increase bone density, decreasing the risk of developing osteoporosis.

have been told since you were a child that exercising is good for you because it helps you develop stronger bones. Well, that is true, and it is important that you understand why. When you engage in activities that stress the bones, they demand that the bones strengthen their structures. We know that when muscles work, they pull on

Bioavailability Synonymous with *absorbability*; refers to the individual differences in ease of absorption of nutrients.

the bones and signal the bones that more tissue needs to be developed. Simultaneously, the hormones that promote increases in bone mineralization also promote the making of new muscle tissue.

Athletes who participate in weight-bearing exercises have exhibited as much as a 40 percent increase in bone mineralization when compared to sedentary controls. Bone density is increased by weight-bearing activities such as jogging, walking, aerobics, stairmaster exercise, stair climbing, dancing, calisthenics, and even swimming. From this wide range of activities, it is obvious that you can increase bone density by participating in aerobic and anaerobic exercises. To reduce bone loss after reaching peak bone mass, however, you should engage in aerobic activity for at least 30 minutes at least three times per week.

Calcium Nutrition Calcium is essential for bone and tooth formation. In fact, 99 percent of all the calcium in your body is used for these two purposes. One factor that leads to confusion in terms of setting dietary recommendations for calcium intake in relation to minimizing your risk of osteoporosis is the principle of **bioavailability.** This principle is important to your understanding of all vitamins and minerals because the amount of a mineral such as calcium obtained from your diet or even in supplements is not always absorbed. We know that the typical rate of absorption for calcium is 60 percent for infants and children, and that it decreases to 50 percent during pregnancy and to a startling 10–30 percent for adults. The rate of absorption depends on several factors. Your total dietary intake of calcium is one factor affecting bioavailability. For example, if you take in only 400 milligrams of calcium per day and your RNI is 800 milligrams, you may absorb a much higher percentage of the ingested calcium than a person who ingests 1400 milligrams per day. Thus, low dietary intake of calcium leads to a higher absorption rate in some people. As can be seen, the principle of bioavailability can often make it difficult to determine just how much calcium is needed to prevent or retard osteoporosis.

We also cannot say that osteoporosis is a calcium-deficiency disease. This is because, although chronically low levels of dietary calcium prior to age 24 are a strong risk factor for osteoporosis, high calcium intake during adulthood is not effective in reversing bone loss when no other measures are taken. Some research suggests that continued high intake of calcium after age 24 slows down bone loss but is still insufficient to prevent bone loss completely. A disease such as iron-deficiency anemia can be totally reversed when sufficient amounts of iron are added to the diet. Yet research has not demonstrated that increasing calcium intake will reverse osteoporosis.

Recently, researchers have found that people with high blood pressure have lower calcium intake than those with normal blood pressure. If your calcium intake is less than 300 milligrams per day, you have a two to three times greater risk of developing high blood pressure than individuals with a daily calcium intake exceeding 1200 milligrams. Thus, if you are at risk of developing hypertension, we recommend that you at least meet the current RNI for calcium (see Table 14.7).

Finally, we recommend that you concentrate on meeting the RNI for calcium each day. Regardless of your rate of absorption or bone loss, meeting the RNI is your best protective measure from a dietary perspective. Unfortunately, most girls and adult women fail to meet the RNI for calcium during their bone-building years.

Table 14.7 ✦ The Osteoporosis Society of Canada's Recommended Daily Nutritional Intake of Calcium

AGE	DAILY CALCIUM REQUIREMENT
4–8	800 mg
9–18	1300 mg
19–50	1000 mg
50+	1500 mg
Pregnant or lactating women 18+	1000 mg

Source: Reprinted with permission of the Osteoporosis Society of Canada. "How Much Calcium Do We Need?" off *Osteoporosis Society of Canada* Web page, accessed January 8, 2003, **www.osteoporosis.ca**

Such girls are at a disadvantage because they will begin their adult lives with a lower bone mass and will be more prone to osteoporosis in later years. Complete Lab Activity 14.1: Osteoporosis Risk Assessment at the end of this chapter. If you are not meeting the RNI and answer yes to three or more questions in this Lab, you are susceptible to developing osteoporosis in later years.

Suggestions for increasing the intake of calcium in your diet are given in Table 14.8. If you have problems drinking milk or eating dairy products, you can see that several kinds of meat, fruits and vegetables, and grains are excellent sources of calcium. Strive to meet the RNI for this all-important mineral each day, and add quality to your life as you grow older.

Table 14.8 ✦ Suggestions for Increasing Dietary Intake of Calcium

1. Drink low-fat milk with meals or as a snack.
2. Drink orange juice that has added calcium.
3. Eat canned sardines or canned fish prepared with the bones.
4. Use milk, instead of water, when you prepare creamed soups.
5. Add grated cheese to salads, tacos, spaghetti, and lasagna.
6. Increase intake of broccoli and turnip greens.
7. Add powdered nonfat milk to soups, casseroles, sauces, and beverages such as cocoa.
8. Eat low-fat yogurt as a snack.
9. If you are a postmenopausal woman, drink 3–5 cups of milk daily (1 cup = 227 mL).
10. Drink buttermilk with meals or as a snack.
11. Make dairy products a part of your meals, especially low-fat and nonfat cheeses.
12. Increase intake of pork and beans and other legumes.
13. Eat cheese as a snack, or add a slice to your sandwiches.
14. Drink cocoa occasionally instead of drinking hot tea or coffee.
15. If you are a teenager, drink 4 or more cups of milk daily.
16. Use low-fat or nonfat yogurt to make a low-calorie salad dressing.
17. Choose calcium-rich desserts, such as ice cream, custard, or pudding.
18. If you are a pregnant or lactating woman, drink 3–4 cups of milk daily.
19. Increase intake of tofu (bean curd).
20. Drink fluoridated water.
21. Eat fortified breakfast cereals with skim milk.
22. Add cheese to casseroles.

IRON-DEFICIENCY ANEMIA

Have you ever experienced a period of several weeks when you felt chronically tired and apathetic and had a tendency to feel cold in a room where everyone else seemed to be comfortable with the temperature? **Iron-deficiency anemia** is one of the most frequently recurring nutritional problems among younger women of childbearing age. Iron deficiency occurs when the amount of iron ingested from the diet and/or absorbed from foods is less than the amount of either iron lost or iron needed to maintain all bodily functions.

Women are usually diagnosed as having **anemia** when they have a hemoglobin level of less than 12, and men when they have a level less than 14. The normal hemoglobin value for women is 14 and for men is 16.

Nutritional deficiencies, accelerated iron loss, and low bioavailability of iron affect the body's iron stores, regardless of sex. A woman's average monthly menstrual flow, however, typically results in the daily loss of 1.3 milligrams of iron. This is more than twice the amount of iron that men lose daily, 0.6 milligrams. For this reason, women in particular need to understand the causes of iron-deficiency anemia and be aware of dietary methods of increasing their iron intake.

Functions of Iron in the Body

Iron is used in four major ways in the body: as hemoglobin, myoglobin, ferritin, and transferrin. Approximately 75 percent of all iron in the body is a component of the proteins hemoglobin and myoglobin. Maintaining normal **hemoglobin** levels is especially important for endurance-type athletes because oxygen delivery plays a paramount role in aerobic enery production. **Myoglobin** is another iron-containing protein that helps transport oxygen directly into the muscles for the production of energy. Nearly 20 percent of iron in the body is in the form of **ferritin**; the remaining iron is in the form of **transferrin**.

Causes of Iron-Deficiency Anemia

The primary cause of iron-deficiency anemia is usually inadequate iron intake, either because the total caloric intake is too low or because too much of the wrong kinds of food are consumed. Most people in Canada suffer from iron deficiency because they eat foods that are high in fats and sugar but are poor sources of iron. Also, with the increase in the number of vegetarians and red-meat abstainers, many people are planning their meals without including enough sources of absorbable iron

and eventually become prone to anemia. Examples of dietary sources of iron can be found in Table 14.9.

Another major cause of iron deficiency may be poor absorption, also referred to as low bioavailability, of the iron in foods eaten. There are two types of iron in foods. **Heme iron** (the form of iron found in most meats, fish, and poultry) is the most absorbable form. Nearly 40 percent of the iron in heme sources is absorbed by the body. Typically, only 10–20 percent of the iron found in **nonheme iron** (plant) sources is absorbed by the body. For this reason, foods such as meats are recommended several times per week if you are diagnosed as being anemic.

Several factors decrease the amount of iron that is absorbed from the foods eaten. Tea and coffee contain a substance called tannic acid, which decreases iron absorption. Also, a high intake of wheat bran, calcium supplements, phosphates in cola drinks, and excessive fibre is known to impair iron absorption. Fortunately, certain substances will enhance iron absorption from foods, especially from nonheme food sources. These include ingesting any source of vitamin C at the same time that foods containing iron are ingested. Vitamin C ingested with nonheme iron sources can triple the amount of iron absorbed. Table 14.10 gives several sources of vitamin C. Remember, when you include any heme iron source with a meal, a higher percentage of the nonheme iron is also absorbed.

Table 14.9 ✦ Dietary Sources of Iron

FOOD	SERVING SIZE	IRON (mg)
Beef liver	85 mL	5.3
Beef pot roast	85 mL	3.3
Chick peas	227 mL	4.7
Chicken breast	85 mL	0.9
Chicken liver	1 each	1.7
Clams	85 mL canned	23.8
Hamburger	85 mL	2.0
Kidney beans	227 mL	3.2
Oysters	227 mL	16.6
Pinto beans	227 mL	4.5
Prune juice	227 mL	3.0
Prunes	10 medium	2.1
Raisins	227 mL	3.0
Spinach	227 mL	6.4
Total (cereal)	227 mL	21.0
Tuna, canned	85 mL	2.7
Turkey, roasted	85 mL	1.7

Table 14.10 ✦ Dietary Sources of Vitamin C

FOOD	SERVING SIZE	VITAMIN C (mg)
Banana	1 whole	10
Broccoli spears	1 each	141
Brussels sprouts	227 mL	100
Cabbage	227 mL	25
Cantaloupe	½	113
Cranberry juice	227 mL	90
Grapefruit juice	227 mL	80
Orange	1 medium	70
Orange juice	227 mL	120
Potato, baked	1 each	26
Pink grapefruit	1 each	47
Snow peas	227 mL	84
Strawberries	227 mL	84
Tomatoes	227 mL	34
Tomato juice (canned)	227 mL	45
Whole milk	227 mL	2
1% milk	227 mL	2

It is also possible to become anemic from causes other than lack of iron in the diet. Any condition that causes increased blood losses will eventually result in anemia. The monthly menstrual cycle is thus partially responsible for the higher incidence of anemia among women. Ulcers can cause anemia when blood loss is uncontrolled. Some vitamin deficiencies can also cause anemia in an individual.

Who Is at Risk of Developing Iron-Deficiency Anemia?

Certain groups of people typically need more iron than others. Anybody experiencing a period of growth in the body usually needs more iron. Therefore, infants, children, adolescents, and pregnant women have increased iron needs. Because of the special role of iron in the formation of hemoglobin, some athletes also have increased iron needs. Several groups of athletes may be at risk for developing iron-deficiency anemia. These include endurance athletes, teenage athletes, athletes who do not eat red meat, female athletes, and low-body-weight athletes. If you fall into one of these categories, you should examine your diet periodically to assess whether you are ingesting adequate amounts of iron. Complete Lab Activity 14.2: Assessing Your Daily Iron Intake at the end of this chapter to estimate your daily iron intake.

Were you surprised at your iron intake? Experts recommend that women consume 15 milligrams of iron daily until menopause and that men and postmenopausal women consume 10 milligrams per day. If your intake is below these norms, you may be at risk of depleting your body's iron stores even if a blood test shows that you have a normal hemoglobin level. Include more iron-rich foods in your diet from both animal and vegetable sources.

Although some people may need to take iron supplements, the best way to ensure that you meet your daily iron needs is to increase food sources. Table 14.9 listed several sources of dietary iron, and Table 14.11 includes recommendations for boosting the amount of iron in your diet. The normal Canadian diet provides approximately 5–6 milligrams of iron for every 1000 calories ingested, so a woman with very restricted caloric intake may have problems getting enough iron from the diet alone. We recommend that women double the iron-to-calorie ratio daily by choosing iron-rich foods that are also low in calories. If you follow these guidelines, you should not have to worry about developing iron-deficiency anemia.

Iron-deficiency anemia A condition that occurs when the red blood cells do not contain enough hemoglobin and consequently do not deliver enough oxygen to the tissues.

Anemia Occurs when the hemoglobin level falls below the normal reference range for individuals of the same sex and age.

Hemoglobin An iron-containing protein responsible for carrying oxygen through the bloodstream to body tissues, such as muscle, where it is used to provide energy for all forms of physical work.

Myoglobin Another iron-containing protein that helps transport oxygen directly into the muscles for the production of energy.

Ferritin A protein-rich compound that contains iron and constitutes the form in which iron is stored in the liver, spleen, and bone marrow.

Transferrin Another protein-rich compound that transports iron in the bloodstream.

Heme iron The form of iron found in most meats, fish, and poultry; has a high rate of absorption.

Nonheme iron The form of iron found in most plant sources of iron; has a much lower absorption rate than heme iron does.

Table 14.11 ✦ Suggestions for Increasing Dietary Intake of Iron

1. Eat iron-rich foods along with foods containing vitamin C to increase absorption.
2. Decrease caffeinated and decaffeinated coffee intake.
3. Decrease hot tea and iced tea intake.
4. Eat beef liver.
5. Use cast-iron skillets when you cook whenever possible.
6. Purchase only fortified or iron-enriched breakfast cereals.
7. Increase intake of green, leafy vegetables.
8. Eat dry iron-enriched cereals as snacks.
9. Buy iron-enriched or fortified breads.
10. Increase intake of legumes such as kidney beans, chick peas, and lima beans.
11. Combine animal sources of iron with vegetable sources of iron to increase absorption.
12. Eat limited amounts of oysters (be careful of high dietary cholesterol intake).
13. Increase intake of spinach.
14. Eat chicken livers.

Stages of Iron Depletion

As has been already mentioned, you can have a normal hemoglobin level but still be depleting your body's iron stores. To explain how this is possible, we need to briefly discuss the three stages of iron depletion. The first stage is **depleted iron stores**. Many menstruating women, growing children, or even healthy individuals experience this initial phase of iron depletion. Researchers estimate that nearly 20 percent of all women and 3 percent of all men have no iron in their body stores.

It is estimated that millions of people suffer from iron deficiency without the benefit of a diagnosis. This second stage of iron depletion is **iron deficiency without anemia**. The hemoglobin may begin to fall to the low end of the normal range of values at this point. Because the hemoglobin level may still be considered normal, anemia is not diagnosed.

The final stage of iron depletion is iron-deficiency anemia. Approximately 8 percent of women and 1 percent of men have progressed to this final stage of anemia. A peculiar symptom of iron-deficiency anemia is **pica**. Sometimes when people become anemic, they develop an appetite for such items as ice, paste, and/or clay. In particular, women from low-income families are often

initially diagnosed as being anemic because of the reported symptom of eating ice all the time. As soon as the hemoglobin level returns to normal, the appetite for ice or other nonnutritious items disappears. In correctly diagnosed cases of iron-deficiency anemia, supplemental iron will be required in order to improve iron status. Large supplements of iron should only be taken under medical supervision because excesses can be toxic. If your hemoglobin level is normal, you have no history of anemia, and you ingest adequate amounts of iron in your daily caloric intake, we recommend that you avoid taking iron supplements to reduce the danger of iron toxicity.

Early diagnosis of iron-deficiency anemia is crucial because chronic anemia causes people to work less, play less, or simply do less because they do not seem to have the energy. As their level of physical activity drops, many chronic problems such as obesity can arise simply because they are too tired to exercise. Also, anemic children are less productive in school and may be perceived as lazy by teachers. Teachers become reluctant to spend additional time aiding them, and the children fall further behind in school. This is a tragic scenario because many such problems could be avoided by simply increasing the amount of iron in the diet.

SPORTS ANEMIA

Researchers have found that female endurance athletes are especially prone to periods of iron deficiency. This type of anemia is often called *sports anemia* because of its nature. There are several proposed causes of this transient anemia that occurs in female and other endurance athletes, particularly during the early phases of a training program. One suspected factor is **hemodilution**. When a person begins a very heavy aerobic training program, there is an increase in both the plasma volume and the total amount of hemoglobin produced. There is a greater proportional increase in the plasma volume, however, than in the hemoglobin; and the hemoglobin level apparently is lower. In simpler terms, the blood is less concentrated, so the athlete has less hemoglobin for every 100 millilitres of blood. Thus, with less oxygen being delivered to the tissues with every heartbeat, the athlete appears anemic. This condition usually is transient and lasts approximately two to eight weeks during the initial training period.

Another possible cause of sports anemia is a diet inadequate in iron, especially heme iron sources. Exercisers who consume large quantities of junk food may meet the caloric requirements to maintain their body weight, in spite of strenuous training schedules. The iron-to-calorie ratio, however, may in fact be very low.

In one report, 42 percent of the female distance runners studied were modified vegetarians, ingesting less than 200 grams of meat a week. This excessively low intake of such a rich source of heme iron partially explains the inability of many female athletes to meet the suggested intake of iron. We recommend that coaches regularly include an assessment of iron status as part of the medical screening for all athletes.

Recent research has shown that exercisers lose significant amounts of iron through sweating. As the level of fitness increases, however, a smaller amount of iron is lost. In spite of this positive training adaptation, exercisers still lose significant amounts of iron through their sweat. Because this is unavoidable, we recommend that endurance exercisers increase dietary iron during heavy periods of training.

Finally, sports anemia may be caused by the rupture of red blood cells. Red blood cells are sometimes destroyed when the soles of the feet, or similar body tissues, make very-high-impact contact with a hard surface.

Any combination of these factors will likely result in the transient anemia that plagues some endurance athletes. Because women often have lower normal values of hemoglobin than men, very strenuous exercise is of some concern. It is important to realize that true sports anemia cannot be reversed with iron supplementation. Sports anemia appears to be a temporary response to exercise; thus, no treatment is required.

MENSTRUATION AND EXERCISE

Exercise and Menstrual Disorders

Many female athletes engaging in intense chronic aerobic exercise have reported abnormal menstrual cycles. Although much research has been conducted to find the causes of this phenomenon, we still are unable to define clearly who will have abnormal menstrual cycles and why. Most women and nonendurance athletes have **eumenorrhea**—regularly occurring cycles. However, with chronic endurance exercise, an increased percentage of female athletes report **oligomenorrhea:** reduced, scanty, or irregular menstruation. Some researchers estimate that 5–40 percent of female athletes, depending on the sport, are oligomenorrheic, as compared to 10–12 percent in the general female population. One research project reported that 45 percent of female track and cross-country runners who ran more than 80 miles per week experienced irregular menstrual cycles. A smaller percentage report amenorrhea. Only 2–3 percent of women in the general population are amenorrheic. Yet in activities such as dis-

tance running, as many as 34 percent of women reportedly are amenorrheic. The incidence of amenorrhea decreases to 23 percent of joggers and to only 4 percent among a nonrunning control group. Runners were defined as running more than 48.3 kilometres per week at very hard intensity. Joggers ran from 8 to 48.3 kilometres per week, but all at low-to-moderate intensity.

As shown in numerous studies, the decrease in menstrual function often is directly related to the intensity and duration of exercise. For women engaging in very intense training programs such as ballet dancing, figure skating, distance running, gymnastics, and cycling, irregular menstruation may be the norm rather than the exception. Some female athletes have reported the absence of menstruation for months or even years while engaging in high-intensity endurance exercise.

Possible Causes of Menstrual Disorders Among Female Athletes

What is it about chronic participation in aerobic exercise that leads to abnormal menstrual function? Actually, neither the cause nor the long-term consequences of oligomenorrhea or secondary amenorrhea are known. Researchers have, however, discovered several possible reasons for this phenomenon. Numerous studies link the intensity of exercise with abnormal menstrual function. Athletes who perform at higher levels of intensity appear to be more susceptible to oligomenorrhea.

Depleted iron stores The initial state of iron depletion whereby you become vulnerable to low iron stores but do not experience any adverse physiological effects.

Iron deficiency without anemia The second phase of iron depletion, in which some adverse physiological effects occur such as chronic fatigue, decreased physical work capacity, and diminished productivity due to a reduced hemoglobin level.

Pica A craving for nonfood substances that occurs as a symptom of iron-deficiency anemia.

Hemodilution An increase in the plasma volume (fluid portion of blood) that exceeds the increase in the total amount of hemoglobin produced, creating symptoms of anemia.

Eumenorrhea Regularly occurring menstrual cycles.

Oligomenorrhea Reduced, scanty, or irregular menstruation.

DIVERSITY ISSUES

Women, Amenorrhea, and Stress Fractures

Amenorrhea and stress fractures can occur together in active young women. The sports most commonly associated with amenorrhea are ballet, distance running, gymnastics, cycling, rowing, and Nordic skiing. Stress fractures are also commonly found in these same sports. Amenorrhea is typically a symptom of an underlying problem and requires looking at more than simply an athlete's level of activity. When possible, athletes showing symptoms of amenorrhea and stress fracture should observe the following guidelines, under the direction of a physician:

1. Decrease the level of activity when possible, and allow weight gain until normal menstrual cycles occur.
2. Begin or continue calcium supplementation.
3. Consider estrogen–progesterone supplementation.

Proper diagnosis of female athletes at risk for amenorrhea should include a nutrition evaluation, exertion evaluation, estrogen evaluation, and bone-density measurement. The history, physical examination, and laboratory assessment can lead to an effective diagnosis and treatment regimen. Finally, sound nutritional practices are essential for optimal performance in all female athletes. ◆

Athletes who lose large amounts of weight through the reduction of body-fat stores are more prone to amenorrhea. Researchers report that a loss of 33 percent body fat or even a 10–15 percent reduction in body weight will induce amenorrhea. As discussed previously, female athletes in nearly all endurance sports have much lower body-fat percentages than the general nonathletic population. For example, body-fat levels of less than 12 percent have been reported for world-class marathon runners.

The storage and metabolism of the female sex hormone estrogen is related to the amount of body fat stored. Thus, as body-fat stores decrease, so does estrogen production. With low levels of estrogen available, the follicular phase of the menstrual cycle is affected,

Dysmenorrhea Painful menstrual cycles.

and menstruation may be abnormal or may cease totally. Menstrual irregularities may therefore be caused by changes in the levels of circulating sex hormones as the level of body fat decreases.

It is difficult to separate the effects of exercise from those of the emotional stresses associated with intense physical training. We know that the athletes who train hardest tend to perform at a higher level. This higher level of performance and competition generally leads to more stress. When the athlete is exposed to more psychological stress, hormone production is also affected.

You can easily see that explaining the causes of amenorrhea can be complicated. High levels of training lead to low body-fat stores. High levels of training also lead to increased psychological stress. Low fat stores cause reductions in hormone production. High levels of psychological stress also cause changes in levels of circulating hormones. These factors combined have all been associated with menstrual irregularities. However, it is impossible to determine the relative contribution of each factor.

Performance and Competition During Menstruation

Surveys show that many female athletes are concerned about the potential effects of the menstrual cycle on performance during competition. Several studies report considerable individual variation in these effects. Some women are totally unaffected by their menstrual cycle, but others have problems during the premenstrual and initial-flow phases. **Dysmenorrhea** was more often reported by those women.

Some women have even reported improvement in performance in the immediate period postflow. The number of women who report difficulties with performance is approximately equal to those who report no effect of menstruation on their level of performance. Thus, individual variations must always be considered. In general, most young athletes are unaffected by menstruation. Endurance athletes tend to report more adverse effects of the menstrual cycle on their levels of performance. Track and field athletes, especially sprinters, appear to be least affected by menstruation during performance.

Physiologically, no research projects report significant cardiorespiratory or metabolic changes either at rest or during maximal exercise in any phase of the menstrual cycle. A limited number of studies report minor changes at rest during certain phases of the cycle. None, however, report any physiological fluctuations during exercise.

Some physicians advise women not to swim while menstruating. Yet there is no physiological basis supporting this advice. Researchers have shown that there is no bacterial contamination of the pool water when women swim while menstruating. We also know that no signs of bacterial infections have appeared in the reproductive organs. When women use tampons while swimming, all indications are that they are not susceptible to contracting bacterial infections, and no one is susceptible to contracting infections as a result of their menses.

In conclusion, on the basis of current data, we have no reason to suggest that women avoid physical activity of any type during any phase of the menstrual cycle. If a woman feels any physical discomfort, she should not feel compelled to exercise. She should experience no physiological fluctuations during performance as a result of menstruation.

PREGNANCY, LACTATION, AND EXERCISE

Exercise During Pregnancy

The Canadian Society for Exercise Physiology (CSEP) advocates that healthy women with uncomplicated pregnancies can integrate physical activity into their daily living and can participate without significant risks either to themselves or to their unborn child. Postulated benefits of such programs include improved aerobic and muscular fitness, promotion of appropriate weight gain, and facilitation of labour. Regular exercise may also help to prevent gestational glucose intolerance and pregnancy-induced hypertension. Because the safety of prenatal exercise programs depends on the physiological health of the mother and fetus, CSEP has developed a Physical Activity Readiness Medical Examination for Pregnancy (PARmed-X for Pregnancy), which physicians use to decide if physical activity is recommended or contraindicated for pregnant women. When such activity is recommended, PARmed-X for Pregnancy provides prescriptions for aerobic activity and muscle conditioning (see Appendix D).

There is still some debate about whether participation in athletics has an adverse effect on childbirth. A recent extensive review by Lokey and associates (1991) of all major research papers concerning pregnant women summarized several findings with respect to the safety of exercise during pregnancy, effects of exercise on delivery, and guidelines for participation in exercise. Most of the studies support the finding that athletes had fewer complications of pregnancy than nonathletes. Also, exercisers who remained active during pregnancy weighed less, gained less weight during pregnancy, and delivered smaller babies than nonexercising women. The exercising women had shorter labour and appeared to tolerate labour pain better than nonexercising women did. Athletes had fewer cesarean sections and fewer tissue ruptures during delivery than nonathletes. Although all women decreased their amount of total work as the pregnancy progressed, many remained active up to the day of delivery.

Although most studies report no adverse effects on pregnancy, especially for women who were already physically active, pregnant women still should seek the advice of their personal physicians before engaging in endurance exercise programs. Because there is the potential for pregnancy-related physiological changes to affect the ability to engage safely in some forms of exercise, the Society of Obstetricians and Gynecologists of Canada advises pregnant women to participate in physical activities that use large muscle groups, such as walking, swimming, stationary cycling, and low impact aerobics. Also, women should be aware of safety considerations.

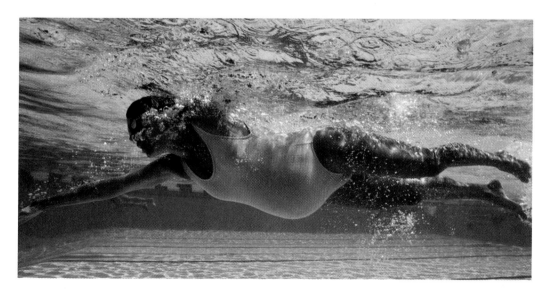

Normal pregnancy is not a condition that requires a sedentary lifestyle, and pregnant women can exercise so long as they heed the appropriate safety considerations.

Benefits of Exercise on Weight ◼ Reduction After Pregnancy

Have you ever heard a woman complain of developing "thunder thighs" that she seemed unable to get rid of after having a baby? It is true that women tend to store more body fat in the hips and thighs while they are pregnant. When they do not become physically active and do not breastfeed their babies, it is very difficult for many of them to lose all the weight they gained during the pregnancy. Researchers have found that women who maintain an exercise program during and after pregnancy are much more likely to reduce the thunder thighs than those who are not active. What role does physical activity play in this puzzle?

When we eat fat, it is broken down and packaged in the liver in the form of a triglyceride. Triglycerides are combined with lipoproteins (fat carriers) because triglycerides cannot dissolve directly in the blood. Lipoproteins carry the triglycerides through the bloodstream to the fat cells all over the body. At the entrance to each fat cell is an enzyme called lipoprotein lipase (LPL) whose job is to break apart the lipoprotein and triglyceride. The triglyceride, or fat, is then transported to the fat cell where it is stored, and the lipoprotein continues travelling through the bloodstream.

The enzyme LPL plays a major role in increased fat stores during pregnancy. When the body-fat stores get low, the activity of this enzyme increases so that more fat is stored in the fat cells. In addition, during the early stages of pregnancy, LPL activity in the thighs increases so that more fat is stored in these areas. This is a protective mechanism for the mother because more fat will be needed in these areas to provide the energy to make milk when the mother begins breastfeeding her baby. Milk production actually requires a great deal of energy. So this extra body fat is constantly being broken down to provide energy as long as the baby continues breastfeeding. Thus, when women breastfeed babies, they break down more of the fat that is stored in the hips and thighs and lose weight quicker.

Also, endurance exercise will trigger the breakdown of fat in the hips and thighs for women who have delivered babies. As you get involved in an exercise program, more fat is released from those fat stores to provide the energy for long-duration activity. But simply dieting in order to lose thunder thighs is totally ineffective because cutting down on your calories without exercising will not trigger the stubborn fat cells to burn the fat stored within them. Remember to encourage women who are considering getting pregnant or who have recently had a baby to get involved in a physical activity program in order to maintain their body-fat percentage.

SUMMARY

Physiological Differences Between Women and Men Related to Athletic ◼ Performance and Physical Fitness

On average, women weigh less and are shorter than men but have more fat tissue and less muscle mass. This remains true even when female athletes are matched against male athletes for any given sport. There are many differences in the energy systems and physical stature of women and men.

The two anaerobic energy systems are called ATP and PC, which make up the immediate energy and the lactic acid or anaerobic glycolysis systems. No sex differences exist with the immediate energy system in terms of the muscle concentrations of ATP and PC. Because women tend to have a smaller total muscle mass than men do, their anaerobic capacity is less.

Women also have lower levels of lactic acid than men do at the end of maximal exercise. This is primarily because they have smaller muscle mass. Thus, there are no significant biological differences between males and females with respect to anaerobic performance.

After puberty, men tend to have an average of 20 percent higher VO$_2$max. This is primarily because women have smaller hearts and less blood volume, so they are not able to deliver as much oxygen to the tissues. Also, women have smaller muscle mass, so they are able to draw less oxygen from the blood to be used aerobically.

After puberty, women have a higher percentage of essential body fat than men do because of increased estrogen production. This increased fat is stored in the hips and thighs and most internal organs of the body. Women also have high subcutaneous body-fat stores. An optimal body-fat percentage can be determined on the basis of individual differences and level of performance.

In general, the muscular strength of women is about two-thirds that of men. Although there is no genetic difference in the percentage of muscle fibres between the sexes, there is a difference in the size of the muscle fibres. Men tend to have larger muscle fibres than women, and this leads to greater strength.

◼ Special Considerations for Women

Women are more susceptible than men to certain conditions, including osteoporosis, iron-deficiency anemia, sports anemia, and menstrual disorders. All such conditions can have a debilitating effect on exercise capacity. Also, pregnancy and lactation cause physiological changes that may affect exercise tolerance. Still, exercise is beneficial for regaining fitness and restoring physique after pregnancy.

Osteoporosis is more commonly known as adult bone loss. Many postmenopausal women are plagued with this disease. Peak bone mass is developed up to age 24. After age 30, bone loss begins to occur, regardless of how dense the bones are. Risk factors such as being female, growing older, being amenorrheic, being of northern European ancestry, being underweight, smoking cigarettes, drinking alcohol, and leading a sedentary lifestyle make individuals more prone to developing osteoporosis.

It is important to maintain the RNI for calcium, especially in the bone-building years. Women should ingest at least 1200 milligrams per day up to age 24, and men and women past age 24 should ingest 1000 milligrams per day. Weight-bearing activities have been shown to increase bone density. Thus, maintaining a lifetime physical activity program is crucial to retarding and preventing this disease.

In iron-deficiency anemia, the red blood cells do not contain enough hemoglobin. Most of the iron in the body is a component of the protein hemoglobin. Hemoglobin is used to carry oxygen throughout the bloodstream to the body tissues, where it provides energy for all forms of physical work.

The major cause of iron-deficiency anemia is usually inadequate iron intake. Increased blood loss also leads to such deficiency, as does poor absorption of the iron in foods. Heme iron is found in most meats, fish, and poultry and has the highest rate of absorption. Nonheme iron is in most plant sources and has a much lower absorption rate.

Infants, children, adolescents, and pregnant women usually have increased iron needs. Premenopausal women need to consume 15 milligrams of iron daily. Men and postmenopausal women need to consume 10 milligrams per day.

Iron-deficiency anemia occurs in three stages. The first stage is depleted iron stores. During this stage, there are no adverse physiological effects. The second stage is iron deficiency without anemia. At this point, the hemoglobin level may be reduced to the low end of normal. In the final stage, iron-deficiency anemia, hemoglobin levels drop and chronic fatigue is induced. Some women experience symptoms called *pica*. They have a desire to eat ice, clay, and/or paste as a result of the iron deficiency.

This transient anemia is not treatable by iron supplementation and often occurs during the early phases of a strenuous endurance-training program. True sports anemia is reversible by the end of the ninth week of training. Athletes who experience decreased iron absorption and increased iron loss through the menstrual cycle are more susceptible to both iron-deficiency and sports anemias.

Amenorrhea is a common occurrence among many female endurance athletes. It occurs in approximately one-third of female distance runners. Its exact cause is unknown but it is suspected to be related to the intensity of exercise. As weekly training mileage increases, so does the prevalence of amenorrhea. At higher levels of competition, more psychological stress occurs, which affects hormone production. As the level of hormones such as estrogen is reduced, menstrual disorders are more likely to occur. Menstruation itself has not been shown to adversely affect physical training or competition. In many cases, oligomenorrhea and amenorrhea are reversed as training intensity decreases.

More and more physicians are advising women to remain physically active during pregnancy. Women may have shorter labour and tolerate the pain better. Athletes may have fewer complications of pregnancy than nonathletes. Exercisers may weigh less and be less likely to need cesarean sections than nonexercisers. A woman should seek the advice of her physician before initiating an exercise program.

During the early stages of pregnancy, the fat cells in the body are stimulated to increase the amount of fat stored, especially in the hips and thighs. If women fail to breastfeed their babies and do not exercise, many of them end up with thunder thighs, which cannot be reduced through dieting alone.

STUDY QUESTIONS

1. What are the main differences between fast- and slow-twitch muscle fibres? In which types of sports are each mainly used?

2. How does Type I osteoporosis differ from Type II osteoporosis?

3. What are the risk factors for osteoporosis?

4. What types of foods would be recommended to alleviate iron-deficiency anemia and why?

5. What are the causes of sports anemia?

6. What are the benefits of exercising during and after pregnancy?

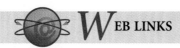

WEB LINKS

Clinical Practice Guidelines for the Diagnosis and
Management of Osteoporosis
www.cma.ca

Canadian Association for the Advancement of Women in
Sport and Physical Activity
www.caaws.ca

Health Canada (A–Z index, pregnancy and maternal health)
www.hc-sc.gc.ca/

Health Promotion Online (choose: Health Topics,
Women's Health Bureau)
www.hc-sc.gc.ca/english/for_you/hpo/index.html

Sport Canada
www.pch.gc.ca/sportcanada/

REFERENCES

International Working Group on Women and Sport. The
Montreal Tool Kit; A Legacy of 2002 World Conference.
www.canada2002.org

Lokey, E. A., Z. U. Tran, C. L. Wells, B. C. Myers, and A. C.
Tran. "Effects of Physical Exercise on Pregnancy Out-
comes: A Meta-Analytic Review." *Medicine and Science in
Sports and Exercise* 23, 11 (1991): 1234–1239.

Society of Obstetricians and Gynecologists of Canada
(SOGC). *Healthy Beginnings: Guidelines for Care During
Pregnancy and Childbirth.* Ottawa: SOGC, 1995.

Lab Activity 14.1

Osteoporosis Risk Assessment

✦ **Step 1** Write in the number of servings of the following foods you consume daily (1 cup = 8 oz = 227 mL). Multiply the number of servings (column 1) by the given number of milligrams of calcium per serving (column 2). Now total the numbers in the last column. This number is your daily calcium intake from dairy products.

Food	Serving Size	(1) Number of Servings	(2) Calcium (mg) per Serving	(1) × (2) Daily Calcium Intake
Milk	1 cup	_____	× 300 =	_____
Yogurt	1 cup	_____	× 300 =	_____
Cheese	1 slice	_____	× 200 =	_____
Cottage cheese	½ cup	_____	× 70 =	_____
Ice cream	1 cup	_____	× 180 =	_____

Daily calcium intake from dairy products: _____

✦ **Step 2** Write in the number of servings of the following foods you consume weekly (column 1). Multiply that number by the given number of milligrams of calcium (column 2) and add these amounts to get a total. This number is your weekly calcium intake from nondairy products.

Food	Serving Size	(1) Number of Servings	(2) Calcium (mg) per Serving	(1) × (2) Weekly Calcium Intake
Broccoli	½ cup	_____	× 65 =	_____
Baked beans	½ cup	_____	× 65 =	_____
Pizza	1 slice	_____	× 100 =	_____
Soup (made with milk)	1 cup	_____	× 170 =	_____
Sardines	3 oz	_____	× 375 =	_____
Canned salmon	4 oz	_____	× 300 =	_____
Shrimp	3 oz	_____	× 100 =	_____

Weekly calcium intake from nondairy foods (except soup base): _____

Now divide your weekly calcium intake from nondairy foods by 7: $\dfrac{}{7}$ = _____

(continued)

Lab Activity 14.1 *(continued)*
Osteoporosis Risk Assessment

✦ **Step 3**   Add your daily calcium intake from section 1 and your weekly calcium intake divided by 7 from section 2. The total of these two figures is your average daily calcium intake.

Daily calcium intake from dairy foods   = _____

+ Weekly calcium intake from other foods divided by 7 = _____

Average daily calcium intake   = _____

✦ **Step 4**   Compare your average daily calcium intake to:

Women and men aged 11 to 24 years = 1200 mg/day

Women and men aged 25 years and older = 800 mg/day

Some researchers recommend that premenopausal women ingest 1000 milligrams of calcium per day and that postmenopausal women ingest 1500 milligrams of calcium per day. Seek the advice of your personal physician before taking amounts in excess of the RNI.

✦ **Step 5**   Answer the following questions. If you answer Yes to three or more, you are at risk for developing osteoporosis.

1. Has anyone in your family ever suffered a hip or vertebral (back) fracture?

    Yes _____   No _____   Relationship: _____

2. Is your ethnic background northern European?

    Yes _____   No _____

3. Do you exercise less than 3 times a week for 30 minutes each time?

    Yes _____   No _____

4. Do you regularly take antacids? (Aluminum increases calcium excretion. Anyone who takes an aluminum-containing antacid regularly should switch to one with no aluminum.)

    Yes _____   No _____   Brand name: _____

5. Do you consume carbonated beverages? Yes _____   No _____

    Number per day: _____   Type: _____

    A calcium-to-phosphorus ratio of 1:1 is needed to avoid calcium depletion. Some research has shown that because of significant changes in the North American diet, most people's calcium-to-phosphorus ratio is now close to 1:2. This excessive consumption of phosphorus is thought to leach more calcium out of the bones, resulting in increased bone loss.

    One significant source of phosphorus is most carbonated beverages. Excessive consumption of these must be considered when assessing dietary risk of osteoporosis. Check labels for phosphorus content, and substitute skim or whole milk when possible.

6. Do you not take any calcium supplements?

    Yes _____   (I do *not* take calcium supplements.)

    No _____   (I *do* take calcium supplements.)

    Number per day: _____   Type: _____

Source: A. Larson and S. Shannon, "Decreasing the Incidence of Osteoporosis-Related Injuries Through Diet and Exercise," *Geritopics* 8 (1985): 2, 5–9. Reprinted from *Geritopics* with the permission of the American Physical Therapy Association.

Lab Activity 14.2

Assessing Your Daily Iron Intake

✦ **Step 1** For each item on this list of several sources of heme and nonheme iron, write in the number of servings you consume daily (1 cup = 8 oz = 227 mL). Multiply the number of servings (column 1) by the given number of milligrams of iron per serving (column 2). Now total the numbers in the last column. This number is your daily iron intake from heme and nonheme food sources.

Food	Serving Size	(1) Number of Servings	(2) Iron (mg) per Serving	(1) × (2) Daily Iron Intake
Good Sources of Iron				
Beef liver	3 oz	_____	5.3	_____
Chicken liver	1 each	_____	1.7	_____
Clams	3 oz canned	_____	23.8	_____
Oysters	1 cup	_____	16.6	_____
Corned beef	3 oz	_____	1.8	_____
Pork loin	3 oz	_____	1.0	_____
Prune juice	1 cup	_____	3.0	_____
Prunes	10 medium	_____	2.1	_____
Raisins	1 cup	_____	3.0	_____
Lima beans	1 cup	_____	4.5	_____
Kidney beans	1 cup	_____	3.2	_____
Pinto beans	1 cup	_____	4.5	_____
Black-eyed peas	1 cup	_____	4.3	_____
Chick peas	1 cup	_____	4.7	_____
Soybeans	1 cup	_____	8.8	_____
Sunflower seeds	¼ cup	_____	2.4	_____
Almonds	1 cup	_____	5.0	_____
Cashews	1 cup	_____	6.0	_____
Total cereal	1 cup	_____	21.0	_____
Most cereal	⅔ cup	_____	9.0	_____
Raisin bran	½ cup	_____	4.5	_____
Cheerios	1 cup	_____	3.6	_____

(continued)

Lab Activity 14.2 (continued)
Assessing Your Daily Iron Intake

Food	Serving Size	(1) Number of Servings	(2) Iron (mg) per Serving	(1) × (2) Daily Iron Intake
Fair Sources of Iron				
Tuna, canned	3 oz	_____	2.7	_____
Salmon	3 oz	_____	0.9	_____
Shrimp	6 medium	_____	2.6	_____
Sardines	3 oz	_____	2.5	_____
Veal	3 oz	_____	1.0	_____
Chicken, breast	3 oz	_____	0.9	_____
Turkey, roasted	3 oz	_____	1.7	_____
Rabbit	3 oz	_____	2.0	_____
Liverwurst	1 oz	_____	1.5	_____
Beef pot roast	3 oz	_____	3.3	_____
Hamburger	3 oz	_____	2.0	_____
Ham	3 oz	_____	1.2	_____
Hot dog	1 each	_____	0.7	_____
Fish stick	1 oz	_____	0.1	_____
Walnuts	1 cup	_____	3.0	_____
Pecans	1 cup	_____	2.3	_____
Peanuts	1 cup	_____	2.6	_____
Peanut butter	1 tbsp	_____	0.3	_____
Apricots, dried	¼ cup	_____	1.2	_____
Bananas	1 each	_____	1.1	_____
Strawberries	1 cup	_____	0.6	_____
Watermelon	1 slice	_____	0.8	_____
Canned peaches	1 cup	_____	0.7	_____
Nectarines	1 each	_____	0.2	_____
Potato	1 medium	_____	2.8	_____
Green beans	1 cup	_____	1.1	_____
Green peas	1 cup	_____	2.6	_____
White rice	½ cup	_____	0.9	_____
Whole wheat bread	1 slice	_____	1.0	_____
Egg noodles	1 cup	_____	2.5	_____
Corn flakes	1¼ cup	_____	1.8	_____
Oatmeal, cooked	1 cup	_____	1.6	_____
Bagel	1 each	_____	1.8	_____
Collard greens	1 cup	_____	0.2	_____

Food	Serving Size	(1) Number of Servings	(2) Iron (mg) per Serving	(1) × (2) Daily Iron Intake
Spinach	1 cup	_____	6.4	_____
Mustard greens	1 cup	_____	1.7	_____
Turnip greens	1 cup	_____	1.7	_____
Broccoli	1 cup	_____	1.3	_____
Corn	1 ear	_____	0.5	_____
Eggs	1 each	_____	0.7	_____
Flour, enriched	1 cup	_____	3.2	_____
Flour, unenriched	1 cup	_____	0.9	_____
Others				
_____	_____	_____	_____	_____
_____	_____	_____	_____	_____
_____	_____	_____	_____	_____
_____	_____	_____	_____	_____
_____	_____	_____	_____	_____
_____	_____	_____	_____	_____

*The number of milligrams of iron per serving is calculated by using the average values from several nutrition textbooks.

This is your daily intake from iron (heme and nonheme) sources: _____ mg/day

✦ **Step 2**　Review your food sources of iron and make a list of heme compared to nonheme sources in the space provided.

Heme Iron		Nonheme Iron	
Source	Amount (mg)	Source	Amount (mg)
_____	_____	_____	_____
_____	_____	_____	_____
_____	_____	_____	_____
_____	_____	_____	_____
_____	_____	_____	_____
_____	_____	_____	_____
Total (mg)　_____		Total (mg)　_____	

(continued)

Lab Activity 14.2 *(continued)*
Assessing Your Daily Iron Intake

1. From which source are you obtaining most of your dietary iron?

   Heme _____   Nonheme _____

2. What is the significance of differentiating between heme and nonheme sources of iron in your diet?

   _____

   _____

   _____

   _____

✦ **Step 3**   Compare your average daily iron intake with:

Premenopausal women   = 15 mg/day
Postmenopausal women = 10 mg/day

Men aged 11 to 18 years = 12 mg/day
Men aged 18 and older   = 10 mg/day

✦ **Step 4**   Answer the following questions. If you answer Yes to three or more, you may need to take an iron supplement. Please seek the advice of your personal physician before doing so.

		Yes	No
1.	Does most of your daily iron come from nonheme sources?	_____	_____
2.	Does anyone in your family have a history of iron-deficiency anemia?	_____	_____
	Relationship: _____		
3.	Do you exercise more than 3 times a week for 45 minutes or longer?	_____	_____
4.	Do you drink more than two glasses of iced tea each day?	_____	_____
5.	Do you drink more than two carbonated sodas each day?	_____	_____
6.	Do you take calcium supplements?	_____	_____
7.	Do you have heavy menstrual cycles?	_____	_____

15

Designing a Program Unique for You: A Physically Active Lifestyle for a Lifetime

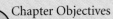

Chapter Objectives

By the end of this chapter, you should be able to:

1. Identify your physical activity goals.

2. Select physical activities to meet your goals.

3. Design an exercise program that is appropriate for you now and that can be continued and/or adapted for many years to come.

4. List criteria for evaluating an exercise club and selecting exercise equipment to purchase.

5. Describe how you can keep active and fit as you age.

WHEN MANDY WAS an infant, she crawled around her playpen and on the carpet endlessly. A full day of that type of exercise tired her out, and she had no problem sleeping through the night. When she started school, Mandy participated in physical education and soon learned sports skills she used to become physically fit and healthy. She became enamoured of soccer, in particular, and joined a recreational soccer league that played on the weekends. By the time she enrolled in college, Mandy was interested in weight training and aerobic dance classes. She used the college's exercise room to lift weights and signed up for an aerobic dance class to meet the physical-education course requirement before graduation. Mandy is now in her 60s and no longer interested in aerobic dance, is not in condition to play soccer, and cannot lift the amount of weight she could when younger. Yet she still exercises regularly. She walks daily and joins her contemporaries in the pool for aqua aerobics four days a week. She found that the local Y has a weight room with a staff person qualified to advise her on the best type of weight training for someone of her age and in her condition, so she even weight-trains three days a week. In a very real sense, Mandy is still enrolled in physical education, only this time with a different type of instructor.

Today, there are some excellent physical-education instructors who understand the nature of physical fitness and how it relates to health and wellness. Unfortunately, there are also many inadequate instructors who force individuals to run long distances even though they are not in shape to do so or who only teach how to play softball, basketball, or football. These instructors teach individuals to hate running as it tires them out for the rest of the day and creates needless aches and pains. The team sports, on the other hand, may be great fun, but once the class is over, it is difficult to get enough people together to play football, softball, or basketball. Of course, there are coed softball leagues and pick-up basketball games at the local YMCA or community centre, and some people still meet on the weekends to play touch football. And yet, most of us would prefer physical activities that require less organization. That may be why we join health clubs and weight-train. Or why we take up jogging and swimming. Or why we play tennis or golf. These lifetime sports activities can be done alone or at most require only one other person. And our bodies can withstand the activity even into our later years.

Today, more and more physical-education courses of study include instruction on tennis, golf, weight training, and badminton, while not neglecting more aerobically intensive physical activities such as basketball, soccer, football, and jogging. What is more, they sometimes even add a broader health and wellness perspective to the courses.

In this concluding chapter, we provide you with the information you need to continue your physical-activity program for the rest of your life. We do this by helping you determine your fitness and physical-activity goals and by then showing you how to achieve them. We even help you evaluate fitness and health clubs and identify what you should look for when purchasing exercise equipment.

IDENTIFYING YOUR FITNESS AND PHYSICAL-ACTIVITY GOALS

Why do you want to engage in physical activity? Some people simply want to be healthy. Others want to look good, to have energy, to develop strength, or to compete for the sake of competing. It stands to reason that if you do not know why you participate in physical-fitness activities, you cannot select activities that will help you meet your goals. Determine your fitness goals by completing Lab Activity 15.1: Why I Want to Be Physically Fit at the end of this chapter.

HEALTH PROMOTION AND DISEASE PREVENTION

One of your physical-activity and fitness goals is probably to maintain good health. We have already discussed the fact that this requires more than simply exercise. For example, you know that in order to remain healthy, you need to eat nutritious food, to use stress-management techniques to prevent illness and disease, and to refrain from using chemical substances that can harm you (such as tobacco and illicit drugs). When you do all this, you can prevent, or at least postpone, the onset of cardiovascular diseases (such as coronary heart disease and stroke) as well as precursors of these diseases (such as high blood pressure). You can also decrease your risk of contracting cancer or other life-threatening diseases. But beyond merely preventing illness and disease, you can also enhance your well-being by engaging in a variety of lifestyle behaviours. Although we will now focus on exercise behaviours, do not neglect to consider other lifestyle behaviours when designing a total fitness program for yourself. We will return to this at the conclusion of this chapter.

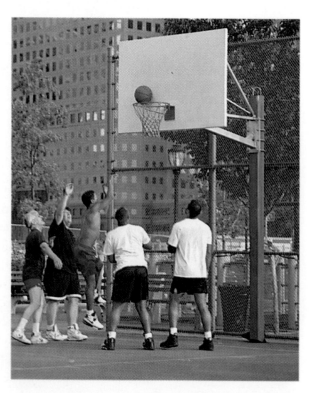

Exercise is important for people of all ages who wish to promote health and prevent disease.

PHYSICAL ACTIVITIES TO HELP YOU ACHIEVE YOUR GOALS

There is a seemingly endless array of physical activities in which you can participate. Now that you have completed Lab Activity 15.1 and have a better idea of why you want to exercise, it will be easier for you to choose one of these activities. Refer to Figure 15.1 to see if your favourite physical activity is among the favourites of other Canadians. We will describe several of the more popular and effective exercise options in this section. If we skip your favourite activity, we apologize, but be comforted by knowing that a trip to the library will probably disclose all you ever wanted to know about it.

■ Walking

Walking is an excellent way to keep fit without putting undue stress on your connective tissue and bones. Studies have shown that adults who walk for exercise 2½–4 hours a week tend to have less than half the prevalence of elevated serum cholesterol of those who do not walk or exercise regularly. Walking can develop cardiores-

piratory endurance (especially if done at a brisk speed) and is effective as a calorie burner. What's more, it is an activity in which people of all ages can participate, and it can have psychological benefits, helping to reduce anxiety and depression.

Here are some tips to help you develop an efficient walking style:

1. Hold your head erect and keep your back straight and abdomen flat. Your toes should point straight ahead and your arms swing loosely at your sides.

2. Land on the heel of your foot and roll forward to drive off the ball of your foot. Walking only on the balls of your feet or flat-footed may cause fatigue and soreness.

3. Take long, easy strides, but do not strain for distance. When walking up or down hills or at a very rapid pace, lean forward slightly.

4. Breathe deeply (in through the nose and out through the mouth).

To help you to begin a walking program, follow the regimen in Table 15.1.

Figure 15.1 ✦ Popularity of Physical Recreation Activities in Canada, Age 20+

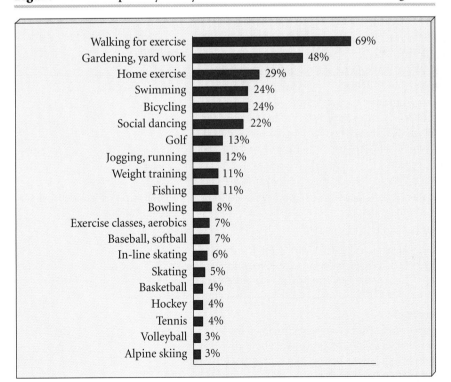

Source: Data from National Population Health Survey 1998/99, available at **www.cflri. ca/cflri/pa/surveys/2001survey/2001survey.html**. Accessed March 14, 2003. Reprinted with permission of the Canadian Fitness and Lifestyle Research Institute.

Table 15.1 ✦ Walking

WEEK	AEROBIC TRAINING PROGRAM	COMMENTS
I. Very Beginning		
1st week	Walk at a slow-to-average pace for the first 5 minutes of your workout, then walk at a brisk pace for 1.6 kilometres. Do three workouts per week.	Avoid doing too much the first few weeks by walking slowly when fatigued and walking briskly when fresh. After several weeks, you should be able to keep walking at a brisk pace for the entire distance.
3rd week	Increase the distance covered to 2.4 kilometres. Do not be concerned about time. Be sure to cover the proper distance each workout.	—
6th week	Test yourself in the 2.4-kilometre test. If your category has changed, move on to the program for rating II. If there was no change, continue adding 0.16 kilometre per workout until the distance covered is 3.2 kilometres.	—
II. Beginning		
1st week	Walk at a brisk pace for 3.2 kilometres. Do three workouts per week.	Instead of one 3.2-kilometre session, you may do two workout sessions of 1.6 kilometres—that is, 1.6 kilometres in the morning and 1.6 kilometres in the evening.
3rd week	Increase your distance to 4 kilometres three times per week.	—
6th week	Test yourself in the 2.4-kilometre test. If your category has changed, move on to the program for rating III. If there is no change, continue adding 0.16 kilometre per workout until the distance covered is 4.8 kilometres.	—
III. Intermediate		
1st week	Walk at a brisk pace for 4.8 kilometres. Do three workouts per week.	Time your walk and aim at a time of 45–60 minutes.
3rd week	Add one workout for a total of four per week. Keep your distance the same.	—
6th week	Test yourself in the 2.4-kilometre test. If your category has changed, move on to the program for rating IV. If there is no change, continue adding 0.16 kilometre per workout until the distance covered is 6.4 kilometres.	—
IV. Advanced		
1st week	Walk at a brisk pace for 7.2 kilometres. Do four workouts per week.	Time your walk and aim at a time of 1 hour and 30 minutes.
3rd week	Walk 7.2 kilometres five times each week.	—
6th week	Test yourself in the 2.4-kilometre test. If your category has changed, move on to the program for rating V. If there is no change, add 0.16 kilometres per workout until the distance covered is 8 kilometres.	—
V. Excellent/Superior		
1st week	Begin walking for 10 minutes, then jog for as long as possible. Do not be concerned about distance, but try to jog nonstop for 20 minutes. Do three of these workouts per week.	—
3rd week	Continue jogging three times per week and add 1 minute to each workout until you can jog for 30 minutes.	—
6th week	Test yourself in the 2.4-kilometre test.	—

Jogging and Running

If walking is too slow for you, try **jogging** or **running**. With either, you can get a comparable workout in a shorter period of time. Unfortunately, jogging puts stress on your body, subjecting you to a greater chance of injury than walking does. Foot, ankle, knee, and back problems can develop. Yet with the proper precautions (good shoes and not doing more than you are in condition to do), jogging injuries can be minimized.

Having the right running shoes is important if you choose to jog. There are many shoes from which to choose. We will discuss how to purchase shoes in which to run or jog later in this chapter. Personnel in stores selling running shoes can help you select a shoe right for you, but *you* need to be the final judge. If the shoe feels comfortable and provides enough support, that is probably the right shoe for you.

Running for fitness is different from running for speed and power. When you run for fitness, you should maintain a comfortable, economical running style:

1. Run upright, avoiding excessive forward lean. Keep your back as straight as you comfortably can and keep your head up. Do not look down at your feet.
2. Carry your arms slightly away from your body, with your elbows bent so your forearms are roughly parallel to the ground. Occasionally shake and relax your arms to prevent tightness in your shoulders.
3. Land on the heel of your foot and rock forward to drive off the ball of your foot. If this proves difficult, try a more flat-footed style. Running only on the balls of your feet will tire you quickly and make your legs sore.
4. Keep your stride relatively short. Do not force your pace by reaching for extra distance.
5. Breathe deeply with your mouth open.

One concern about either walking or running is safety. Recognizing the need to advise runners how to exercise to limit vulnerability, the Road Runners Club of America offers these tips in their booklet entitled *Women Running: Run Smart. Run Safe:*

1. Stay alert.
   a. Do not wear headphones. If you wear them, you will not hear an approaching car or an approaching attacker.
   b. Run against traffic so that you can observe approaching vehicles.
   c. Practise identifying characteristics of strangers and memorizing licence plates.
   d. Tune in to your environment, not out of it.

2. Avoid isolation.
   a. Run in familiar areas.
   b Run with a partner or dog.
   c. Write down or leave word about the direction of your run. Tell friends and family of your favourite running routes.
   d. Befriend neighbours and local businesses.
3. Use your intuition.
   a. Trust your intuition about an area or a person, avoiding any place or person you are unsure of.
   b. Use discretion in acknowledging verbal harassment by strangers. Look directly at others and be observant, but keep your distance and keep moving.
   c. Call police immediately if something happens to you or someone else or if you notice anyone out of the ordinary.
4. Be prepared.
   a. Carry identification or write your name, phone number, and blood type on the inside of your running shoe.
   b. Do not wear jewellery.
   c. Carry a noisemaker.
   d. Be prepared to scream and break the silence.
   e. Wear reflective material.
   f. Know the location of telephones.
   g. Vary your route.

Jogging or running costs relatively little (good running shoes are the only major expense), can be done almost anywhere (indoors or outdoors), and is an excellent aerobic exercise. To help you begin a jogging and running program, follow the regimen in Table 15.2.

Rope Jumping

When one of the authors was 13, he fell head over heels in love with 12-year-old, blonde-haired, adorable, vivacious Jill—heart-poundingly, palm-perspiringly, any-spare-time-spent-with-her love. The problem was that Steven was also in love with Jill. In the competition to win Jill's heart, he and Steven learned how to jump rope that summer. While their friends played basketball and softball, they jumped rope with Jill. They were frantic not to be seen by their friends in this sissy activity. If their other friends had seen them, they would have died.

Jogging Running at a 5.6-minute-per-kilometre pace or slower.

Running Running faster than 5.6 minutes per kilometre.

Table 15.2 ✦ Jogging and Running

WEEK	AEROBIC TRAINING PROGRAM	COMMENTS
I. Very Beginning		
1st week	On a track, begin running at a comfortable pace until you sense the onset of mild fatigue. Stop immediately and note the distance covered. Walk at an average pace until fatigue symptoms subside. Note the distance. Return to running until fatigue symptoms reappear. Stop. Record the total distance covered during the two running phases and one walking phase. This is your first target. Until you can run this distance nonstop, do not add any distance to your workout.	This is a run/walk workout. Do not overdo it on the first day. After several weeks, you should be able to run the target distance nonstop. Work out at least three times weekly.
3rd week	Begin LSD (long/slow/distance) training. Use a pace that permits a pleasant conversation and causes only mild distress. Continue running nonstop for as long as possible. Rather than walk, slow the pace and attempt to finish the workout pleasantly tired but not exhausted. Do not be concerned about time.	Continue LSD training, adding 0.5–1 minute to each workout until you can run nonstop for at least 20 minutes. Work out at least three times weekly.
6th week	Test yourself in the 2.4-kilometre test. If your category has changed, move on to the program for rating II. If there is no change, continue LSD training until you can run 30 minutes nonstop.	—
II. Beginning		
1st week	Use LSD training as described above, covering a minimum of 1.6 kilometres each workout (nonstop) for several weeks before walking/running 2 or 3 additional kilometres at the end of each workout.	Increase the number of weekly workouts to four.
3rd week	Begin to time each kilometre, running at a 6-minute-per-kilometre pace for as long a distance as possible. Attempt to achieve 3.2 kilometres in 18 minutes or less.	Run a minimum of 10 kilometres weekly.
6th week	Test yourself in the 2.4-kilometre test. If your category has changed, move on to the program for rating III. If there is no change, continue LSD training until you can run 1 kilometre in under 6 minutes and 2 kilometres in under 12 minutes.	—
III. Intermediate		
1st week	Continue LSD training at a 6-minute-per-kilometre pace.	Increase to 16–20 kilometres weekly.
3rd week	Increase your nonstop run to 4.8 kilometres.	—
6th week	Test yourself in the 2.4-kilometre test. If your category has changed, move on to the program for rating IV. If there is no change, continue to increase weekly distance by 3.2–4.8 kilometres.	—

Table 15.2 ✦ Jogging and Running *(continued)*

Week	Aerobic training program	Comments
IV. Advanced		
1st week	Increase your nonstop run to 9.7 kilometres. Continue LSD training at a 5.6-to-5.8-minute pace.	—
3rd week	Continue LSD training, picking up the pace by 3–7 seconds per kilometre.	—
6th week	Test yourself in the 2.4-kilometre test. If your category has changed, move on to the program for rating V. If there is no change, continue the above training for 2 additional weeks, then retest.	—
V. Excellent/Superior		
—	If this is your test category, continue with whatever program you have been using. Take the 2.4-kilometre test once a month to judge the success of your maintenance program.	—

Note: Each workout at all levels begins with a slow, 1.6-kilometre warm-up run/walk, and ends with a 1-to-1.6-kilometre slow, cool-down jog.

Well, no longer crippled by that thought, we learned that the sex you were born with need not stop you from participating in any enjoyable activity, and that rope jumping is an excellent way of developing cardiorespiratory endurance, strength, agility, coordination, and a sense of wellness. Here are some pointers for rope jumping:

1. Determine the best length for your rope by standing on the centre of the rope. The handles should reach from armpit to armpit.

2. When you are jumping, keep your arms close to your body with your elbows almost touching your sides. Have your forearms out at right angles, and turn the rope by making small circles with your hands and wrists. Keep your feet, ankles, and knees together.

3. Relax. Do not tense up. Enjoy yourself.

4. Keep your body erect, with your head and eyes up.

5. Start slowly.

6. Land on the balls of your feet, bending your knees slightly.

7. Maintain a steady rhythm.

8. Jump just 3 or 4 centimetres off the floor.

9. Try jumping to music and maintaining the rhythm of the music.

10. When you get good, improvise. Create new stunts. Have fun.

Swimming

Swimming, ranked fourth in popularity in Canada (Figure 15.1), is both an enjoyable and a very good physical-fitness activity. What's more, it enhances physical fitness while diminishing the chances of injury. That is because it limits the amount of weight your body must bear. When you are submerged up to the neck in water, you experience an apparent loss of 90 percent of your weight. If you weigh 59 kilograms, when you are in water up to your neck your feet and legs have to support a weight of only 5.9 kilograms. Therefore, you are less apt to injure your legs and feet.

Many people who use swimming for conditioning do lap swimming—that is, they swim back and forth. When you are lap swimming, you should periodically check your heart rate to determine if you are at your target. But lap swimming is not appropriate for everyone. Backyard pools usually are not large enough. Most residential pools are no bigger than 11 by 5 metres, with approximately 54 square metres of water surface and depths of 0.9–2.4

metres. In a swimming pool of this size, a workout must be adjusted considerably from that usually practised in the typical school, university, or athletic club pool. Otherwise, swimming in the backyard pool becomes largely a matter of diving in, gliding across, and climbing out. For the typical person, it means only inactive bathing. But swimming pools, regardless of size, have a high potential as exercise facilities. This potential can be realized as individuals learn how to exercise in limited water areas.

To help you begin a swimming program, follow the regimen in Table 15.3.

Tennis

As with all fitness activities, duration and intensity will determine how much your tennis game contributes to your physical fitness and wellness. A doubles match generally results in less of a workout than a singles match. In fact, a doubles match will use up to 330 calories per hour, whereas a singles match will use up to 390 calories per hour.

The contribution of tennis to wellness, however, is another matter. As we have stated so often in this book, even if your physical health is improved, if the other components of your health suffer, you have not improved your health. Playing tennis may improve the efficiency of your heart, but if your attitude and behaviour on the court loses you friends, results in your not enjoying yourself, or frustrates you, you would be better off not playing at all. In spite of exercising, you are making yourself *less well.* Two solutions make the most sense to us: Either approach tennis with a different attitude, or select a less competitive exercise in which to engage regularly.

When stroking the ball, if you roll over the shot too much (too much topspin), you can contribute to tennis elbow. Using too much wrist in the shot will lead you to roll over; instead, you should stroke through the ball with your wrist locked. If tennis elbow does develop, you can switch to a lighter racquet to aggravate the elbow less. Applying ice after playing will also help.

A warm-up that includes stretching is a must. Tennis involves dynamic, quick movements with a great deal of stretching to reach the ball. Therefore, if you are not flexible enough, you may be prone to muscle and connective-tissue injuries, such as muscle pulls or sprained ligaments.

Racquetball, Handball, and Squash

The indoor racquet sports can be excellent ways to develop and maintain fitness. That is because they contribute to cardiorespiratory endurance, muscular strength and endurance of the legs, flexibility, agility, balance and coordination, and weight control. They are also usually

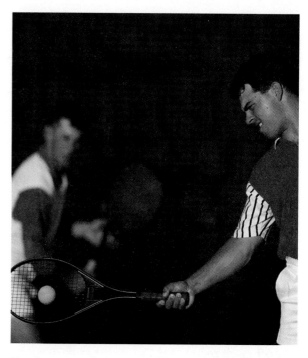

Tennis can contribute to overall fitness, muscular strength, and flexibility.

fun. Yet there is danger involved in these sports. Every year, over 3000 eye injuries result from them. That need not be the case if players wear appropriate eye protectors. Eye protectors should offer a complete shield (do not use the kind with narrow bands with openings between them) and be made of polycarbonate.

Another risk involved in these sports can be found in the environment in which they are played. Exercising in a hot room can be hazardous unless you take certain precautions. You should drink plenty of water before starting to play and intermittently take breaks to replenish the water you lose through perspiration. You should not play longer than you are in condition to play; to overdo it in a hot room can be risky. Know when to stop.

Finally, you must be in good physical condition before engaging in these sports. Because they are highly competitive, they are usually played in a hot environment, and they involve dynamic (stop-and-go) and stretching movements. If you are not in good physical condition, you may injure yourself. If you *are* in good condition, these sports are excellent activities to help you remain fit.

Aerobic Dance

One of the best fitness activities is dance, especially if you're serious about your training. Look at the bodies of dancers. They are remarkably muscular, incredibly supple,

Table 15.3 ✦ Swimming

WEEK	AEROBIC TRAINING PROGRAM	COMMENTS
I. Very Beginning		
1st week	Begin by using any stroke and swim for 12–20 minutes per session at least three times per week.	Swim until out of breath. Continue until swimming is nonstop for the allotted time.
3rd week	Swim three to five times per week. Try to use the freestyle stroke as much as possible.	Swim continuously for 20 minutes.
6th week	Test yourself in the 2.4-kilometre test. If your category has changed, move on to the program for rating II. If there is no change, remain at this point for 2 more weeks, then retest.	—
II. Beginning		
1st week	Begin by using any stroke and swim for 15–22 minutes per session at least three times per week.	Swim until out of breath. Continue until swimming is nonstop for allotted time.
3rd week	Swim daily. Use the freestyle stroke as much as possible.	Swim continuously for 22 minutes.
6th week	Swim daily for 30 minutes. Test yourself in the 2.4-kilometre test. If your category has changed, move on to the program for rating III. If there is no change, remain at this point for 2 more weeks.	—
III. Intermediate		
1st week	Swim freestyle for 500 metres per workout, three times per week.	Begin to time your workouts. Aim for a time of 12 minutes. If you reach 12 minutes, then aim for 10.5 minutes.
3rd week	Continue 500 metres per workout. Add one additional workout each week.	Try to reach the above target times.
6th week	Test yourself in the 2.4-kilometre test. If your category has changed, move on to the program for rating IV. If there is no change, remain at this point for 2 more weeks, then retest.	—
IV. Advanced		
1st week	Swim freestyle for 650 metres per workout, four times each week.	Aim for a time of 15.5 minutes.
3rd week	Add one workout for the next 2 weeks for a total of six workouts per week.	—
6th week	Test yourself in the 2.4-kilometre test. If your category has changed, move on to the program for rating V. If there is no change, remain at this point for 2 more weeks and add 50 metres per workout, then retest.	—
V. Excellent/Superior		
—	Aim to swim freestyle for 1000 metres per workout. Begin with 700 metres per workout and add 50 metres every two workouts.	Aim for a 1000-metres time of under 16.5 minutes.
—	Take the 2.4-kilometre test once monthly to judge the success of your maintenance program.	If you want to improve rather than maintain present level, add 50 metres every three workouts until you reach 2000 metres. Aim for a time of 34 minutes.

and highly prepared to meet the demands strenuous exercise places on their cardiorespiratory systems. Dance is a good way to develop and maintain physical fitness.

The traditional dance programs were tap, ballet, and modern dance. In recent years, a different form of dance has swept the country and become a significant part of the fitness movement. It combines calisthenics and a variety of dance movements, all done to music, and is called aerobic dance. The term, coined by Jacki Sorenson in 1979, involves choreographed routines that include walking, jumping, hopping, bouncing, kicking, and various arm movements designed to develop cardiorespiratory endurance, flexibility, and muscular strength and endurance. Dancing to music is an enjoyable activity for many people who would not otherwise seek to exercise. And because aerobic dance is often done in groups, the social contact makes it even more enjoyable.

To maximize the fitness benefits of aerobic dance, you should maintain the dancing for approximately 35–45 minutes and work out three or four times a week. In addition, you should check periodically to see if you are maintaining your target heart rate (THR). Because many communities offer aerobic dance classes (some may be called dancercise or jazzercise) through YMCAs, Jewish Community Centres, colleges, local schools, and even morning television programs, maintaining a regular dance regimen should not be difficult. The only equipment you will need is a good pair of aerobic dance shoes with good shock absorbency, stability, and outer-sole flexibility and clothes to work out in. One caution: do not dance on a concrete floor, because the constant pounding could result in shin splints. A wooden floor is ideal.

Low-Impact Aerobics

Several factors associated with aerobic dance have led some experts to question the manner in which it is usually conducted. A study by the American Aerobics Association found that 80 percent of instructors and students were getting injured during workouts, and another questionnaire administered to instructors revealed that 55 percent reported significant injuries. Among the causes of these injuries are bad floors (too hard), bad shoes (too little shock absorbency and stability), and bad routines offered by poorly trained instructors. With the popularity of aerobics, it is not surprising what is done in its name. Even a *pet aerobics* routine has been developed for the pudgy dog or cat. It is therefore no surprise that many aerobics instructors are poorly trained and teach routines that are inappropriate and injury producing, using surfaces that cause high-impact injuries.

In response to these concerns, several things have happened. One is the certification of aerobics instructors, who, in Canada, are called "fitness leaders." In response to the proven need for trained and competent fitness leaders across Canada, organizations such as the National Fitness Leadership Advisory Council (NFLAC) have been formed. NFLAC is a Canadian collective/partnership dedicated to collaboratively developing, promoting, and recognizing the use of national guidelines and standards for fitness leadership and certification, leading to improved quality and safety. NFLAC works progressively with its partner organizations to advance fitness leadership in Canada; in conjunction with its member organizations, NFLAC has developed minimum standards against which fitness leaders are measured. To be an NFLAC partner, an organization must be Canadian-based, must have been in existence for more than three years, and must have mandates consistent with those of NFLAC. Health Canada, a number of universities, the YMCA/YWCA, and some private training and certification agencies are examples of NFLAC partners. (See the NFLAC Web site.)

In another attempt to limit the injuries from aerobics, *low-impact* aerobic routines have been developed. Low-impact aerobics feature one foot on the ground at all times and the use of light weights. The idea is to cut down on the stress to the body caused by jumping and bouncing while at the same time deriving the muscle-toning and cardiorespiratory benefits of high-impact aerobics. These routines have become more and more popular as the risk of injury from high-impact aerobics has become better known. Something called *chair aerobics* has even been developed. It involves routines done while the participant is seated in a chair.

Low-impact aerobics are not totally risk-free. Injuries to the upper body caused by the circling and swinging movements with weights are not infrequent. Many of these injuries can be treated at home, however, and are not serious. With any form of physical activity, there is always the chance of injury. The benefits to the cardiorespiratory system and the rest of the body—benefits that we have described in this book—are often worth the slight chance of injury.

A recent aerobic dance development is *step aerobics*, which involves stepping up and down on a small platform (step) to the rhythm of music and the directions of an instructor. The workout can vary from mild to extremely intense depending on the speed, movements, and duration of the exercise. Double-step aerobic routines have been developed that involve the use of two platforms. Step aerobic classes are usually offered at the same places aerobic dance classes are conducted.

Bicycling

In the 1998/99 National Population Health Survey, cycling ranked fifth in popularity (Figure 15.1). To begin a bicycle exercise program, you obviously need a bicycle. A good multispeed bike will cost approximately $400. You can get an adequate multispeed bike or a mountain bike (a sturdier bike) for less, however, if you shop around or buy one secondhand. You will also need a helmet to protect your head from injury should you fall. Gloves with padded palms can also make your ride more comfortable. In addition, think about adding pant clips and/or clothes designed specifically for biking.

Of course, you can exercise with any bike—it need not have multiple speeds or be a mountain bike—if you choose. A good bike will, however, allow you to take trips that add to the enjoyment of biking in addition to enhancing overall health and wellness.

When you are biking, follow this advice:

1. Keep your elbows slightly bent.
2. Lower your upper body for a streamlined position.
3. Do not grip the handlebars too tightly.
4. Wear bright clothing so motorists can easily see you.
5. Obey all traffic laws.
6. Always lean into the turn.
7. Learn and use hand signals that indicate which way you are turning.
8. Leave the radio at home so you can focus on the road and hear cars and other hazards.
9. Keep your bike in good working order, well oiled with grease and dirt removed from around the chain and gears.

10. Make sure your seat is horizontal (to minimize stress on the lower back) and set at a height that allows a slight bend in the knee when your leg is extended.
11. Sit comfortably, so your weight is evenly distributed over the seat, handlebars, and pedals.
12. Always wear a helmet.

Some people bike for terrific exercise and yet go nowhere. They use a stationary bike. Many health clubs have computerized stationary bikes that can be set for various kinds of riding (for example, hilly or high-speed) and for various distances. Other people remove a wheel from their bicycle, raise the frame, and bike indoors during the winter months. You can buy equipment called a wind trainer that does this for you.

As with a regular bike, when you ride a stationary bike, you need to adjust the seat and handlebars to the proper height and angle. To work your leg muscles properly, your knee should be slightly bent when the pedal is in the fully down position (see Figure 15.2). Too great or too little a bend will result in inefficient use of the leg muscles. The handlebars should be adjusted so you are relaxed and leaning slightly forward (see Figure 15.3).

To help you begin a biking program, follow the regimen in Table 15.4.

Selecting the Right Activity

Even if you find an exercise that is enjoyable and helps you meet your fitness goals, that does not mean you will stay with it. It simply means you are *more likely* to maintain your exercise program. It also does not necessarily mean you will even begin the program. One way to

Figure 15.2 ✦ Seat Adjustment When Riding a Stationary Bike

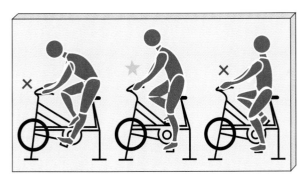

Correct seat height is depicted in the middle drawing. The seat on the left is too high, and the one on the right is too low. Maintain a slight bend in the lower leg when vertical.

Figure 15.3 ✦ Handlebar Adjustment When Riding a Stationary Bike

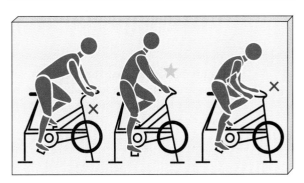

Correct handlebar adjustment is depicted in the middle drawing.

Table 15.4 ✦ Cycling

WEEK	AEROBIC TRAINING PROGRAM	COMMENTS
I. Very Beginning		
1st week	Ride for a distance of 3.2 kilometres, three times per week.	Do not be concerned with time during the first weeks of your program. Cycle at a pace that allows you to finish 3.2 kilometres without undue fatigue.
3rd week	Ride for a distance of 3.2 kilometres, three times per week. Try to finish the distance in 12 minutes or less.	Time your ride and attempt to reach the target time.
6th week	Test yourself in the 2.4-kilometre test. If your category has changed, move on to the program for rating II. If there is no change, add one workout and cycle four times each week.	—
II. Beginning		
1st week	Ride for a distance of 4.8 kilometres, three times per week.	Time your ride and aim for a time of 17 minutes or less.
3rd week	Continue riding for 4.8 kilometres, but work out four times per week.	Try to lower the time for your ride to 14 minutes or less.
6th week	Test yourself in the 2.4-kilometre test. If your category has changed, move on to the program for rating III. If there is no change, add one workout and cycle five times each week.	—
III. Intermediate		
1st week	Ride for a distance of 8 kilometres, three times per week.	Time your ride and aim for a time of 25 minutes or less.
3rd week	Continue riding for 8 kilometres, but work out four times per week.	—
6th week	Test yourself in the 2.4-kilometre test. If your category has changed, move on to the program for rating IV. If there is no change, add one workout and cycle five times each week.	—
IV. Advanced		
1st week	Ride for a distance of 12.8 kilometres, four times per week.	Aim for a time of 35 minutes or less
3rd week	Add one workout and cycle five times per week.	
V. Excellent/Superior		
—	Continue with this workout and try to lower your time to 24 minutes or less. Take the 2.4-kilometre test once a month to judge the success of your program.	—

exercise even when you are not in the mood or when you doubt its benefits is to employ self-talk. This is when you identify your negative thoughts and convert them to positive ones. Lab Activity 15.2: Developing a New Mindset About Exercise at the end of this chapter shows you how to use self-talk.

Furthermore, some sports will better match your personality than others. To identify which sports those are, complete Lab Activity 15.3: Which Sports Match Your Personality? at the end of this chapter.

BEING A FITNESS CONSUMER

To remain physically active and fit your whole life, you need to be an effective fitness consumer. You need to know how to select a health/fitness club and to buy the right equipment.

◗ Selecting an Exercise Club

Joining a health/fitness club is an excellent strategy for beginning and/or maintaining your exercise program. The club will encourage your participation in several ways. First, once you shell out the membership fee, you will want to get your money's worth. Second, after working out a few times, you will probably meet other people at the club whom you would like to get to know better. That social contact is reinforcing, and the subtle peer pressure to be there—"Hey, Betty, where were you last Wednesday?"—may be just enough to get you to the club when you do not feel like working out.

Because a health/fitness club can be expensive, inconvenient to get to, or both, you should carefully select the one you join. It should meet your needs, be safe, and be supportive of your exercise goals. Table 15.5 provides you with a way to evaluate a club and decide whether it is right for you.

◗ Purchasing Exercise Equipment

There are some fitness activities that require little, if any, equipment. A pair of running shoes, shorts, a top, and socks is usually enough for jogging. On the other hand, you cannot play tennis without a tennis racquet or bike without a bicycle.

On average, Canadian adults spend $238 a year on exercise equipment. Men spend almost three times as much as women ($349 versus $133). Equipment is expensive and requires commitment and planning; otherwise, it may simply end up as a dust collector.

In this section, we make brief comments to help you make sensible decisions when you purchase exercise equipment.

Athletic Shoes The major criteria to use when selecting athletic shoes are comfort and support. Here are a few suggestions that will help you purchase the right shoe (and the left one, too, for that matter):

1. Recognize whether you **pronate** or **supinate**. Buy a shoe made specifically for either pronators or supinators.

2. Shop for shoes late in the day. Your feet tend to swell at that time. No sense buying a shoe that fits snugly in the morning when you usually, or even occasionally, exercise in the afternoon.

3. Try shoes on with the kind of socks you usually wear when you are exercising.

4. Buy shoes with uppers made of leather or nylon that breathe.

5. Look for brands of shoes that come in different widths if you have exceptionally narrow or wide feet.

6. Get a shoe with a *last* (the form on which the shoe is made) made for your size foot. That means most women ought to buy shoes made for women, and men shoes made for men, because women's and men's lasts differ.

7. Shop at a store with experienced salespeople. Discuss your particular concerns with them. For example, if you want a shoe with shock absorption, one that is extra wide, or one that will hold up, the salesperson should be able to recommend the appropriate shoe. If you want a shoe for tennis or basketball or some other sport, an experienced salesperson should be able to help with that as well.

8. When trying the shoes on, perform some of the moves you will make when exercising in them. Jump or twist or bend or stretch. Make sure the shoe is comfortable during these movements.

9. Once you decide which shoe you want to buy, check the price at different stores or from several athletic shoe distributors. You can do this by telephone quite easily. Also, check the back of sports magazines for distributors who discount the price of shoes.

Replace athletic shoes regularly, before they wear out. Fifty percent of a shoe's shock-absorbing capacity

---

Pronate Rolling the foot inward when it is pushing off.

Supinate Rocking the foot to the outside when it is pushing off.

Table 15.5 ✦ Is This the Club for Me?

To decide whether a particular fitness facility is the one you want to join, check as many of the following as apply.

A. The Staff

_____ Do professional staff members have the appropriate educational background and/or certification from a nationally recognized professional organization?

_____ Are all staff members certified in cardiopulmonary resuscitation (CPR)?

_____ Does the specialty staff have the appropriate credentials?

_____ Are adequate staff available in the exercise and activity areas?

_____ Are staff members friendly and helpful?

_____ Are all staff in uniform and wearing some type of identification?

_____ Does the staff provide each new member of the facility with an orientation and instruction to using the areas and equipment in the facility?

_____ Does the staff provide an avenue for ongoing communication between members and themselves?

B. Facility and Equipment

_____ Does the facility have the necessary types and quantity of equipment to enable you to achieve your personal program goals?

_____ Does the facility have the necessary activity areas to enable you to achieve your personal program goals?

_____ Does the facility have sufficient equipment so that enough is available at the time of day you'll be using it?

_____ Are all activity areas regularly cleaned and maintained?

_____ Is all equipment regularly cleaned and maintained?

_____ Are all unsafe conditions and equipment malfunctions remedied promptly?

_____ Is the equipment arranged within an activity area in such a way that maximizes its safety and effectiveness?

_____ Are the surrounding outdoor areas that lead to the facility well illuminated?

_____ Does the facility have adequate parking?

_____ Are childcare facilities available if you need them?

C. Programming

_____ Does the facility offer structured exercise activity programs?

_____ Are the structured exercise programs based on sound principles of exercise prescription and exercise physiology?

_____ Does the facility offer personalized exercise programs tailored specifically to your needs and interests?

_____ Does the facility offer structured exercise programs that address the specific fitness component(s) in which you are interested?

_____ If you have a special medical condition, does the facility offer programs that address those needs?

_____ Does the facility offer exercise and recreational programs at convenient times?

(continued)

Table 15.5 ✦ Is This the Club for Me? *(continued)*

_____ Does the facility offer either unstructured or structured recreational programming in an activity in which you are interested?

_____ Does the facility offer programs for specific age groups, such as children and the elderly?

_____ Does the facility offer instruction in an activity you would like to learn?

_____ Does the facility offer specifically focused health promotion programs?

_____ Does the facility provide the option of evaluating your fitness level before you begin an exercise program?

D. Safety Issues

_____ Does the facility refer at-risk individuals to appropriate medical personnel for clearance?

_____ Does the facility have users complete a risk/benefit disclosure form when they initially join the facility?

_____ Does the facility offer ongoing monitoring of all facility users?

_____ Does the facility have a written emergency plan which is available for review?

_____ Does the facility have a first-aid kit that is properly stocked and available at all times?

_____ Are all areas in the facility free from physical hazards?

_____ Are all activity areas in the facility free from environmental hazards?

_____ Is the equipment maintained, suitable for use and well cared for?

_____ Is the staff CPR certified and is at least one first aid certified individual on duty at all times?

E. General Business Practices

_____ Does the facility management provide a grace period in which users can cancel their memberships and receive a full refund on their payments?

_____ Does the facility provide a trial membership or guest pass that allows the prospective user to utilize the facility prior to joining?

_____ Does the facility provide written literature on its facilities, services, programs, and pricing that you can take with you after visiting the club?

_____ Does the facility allow you time to make the decision to purchase a membership?

_____ Does the facility management provide a written set of rules and policies that governs the club's dealings with users?

_____ Does the facility management survey its members periodically to determine their interests and needs?

_____ Does the facility provide a feedback system by which members can express their concerns or needs as they apply to the club?

_____ Does the facility have a system of communication that informs its users of any changes in services, policies, etc. on a periodic basis?

_____ Is the facility a member of a nationally recognized trade organization related to the business?

After completing this checklist, only you can decide if the club is right for you. No club is perfect. Can you live with the club's deficits? Are its benefits worth putting up with its shortcomings?

Source: Reprinted with permission of American College of Sports Medicine, *ACM's Health/Fitness Facilities Consumer Selection Guide.* Indianapolis, IN: American College of Sports Medicine, 1992.

DIVERSITY ISSUES

Active Living for a Lifetime

In past decades, we were encouraged to set aside time for exercise. For many, this meant structured and repetitive activity. All for a noble purpose—to improve physical fitness.

In the 1970s, running was at the forefront of the exercise boom. Participation in fun runs and races was high and rising. Aerobics took over in the 1980s. Leotards and leg warmers were in—going to exercise class was the thing to do. Fashions were important, and high-level fitness was prized above all.

In the 1990s, we branched out. Now, vigorous activity is still important, but there is a growing acceptance of the joys, and values, and benefits of all kinds of activities. Gardening and golfing. Shuffleboard and sailing. Walking and wheeling. Or simply playing in the park with the kids.

"We must learn to appreciate the value of physical activity that has nothing to do with putting on a sweatsuit or counting push-ups," writes Dr. Bryant Stamford, author of *Fitness Without Exercise*. "Scheduled, intense exercise improves work capacity and performance, but if health is the objective, the research shows that regular, light-to-moderate activity does the job."

In fact, the research shows that the biggest health benefits are achieved when those who are least active become even moderately active. There are great benefits to being a modest mover!

As Dr. Stamford extols the virtues of simple activities, he urges us to worry less about kilometres jogged and toes touched. "Why not leaves raked and laundry hung?" he asks. "Or elevators avoided and taxis not taken?" In a world pressed for time, he encourages us to take mini walks (or "long-cuts," as he likes to call them) whenever we can.

There is growing support for this broader and more casual approach to physical activity. "Active living" is the term being used as Fitness Canada, and national and provincial organizations across the country, push beyond the traditional fitness activities and encourage us all to find enjoyment in everyday things.

"Active living" means:

- Valuing physical activity and making it a part of your day
- Pursuing activities you find useful, pleasurable, and satisfying
- Being active in ways that suit your routine, your schedule, and your body

So . . . go ahead. Swing a hockey stick. Go for a stroll. Toboggan with the kids. These are all steps in the right direction. ◆

Source: "Lifestyle Tips," off Web page of *Canadian Fitness and Lifestyle Research Institute*, March 29, 1999, accessed April 3, 1999 **www.cflri.ca/LT/92LT/LT92_01.html**. Reprinted with permission of the Canadian Finess and Lifestyle Research Institute.

---

is gone after 500 kilometres of running or walking or 300 hours of aerobic classes, and 80 percent after 800 kilometres or 500 hours. Exercising with shoes whose shock-absorbing capacity is diminished is a recipe for injury.

Orthotics Some people have problems with their feet that need correcting when they are exercising. They may have leg imbalances (one leg longer than the other), or they may pronate or supinate. Orthotic devices can be placed in athletic shoes to correct these problems and allow people to exercise in comfort. They also diminish the risk of injury. Orthotics come in rigid or soft forms. The rigid orthotic, made of plastic, is usually recommended, but a podiatrist or orthopedic physician may have reason to advise a soft one. Ready-made inserts are available in drugstores and sporting goods shops and may be all that is needed in some cases. Because each foot is different from every other foot, however, if you have a problem, it is wise to consult an expert.

Bicycles There are many different kinds of bikes: city bikes, all-terrain mountain bikes, touring bikes, racing bikes, and so forth. An experienced salesperson can guide you to the right type of bike depending on the use you wish to make of it. When you buy a bike (usually somewhere between $400 and $1200), factor in the cost of a helmet, a water bottle, a repair kit for flat tires, shorts, shoes, and gloves. That means approximately another $300. Purchase the bike at a store that offers good service and is staffed by professionals who *really* know bikes. When you think you are interested in a particular bike, test ride it. Also, test ride others for comparison. Try all the gears. Do they shift easily? Do the brakes work well? How does it corner? Purchasing the right bike is important to the enjoyment you will experience biking and, consequently, to whether you will maintain your exercise program.

HOME EXERCISE EQUIPMENT

Some people prefer to exercise alone. If you can afford to purchase home exercise equipment, you might consider buying a stationary bike (maybe one with a built-in computer), a recumbent bicycle (a stationary bike that is low to the floor so your legs are straight out instead of hanging down), a climber (imitating stair climbing), a rower, a cross-country ski machine, a treadmill, and/or weights. Because this equipment can be quite expensive, you should be careful to buy exercise equipment that will help you meet your physical-activity and fitness goals safely.

Because exercise equipment is constantly being improved, and the cost seems to change every time one turns around, we've decided not to be too specific about particular home exercise equipment in this section. Once you decide you would like to exercise at home, you should consult with an expert in fitness at a local health club, YMCA, or community centre (be sure to speak with someone credentialled in exercise physiology or physical fitness), read articles about selecting home exercise equipment in health and fitness journals and magazines at your local library, and/or speak with a fitness expert at a local university.

The following should be considered when you are deciding what equipment to purchase.

- **What are your fitness goals?** If you are trying to develop cardiorespiratory endurance, you would be better advised to buy a treadmill or stationary bike than weights.

- **Who is going to use the equipment?** If more than one person will exercise with this equipment, it needs to be easily adjustable.

- **How much space do you have?** You might have room for a stationary bike but not if you are going to add a rower. In this case, you will need to decide which piece of equipment you most want.

- **How much can you spend?** In a perfect world, money would not be of concern. But this is not a perfect world, so you will need to decide the best way to spend your limited resources.

Try out the equipment before buying it. Is the seat comfortable? Is the climbing motion smooth? Is the machine sturdy? Is it fun to do? Do you get the type of workout you want?

▪ Stationary Bikes

Your first decision is whether to purchase a standard upright or a recumbent bike. With a recumbent bike, you are seated in a reclined position with your legs

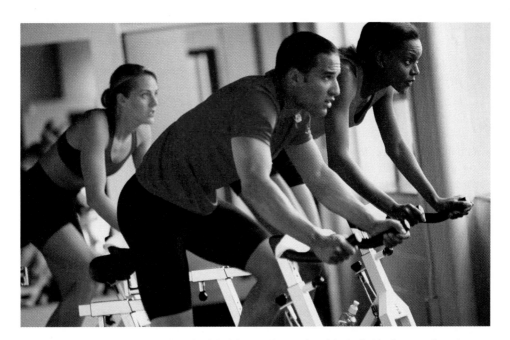

Many exercise machines available at health clubs are also marketed for individuals to purchase for their homes, including stationary bikes, steppers, cross-country ski machines, and others.

outstretched. The recumbent bike works your gluteal muscles more than a stationary bike does, but it requires a little more room to store and operate. Make sure any bike you purchase has a comfortable seat that is adjustable and can lock into place. There should be straps to hold your feet on the pedals. For fast, smooth pedaling, look for a bike with a heavy flywheel (at least 11 kg) and a high gear ratio (at least 4 to 1, and optimally 7 to 1). If you own a road bike, you might think about purchasing a bike trainer or rollers that convert it into a stationary bike for indoor workouts. However, because the front and rear wheels are placed on aluminum drums when using rollers, quite a bit of balance is required. Therefore, you might first try a bike trainer that clamps to the rear axle of the bike, providing resistance via a wind mechanism or a magnetic flywheel.

■ Treadmills

A treadmill costing less than $1000 is usually noisy, wobbly, and difficult to use. In addition, it will not last very long, especially if you use it often. A treadmill should have at least a 0.75-kilowatt motor, adjustable elevation to simulate hills, and a running surface that is wide and long with good traction. Make sure the treadmill has a large, heavy-duty roller that keeps the belt centred. Consider purchasing a treadmill with a two-ply belt because it will last longer. Treadmills come with all sorts of other options. Some have the ability to select different programs for your workout, others have low-impact suspension systems, and still others have a safety feature that shuts the machine down if you lose your balance. Of course, in general, the more features there are, the higher the cost.

■ Steppers

Most people who purchase a stepper for their home buy one with hydraulic shock absorbers rather than the electronic, computer-controlled steppers found in health clubs. These hydraulic steppers are more moderately priced. Some steppers are dual-action—that is, they have the ability to work the arms as well as the legs. An example is the vertical-ascent machine that simulates ladder climbing. Make sure you purchase a stepper that does not wobble (is sturdy) or squeak, that has comfortable foot pedals that are wide enough for your feet, and that provides a smooth and relatively quiet motion. Consider a stepper with a glare-free screen that provides feedback such as elapsed time, step rate, total steps, and estimated calories used.

■ Cross-Country Ski Machines

Some cross-country ski machines have a belt and flywheel for resistance, an abdominal pad for balance, and a friction pulley system threaded with a nylon cord with grips that are held in each hand and pumped during exercise. These machines have independent ski action, with each ski moving independent of the other. Another type has foot pads mounted on ski-type tracks and arm poles that pivot on each side of the machine's base. These machines have dependent ski action—as one ski moves forward, the other moves backward. Dependent ski action makes the machine easier to use; independent ski action is sometimes difficult to get used to. Regardless of which type of ski machine you decide to purchase, make sure that it is solid and stable, that it has separate resistance adjustments for upper- and lower-body movements, and that the display that provides feedback on elapsed time, estimated calories expended, and the like is easy to read.

■ Abdominal Exercise Equipment

If you are up late at night, flipping through the TV channels, you are likely to see someone selling abdominal exercise equipment. If it isn't the Ab Blaster Plus, it's the Abflex, or the Ab Isolator, or the Ab Trainer. The washboard stomach has, unfortunately, become the ultimate symbol of fitness for many people, or at least the most visible. People are willing to pay anywhere from $30 to $200 for the promise of a rippled stomach.

If you are thinking of buying one of these machines, think again. The way to acquire a washboard stomach is through a healthy diet and abdominal exercises for which you do not need any equipment. If you have too much fat around the abdominal area, you can do abdominal exercises until the cows come home with little noticeable effect. Only losing fat and then tightening the abs will work. You would be better advised to take the money you were thinking of spending on abdominal exercise equipment and hiring a trainer or taking a class to learn which abdominal exercises to do and how to do them correctly.

K EEPING FIT AS YOU AGE

The Andean village of Vilcabamba in Ecuador and the community of Abkhagia in Georgia share an unusual reputation. They are places where people supposedly live longer and remain more vigorous in old age than is the case in most places. What factors contribute to the unusual longevity of people in these communities, where men and women who are well beyond 100 years of age are common? In Canada, the average life expectancy is in the 70s (depending on such factors as sex, ethnicity, education, and socioeconomic status), and there are only slightly more than 3 centenarians per 100 000 persons.

Clearly, genetic factors play a major role. This is true in the communities just cited. Many of the elderly had parents who also lived to be quite old. And yet when researchers studied these communities, they found other factors related to longevity. Elders are held in high esteem. They receive encouragement to work and be productive community members. Their efforts are appreciated and valued. These 100-year-olds eat low-calorie diets, about 1800 calories a day compared to the 3300-calorie diet of the average North American. These communities are located in remote and mountainous regions and tend to be agricultural. That means that daily living requires significant climbing and descending steep slopes and vigorous physical activity.

EXERCISE FOR THE ELDERLY

We are generally less physically active than the centenarians just described. Only 50 percent of Canadian residents over 65 years of age exercise regularly. Therefore, we need to plan regular exercise. If we do, we will not only live longer, we will also live better. We will be less ill, less dependent on other people, more pain-free, and more psychologically healthy.

Planning exercise for elderly people requires attention to some special considerations:

- Skeletal structures are more prone to fracture (especially in older women).
- Connective tissue is more dense, and ligaments and tendons less elastic. Range of motion may be significantly limited.
- Muscle mass is somewhat diminished, and reaction and reflex times are slower.

For these reasons, careful assessment should be made before prescribing exercise for an elderly individual. Wrenching and twisting movements should be avoided. So should sudden starting and stopping or changing direction. Slow, rhythmic stretching activities are best, and frequent rests should be built into the program.

Walking is an excellent activity for older people, especially in groups where they can socialize. Supervised swimming or exercises in the water are other good activities because they decrease weight bearing and tend to be fun. Also, do not forget dancing, which can enhance fitness goals when it is done rigorously. See Table 15.6 for one possible program for elders.

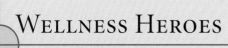

WELLNESS HEROES

Peter Rechnitzer and David Cunningham

The Centre for Activity and Aging at the University of Western Ontario was founded in 1988 to investigate the interrelationship of physical activity and aging and to develop strategies based on research for promoting the independence of older adults. The idea for such a research program was proposed by Dr. David Cunningham to his colleague Dr. Peter Rechnitzer in 1979. These two scientists had been working for many years on the role of physical activity as a rehabilitative and intervention treatment for postcoronary patients.

In 1963, Dr. Rechnitzer was the first Canadian scientist/physician to use exercise as a rehabilitative tool in the treatment of these patients. This unique program was eventually developed, with Dr. Cunningham, into a multi-centred research study of exercise and coronary heart disease known as the Ontario Exercise Heart Collaborative Study. A total of six universities were involved in this groundbreaking research, with Drs. Rechnitzer and Cunningham being the catalysts for our now-widespread understanding of exercise's contribution to heart health.

As the first and second directors of the Centre, Dr. Rechnitzer and Dr. Cunningham built it into the exceptional research institution that it is today. Because of their founding visions and efforts, the Centre for Activity and Aging continues to pursue their mission "to develop, encourage and promote an active, healthy lifestyle for Canadian adults that will enhance the dignity of the aging process." Through the implementation of physical activity programs and the training of leaders to deliver these programs the Centre for Activity and Aging is making a positive difference in the lives of many Canadian adults. ✦

Sources: Adapted from David A. Cunningham, "Centre for Activity and Aging," off *SISA (Sports Information & Science Agency)* Web page, May 17, 1995, accessed April 21, 1999 **www.sportsa.co.za/info/sportstopics/newslet.html.** Additional information received via e-mail communication with Dr. David A. Cunningham, PhD. **Canadian Centre for Activity and Aging** Web page, January 8, 2003, accessed January 9, 2003. **www.uwo.ca**

Table 15.6 ✦ Good Physical Activities for the Elderly

ACTIVITY	FREQUENCY	DURATION
Walking	3 times per week	¾ hour
Swimming	3 times per week	½ hour
Dancing	2 times per week	Sets of 20 minutes with intervals of rest
Stretching/calisthenics	Every day	10–15 minutes
Golf	2 or 3 times per week	As long as necessary to complete 9 or 18 holes
Horseshoe pitching	According to desire	½ hour
Shuffleboard	According to desire	1 hour
Bocce	According to desire	1 hour
Croquet	According to desire	1 hour

■ Benefits of Exercise for Seniors

Exercising will increase longevity and provide older people with a more fulfilling life. It can also enhance their wellness when they exercise with other people (social health), when they exercise out of doors and appreciate the surroundings (spiritual health), when they exercise with family members and learn to control emotions that interfere with performing the activity (emotional health), and when they read and learn about the particular exercise and its benefits (mental health). In addition, exercise can postpone the inevitable changes associated with aging. Table 15.7 shows which physical activities relate to which of these aging changes.

The 2001 Physical Activity Monitor, conducted by the Canadian Fitness and Lifestyle Research Institute, found that inactivity increases with age. By age 65, only 53 percent of men and 47 percent of women in Canada exercise regularly. However, when seniors do exercise, walking and gardening or yard work—excellent means of acquiring the benefits of physical activity—tend to be most popular. Govindasamy and Paterson (1994), researchers at the Centre for Activity and Aging at the University of Western Ontario, offer the following "key messages":

- There is strong evidence that regular exercise, in older adults, reduces cardiovascular risk, decreases resting blood pressure, lowers body fat, improves the blood lipid (cholesterol) profile, and helps with diabetes.

Table 15.7 ✦ Aging Effects and Physical Activities That May Postpone or Reduce Them

EFFECTS	PHYSICAL ACTIVITIES
1. Reduced cardiac output	Aerobic activities, jogging, swimming, cycling
2. Lowered pulmonary ventilation	Exercises that stretch rib-cage joints, aerobic activities of moderate to high intensity
3. Elevated blood pressure	Aerobic activities, jogging, swimming, cycling
4. Decrease in muscular strength	Weight training (resistance training)
5. Decrease in muscular endurance	Aerobic dance, calisthenics
6. Decrease in flexibility	Stretching, bending
7. Increase in percentage of stored body fat	Jogging, running, swimming, cycling
8. Loss of skin elasticity	Weight training (to maintain muscle tone and fill skin out)
9. Reduced calcium resorption	Aerobic activities and weight training
10. Decreased hours of sleep	Aerobic activities

MYTH AND FACT SHEET

Myth	Fact
1. Jogging is a better physical fitness activity than walking.	1. Walking is as good an activity to develop physical fitness as any other. You simply have to walk for a longer time to get comparable benefits.
2. Jogging leads to all sorts of injuries.	2. You can limit injuries from jogging if you take certain precautions. Wear the appropriate athletic shoes and do not overdo your workout.
3. Rope jumping is for wimps.	3. You can get a great workout while having fun if you know several rope-jumping stunts.
4. Most health/fitness clubs are the same.	4. Health/fitness clubs differ in a number of significant ways. Some clubs do not have enough equipment or enough variety of equipment. Others do not have adequately trained staff, do not offer a safe environment in which to exercise, or cost too much.
5. Elderly people do not need to exercise.	5. Everyone can benefit from regular exercise. Not only can exercise help elderly people maintain their physical fitness, it can also enhance their social, mental, emotional, and spiritual health, thereby helping to maintain their overall wellness.

- Carefully conducted research studies report 10–30 percent increases in cardiorespiratory fitness in older adults after one year of training.

- Research has shown that when previously sedentary individuals in their 70s engage in consistent long-term training, they decline physiologically at one-half the expected rate for that age group.

- Maintaining strength with increasing age may contribute to the maintenance of an independent lifestyle and can play a role in the prevention of osteoporosis, as well as in the maintenance of cardiorespiratory fitness.

- Older adults can be expected to increase in strength up to 50 percent after six weeks of strength training (due to neural adaptations early on followed by increases in muscle mass).

- Training with light-resistance exercises represents a safe and practical method for inducing significant improvements in strength in older adults.

- After a couple of months of appropriate training, older adults can show significant improvements in flexibility.

- An increased level of physical activity among seniors may result in a 35 percent reduction in costs of institutionalized care of seniors.

- Scientific evidence suggests that exercise can prevent, slow down, and, in some cases, reverse certain diseases. It is important to note, however, that exercise is just one component of several necessary for disease management.

CONCLUSION: SOME LAST WORDS ON WELLNESS

To help you develop a physical-fitness program, we have provided Lab Activity 15.4: A Guide for Developing a Program Unique for You. Before you complete the Lab, review the following list of considerations to be aware of in establishing the right program *for you*:

1. To be well, pay attention to your body. If you do, you will know when it is doing fine and when it needs special care.

2. Pay attention to your mind. When you choose an activity to include in your fitness routine, choose one that is enjoyable, one you look forward to doing. Not only will this improve the chances of your continuing the activity, it will also increase your wellness by making you feel good.

BEHAVIOURAL CHANGE AND MOTIVATIONAL STRATEGIES

There are many things that might interfere with your ability to maintain a lifetime of physical fitness, health, and wellness. Here are some barriers (roadblocks) and strategies for overcoming them.

Roadblock	Behavioural Change Strategy
There will be occasions when you will decide not to work out. Either you will be too busy, too tired, or too interested in doing something else. It is interesting to note that the most effective behavioural change programs allow for periodic deviation from the goal. That is understandable when you consider a dieter who diets for two months but has an ice cream sundae one weekend. Those who recognize that a deviation is just that, that it need not mean the diet is ruined, are more likely to continue dieting. Those who believe that once they go off their diet they have failed are likely to cease dieting after eating the sundae. It is similar with exercise. It is okay not to exercise when you are supposed to, as long as this does not happen frequently. If it happens often, you need to make an adjustment in your exercise program.	Make a list of the benefits and disadvantages of the exercise(s) that make up your routine. List as many benefits and disadvantages as you can, big ones and little ones. Now go over the list and decide: 1. Are the benefits worth the potential disadvantages? 2. Are there other physical activities that can give me similar benefits with fewer disadvantages? Or less important or significant disadvantages? 3. Are there ways I can decrease the barriers to my engaging in a fitness program? For example, can I exercise closer to home (using chaining to my advantage)? Or exercise with a friend (social support)? 4. What changes do you need to make to maintain an exercise regimen?
You have participated in competitive athletics all your life and have maintained a high level of fitness by doing so. Now you are getting older and the competition is potentially harmful. You are getting bumped around too much and getting injured. In addition, winning is not as important to you as it was when you were younger. Now, maintaining fitness, health, and wellness are your exercise goals.	You need to find noncompetitive physical activities that can help you achieve your new fitness goals. Ask friends who are noncompetitive what they do for exercise. Use their help (social support). You can also use covert techniques. Imagine yourself participating in noncompetitive activities and reward yourself by thinking of a relaxing image or pleasant thought (covert rehearsal). If that is too much unlike you, imagine someone you know who is not competitive engaging in a noncompetitive physical activity and then substitute yourself for that person (covert modelling).
You dislike exercising but know it is good for you. You need to find ways to continue your fitness program. You are afraid you will give it up before too long.	You can use self-monitoring by keeping a record of the times you engage in exercise activities. Then boast to friends in a nice way about sticking with your program. You can also make a contract with yourself that if you exercise at least three times a week for at least 20–30 minutes each time, you will reward yourself. Think up really rewarding rewards. Rewards that are realistic and feasible as well as worth striving for will be most effective. You may also want to question your choice of exercise activity. Exercise should be fun or else you are likely to discontinue it before too long. What other activities can you substitute for what you have been doing that would be more fun but still help you achieve your fitness goals?

Roadblock	Behavioural Change Strategy
List roadblocks interfering with your maintaining a lifetime of physical fitness, health, and wellness.	Cite behavioural change strategies that can help you overcome the roadblocks you just listed. If you need to, refer back to Chapter 3 for behavioural change and motivational strategies.
1. _____	1. _____
2. _____	2. _____
3. _____	3. _____

3. Pay attention to your spirit, too. Gain spiritual health from your fitness selections. Feel closer to nature or to a supreme being. Feel connected to your past and your future. To do so is to move toward high-level wellness.

4. Be aware of the effects of your fitness choices on your mental and social health. Do your choices add to your knowledge? To your learning? Do they improve your relationships or help you establish new ones?

5. Remember that improving one component of your health to the neglect of the others is not being well. Wellness is coordinating and integrating your physical-fitness activities with the mental, social, emotional, and spiritual parts of your life.

We can think of no better image with which to leave you than that of the Special Olympics—athletic competition for the mentally and physically challenged. These athletes try their best, train long and hard, and feel good about participating and competing. What better example of wellness is there? The learning (mental health) that must precede the competition, the good feelings developed between athletes and their coaches and competitors (social health), the satisfaction derived from trying one's best (emotional health), and the sense of oneness and closeness developed in competition (spiritual health), not to mention the physical fitness needed to participate in the first place (physical health), provide evidence of the wellness of these competitors. They may not be totally healthy, but they certainly are *well*.

We wish for all of you the same degree of wellness, and we hope this book helps you achieve it.

SUMMARY

■ Identifying Your Fitness Goals

People engage in physical activity for many reasons. Some do so for their health, others to look good, or to have energy, and still others to develop strength or because they enjoy the competition. In order to select activities to meet your fitness goals, you need to identify why you want to become fit.

■ Fitness Activities to Help You Achieve Your Goals

Many physical activities can contribute to the development of physical fitness; among these are walking, jogging, running, rope jumping, swimming, tennis, racquetball, handball, squash, aerobic dance, low-impact aerobics, and bicy-

cling. Some of these help develop cardiorespiratory endurance; others, muscular strength or muscular endurance; and still others, other components of physical fitness. In choosing an activity in which to engage regularly, make sure it matches your personality. You may be sociable, spontaneous, disciplined, aggressive, competitive, able to concentrate well, a risk-taker, or a combination of two or more of these traits. Because people's personalities differ, their choices of exercise will differ.

■ Being a Fitness Consumer

When you are deciding whether a health/fitness club is right for you, determine if the facility and the equipment are such that they can be used to achieve your fitness goals. The staff should be well trained and the equipment abundant enough that you will not have to wait too long to use it. Safety procedures should be in place so your chances of being injured are minimized. And the club should be easily accessible to you, with adequate parking, not too far from where you live or work, and with a membership fee within your budget.

Purchasing athletic equipment should be done thoughtfully so you do not waste your money. When buying athletic shoes, choose shoes that are comfortable and consistent with any foot problems you may have (for example, if you pronate or supinate). If you need orthotics because of a foot abnormality, you should consult a podiatrist although, in some cases, ready-made shoe inserts are all that is needed. There are many different kinds of home exercise equipment you can purchase. These include stationary bikes, climbers, row-

ers, cross-country ski machines, treadmills, and weights. In deciding what home exercise equipment to purchase, you should determine what your fitness goals are, who is going to use the equipment, how much space you have available to house the equipment, and how much you have to spend.

◼ Keeping Fit As You Age

Exercise can help you live longer and live better. It also staves off some of the effects of aging. For example, it can help with reduced cardiac output, lowered pulmonary ventilation, elevated blood pressure, a decrease in muscular strength and endurance, a decrease in flexibility, an increase in body fat, and a loss of skin elasticity. Furthermore, exercise is an excellent way for elders to enhance their overall wellness.

STUDY QUESTIONS

1. List some short-term and some long-term fitness and wellness goals for you.

2. What kinds of factors do you need to consider before purchasing exercise equipment?

3. What are the "best" kinds of exercise equipment? Justify your answer.

4. What factors are important for youth and older populations in designing exercise programs?

5. Define or describe your ideal of personal fitness and wellness.

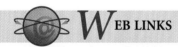

WEB LINKS

The Canadian Association for Health, Physical Education, Recreation and Dance
www.activeliving.ca/cahperd

Canadian Active Living Challenge
www.activeliving.ca/activeliving/calc/

The National Fitness Leadership Advisory Council (NFLAC)
www.activeliving.ca/activeliving/nflac.html#1

The Centre for Activity and Aging
www.uwo.ca/actage/index.html

National Forum on Health
wwwnfh.hc-sc.gc.ca/index.html

1995 Physical Activity Monitor
www.cflri.ca/cflri/95survey.html

Canadian Active Living
**http://www.canadian-health-network.ca/
1active_living.html**

Physical Activity Guides for Children and Youth (downloadable)
www.hc-sc.gc.ca/hppb/paguide/youth.html

Health of Canadians
www.hc-sc.gc.ca/hppb/phdd/report/subin.html

Canadian health promotion
**www.hc-sc.gc.ca/english/for_you/hpo/
index.html**

Life Fitness Academy
www.lifefitness.com/com_edu_main.asp

Buying exercise equipment
www.ftc.gov/bcp/conline/edcams/exercise/

Fitness Training Programs
www.netfit.co.uk/wkmen.htm

REFERENCES

Govindasamy, D., and D. Patterson. *Physical Activity and the Older Adult: A Knowledge Base for Managing Exercise Programs.* A Stipes Monograph. Champaign, IL: Stipes Publishing Company, 1994.

Katz, Jane. "The W.E.T. Workout." *Shape* (June 1986): 82–88.

U.S. Public Health Service. *Physical Activity and Health: A Report of the Surgeon General: Executive Summary.* Washington, DC: U.S. Department of Health and Human Services, 1996.

Winters, Catherine. "For Step Aerobic Addicts, a Challenging New Workout: Doing the Two-Step." *American Health* (May 1993): 92.

Lab Activity 15.1

Why I Want to Be Physically Fit

INSTRUCTIONS: *There are many reasons people engage in physical activity in an effort to become physically fit. If you know why you exercise, you will be able to choose activities that help you achieve your goals. To determine the reason(s) you exercise, rank-order the statements below.*

✦ **I Exercise Because:**

1 ✓ I want to lose, maintain, or increase my weight.

2 ✓ I want to look good.

9 _____ I want to have a healthy heart and lungs.

3 ✓ I want to be strong.

10 _____ I want to make new friends or socialize with my present friends.

5 ✓ I want to channel my aggression positively.

8 _____ I like competition.

11 _____ I like to be out in natural surroundings.

6 _____ I want to develop enough energy not to be tired during the day.

7 _____ I want to be flexible.

4 ✓ I want to have fun.

✦ **Interpretation of Results**

Consult Table 4.2 to match the reasons you exercise with the benefits of the various physical activities. For example, if you exercise to lose weight, consider activities such as aerobic dance, basketball, or bicycling. If you exercise to make friends, play softball or volleyball. If you exercise to look good, weight-train. Matching your fitness goals with activities that can help you achieve those goals is the best way of ensuring you will maintain your exercise program. Conversely, if you exercise regularly but do not achieve your goals because you have chosen the wrong physical activities, you will probably not continue with your program.

Mix and match activities so you achieve more than one of your goals. That way you will further increase the probability that you will become a lifetime participant in physical fitness activities.

Name Ang Chaffey

Date 05/04/06

Lab Activity 15.2

Developing a New Mindset About Exercise

INSTRUCTIONS: *When people try to develop a new habit, they are often plagued by thoughts of failure. During the early stages of your new exercise program, you can become your own worst enemy. Examine the list of excuses. Do any of these look familiar to you? Take a minute to prepare your own list of self-defeating thoughts about exercise. Prepare a list of positive thoughts, too.*

Learn to use these lists wisely. When self-defeating thoughts enter your mind, counteract them immediately with positive ones. Write your list of positive thoughts on a card, and carry it in your wallet or purse so you can refer to it when you are about to avoid a scheduled exercise session. List both long-term benefits (such as more energy, weight loss, and prevention of disease) and more immediate benefits (such as using up calories and feeling good).

Negative Thoughts About Exercise	Positive Thoughts About Exercise
1. I'm too busy to exercise today. I'm working too hard anyway and need a break.	1. I can find time to exercise today. I just have to think about my routine and plan carefully.
2. I'm too tired to exercise today, and if I do work out, I won't have enough energy to do other things I must do.	2. I may feel tired today, but I will do a light exercise routine instead of the heavy one I usually do. If I keep working out on a regular basis, I will build my stamina so I will not feel so tired during the day.
3. I missed my workout today. I might as well forget all this fitness stuff. I do not have the self-control to keep at it.	3. Just because I missed one exercise session does not mean that I should give up. I'm not going to let this small setback ruin everything I've accomplished.
4. None of my friends are fit or trim and they don't worry about it. I am not going to worry either.	4. What my friends do about exercising has nothing to do with my exercise habits. I'll make additional friends who do exercise.
5. I am already over the hill. I should just let myself go and enjoy life more.	5. I can get in shape and stay there. All I have to do is stick to my schedule. Knowing I can control my behaviour is something I can enjoy every day.

(continued)

Lab Activity 15.2 *(continued)*
Developing a New Mindset About Exercise

Negative Thoughts About Exercise	Positive Thoughts About Exercise
1. Too busy	1. Prioritize better
2. Too tired	2. Will help feel more awake
3. Don't feel like it	3. Endorphins will make you feel better
4. Too cold to go	4. Bundle up, invigorating

Source: Jerrold S. Greenberg and George B. Dintiman, and Barbee Myers-Oakes, *Wellness: Creating a Life of Health and Fitness* (Needham Heights, MA: Allyn & Bacon, 1997).

Lab Activity 15.3

Which Sports Match Your Personality?

INSTRUCTIONS: *Fitness experts tell us that if you match your personality with your choice of exercise, the chances are you will stay with your program. Here is a way to do that. Read the description of each psychosocial personality variable, and then rate yourself on the scorecard that follows.*

Sociability: Do you prefer doing things on your own or with other people? Do you make friends easily? Do you enjoy parties?

Spontaneity: Do you make spur-of-the-moment decisions, or do you plan in great detail? Can you change direction easily, or do you get locked in once you make up your mind?

Discipline: Do you have trouble sticking with things you find unpleasant or trying, or do you persist regardless of the obstacles? Do you need a lot of support, or do you just push on alone?

Aggressiveness: Do you try to control situations by being forceful? Do you like pitting yourself against obstacles, or do you shy away when you must assert yourself physically or emotionally?

Competitiveness: Are you bothered by situations that produce winners and losers? Does your adrenaline flow when you're challenged, or do you back off?

Mental Focus: Do you find it easy to concentrate, or do you have a short attention span? Can you be single-minded? How good are you at clearing your mind of distractions?

Risk-Taking: Are you generally adventurous, physically and emotionally, or do you prefer to stick to what you know?

Scorecard					
Fill in the appropriate circles and connect them with a line.					
	Very High ◄────		────► Very Low		
Sociability	○	◉	○	○	○
Spontaneity	○	○	◉	○	○
Discipline	○	○	○	◉	○
Aggressiveness	○	◉	○	○	○
Competitiveness	○	◉	○	○	○
Mental Focus	○	○	◉	○	○
Risk-Taking	○	◉	○	○	○

(continued)

Lab Activity 15.3 *(continued)*
Which Sports Match Your Personality?

 Walking

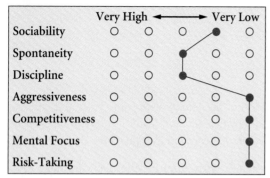

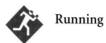 Running

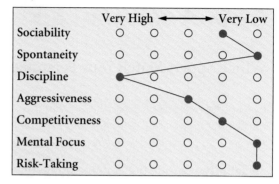

 Cycling

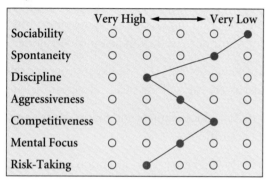

 Weight Training

✦ Understanding Your Score

To see how well your profile matches your sport or exercise activity, look at the four sample profiles in this Lab Activity. If you have the typical personality of a runner, walker, cyclist, or bodybuilder, your profile should look similar to one of these profiles. If your athletic preference lies elsewhere, turn to the "Your Personality/Your Sport" chart that follows to see where your activities rank on each characteristic. Then compare these rankings with how you scored yourself.

Compared to running, for example, walking is more spontaneous and less aggressive. (It is also safer, in terms of physical stress.) Racquet sports are high in sociability, spontaneity, competitiveness, and focus but low in discipline. Swimming is fairly high in discipline and low in sociability, spontaneity, and aggressiveness.

If you've been having trouble sticking to a fitness program, these charts may help explain why. If you're still looking for a sport, use your findings as a guide.

Source: James Gavin, "Your Brand of Sweat," *Psychology Today*, March 1989, pp. 50–57. Reprinted with permission from *Psychology Today* magazine, © 1989 (Sussex Publishers, Inc.).

← Higher   Lower →

SOCIABILITY

Tennis	Running	Weight Training	Golf	Tennis	Martial Arts	Downhill Skiing	Aerobics	Dance	Weight Training	Cross-Country Skiing	Walking	Running	Cycling	Yoga	Swimming

SPONTANEITY

Cycling	Swimming	Martial Arts	Martial Arts	Dance	Walking	Cross-Country Skiing	Cycling	Yoga	Running	Golf

DISCIPLINE

Weight Training	Cross-Country Skiing	Yoga	Cross-Country Skiing	Martial Arts	Aerobics	Walking	Swimming	Golf	Downhill Skiing

AGGRESSIVENESS

Martial Arts	Weight Training	Tennis	Golf	Cycling	Running	Cross-Country Skiing	Aerobics	Dance	Walking

COMPETITIVENESS

Tennis	Downhill Skiing	Martial Arts	Dance	Running	Weight Training	Cycling	Cross-Country Skiing	Swimming	Walking	Yoga

MENTAL FOCUS

Golf	Downhill Skiing	Yoga	Weight Training	Cycling	Aerobics	Cross-Country Skiing	Swimming	Walking	Yoga

RISK-TAKING

Downhill Skiing	Martial Arts	Tennis	Golf	Cycling	Weight Training	Dance	Cross-country Skiing	Aerobics	Swimming	Yoga	Running	Walking

Lab Activity 15.4

A Guide for Developing a Program Unique for You

INSTRUCTIONS: *Now that you are at the end of this book, you have learned a great deal about physical fitness, wellness, and health, and your own fitness needs and motivations. You are now ready to use this knowledge to develop a fitness program unique to you and, therefore, likely to be successful. To do so, complete each of the following items.*

1. My physical fitness needs include:

    a. _____

    b. _____

    c. _____

    d. _____

    e. _____

2. My present level of physical fitness can be described as:

    _____

    _____

3. The behavioural change techniques I can use to *adopt* a program of regular exercise are:

    a. _____

    b. _____

    c. _____

    d. _____

    e. _____

4. The ways I can use these behavioural change techniques to *adopt* an exercise program are:

    a. _____

    b. _____

    c. _____

    d. _____

    e. _____

(continued)

Lab Activity 15.4 *(continued)*
A Guide for Developing a Program Unique for You

5. The behavioural change techniques I can use to *maintain* my exercise program are:

    a. _____

    b. _____

    c. _____

    d. _____

    e. _____

6. The ways I can use these behavioural change techniques to *maintain* my program are:

    a. _____

    b. _____

    c. _____

    d. _____

    e. _____

7. The specific components of my exercise program will include:

Exercise	Duration	Intensity	Frequency
a.			
b.			
c.			
d.			
e.			
f.			
g.			
h.			
i.			
j.			

8. I will evaluate the effectiveness of my exercise program according to those criteria (remembering to assess adherence to my program and psychosocial and spiritual benefits, as well as changes in the specific components of physical fitness):

a. _____

b. _____

c. _____

d. _____

e. _____

Appendix A

Nutritional Information for Selected Foods

Food item	Serving size	Grams	Calories	Protein (g)	Carbohydrate (g)	Fat (g)	Cholesterol (mg)	Sodium (mg)
Beverages								
Alcoholic								
Beer								
Regular	12 fl oz	360	150	1	13	0	0	18
Light	12 fl oz	355	95	1	5	4	4	11
Gin, rum, vodka, whiskey								
80-proof	1½ fl oz	42	95	0	Tr	0	0	Tr
86-proof	1½ fl oz	42	105	0	Tr	0	0	Tr
90-proof	1½ fl oz	42	110	0	Tr	0	0	Tr
Wines								
Dessert	3½ fl oz	103	140	Tr	8	0	0	9
Table								
Red	3½ fl oz	102	75	Tr	3	0	0	5
White	3½ fl oz	102	80	Tr	3	0	0	5
Carbonated								
Club soda	12 fl oz	355	0	0	0	0	0	78
Cola type								
Regular	12 fl oz	369	160	0	41	0	0	18
Diet, artificially sweetened	12 fl oz	355	Tr	0	Tr	0	0	32 [a]
Ginger ale	12 fl oz	366	125	0	32	0	0	29
Grape	12 fl oz	372	180	0	46	0	0	48
Lemon-lime	12 fl oz	372	155	0	39	0	0	33
Orange	12 fl oz	372	180	0	46	0	0	52
Pepper type	12 fl oz	369	160	0	41	0	0	37
Root beer	12 fl oz	370	165	0	42	0	0	48
Fruit drinks, noncarbonated								
Canned								
Fruit punch drink	6 fl oz	190	85	Tr	22	0	0	15
Grape drink	6 fl oz	187	100	Tr	26	0	0	11
Pineapple-grapefruit juice drink	6 fl oz	187	90	Tr	23	Tr	0	24
Frozen lemonade concentrate, diluted with 4⅓ parts water by volume	6 fl oz	185	80	Tr	21	Tr	0	1

Tr = trace amount.

na = information not available.

[a]Blend of aspartame and saccharin; if only saccharin is used, sodium is 75 mg; if only aspartame is used, sodium is 23 mg.

Source: Information summarized from Superintendent of Documents, *Nutritive Value of Foods* (Washington, DC: U.S. Government Printing Office, 1981).

Food item	Serving size	Grams	Calories	Protein (g)	Carbohydrate (g)	Fat (g)	Cholesterol (mg)	Sodium (mg)
Dairy products								
Butter. See **Fats and Oils**								
Cheese								
Cheddar								
Cut pieces	1 oz	28	115	7	Tr	9	30	176
	1 in	17	70	4	Tr	6	18	105
Shredded	1 cup	113	455	28	1	37	119	701
Creamed (cottage cheese, 4% fat)								
Large curd	1 cup	225	235	28	6	10	34	911
Small curd	1 cup	210	215	26	6	9	31	850
With fruit	1 cup	226	280	22	30	8	25	915
Lowfat (2%)	1 cup	226	205	31	8	4	19	918
Cream	1 oz	28	100	2	1	10	31	84
Feta	1 oz	28	75	4	1	6	25	316
Mozzarella, made with								
Whole milk	1 oz	28	80	6	1	6	22	106
Part skim milk (low moisture)	1 oz	28	80	8	1	5	15	150
Muenster	1 oz	28	105	7	Tr	9	27	178
Parmesan, grated	1 oz	28	130	12	1	9	22	528
Provolone	1 oz	28	100	7	1	8	20	248
Swiss	1 oz	28	105	8	1	8	26	74
Pasteurized process cheese								
American	1 oz	28	105	6	Tr	9	27	406
Swiss	1 oz	28	95	7	1	7	24	388
Pasteurized process cheese food, American	1 oz	28	95	6	2	7	18	337
Pasteurized process cheese spread, American	1 oz	28	80	5	2	6	16	381
Cream, sweet								
Half-and-half (cream and milk)	1 cup	242	315	7	10	28	89	98
	1 tbsp	15	20	Tr	1	2	6	6
Light, coffee or table	1 cup	240	470	6	9	46	159	95
	1 tbsp	15	30	Tr	1	3	10	6
Cream, sour	1 cup	230	495	7	10	48	102	123
	1 tbsp	12	25	Tr	1	3	5	6
Ice cream. See **Milk Desserts, Frozen**								
Milk								
Whole (3.3% fat)	1 cup	244	150	8	11	8	33	370
Low-fat (2% fat)	1 cup	244	120	8	12	5	18	377
Low-fat (1% fat)	1 cup	244	100	8	12	3	10	381
Nonfat (skim)	1 cup	245	85	8	12	Tr	4	406

Food item	Serving Size	Grams	Calories	Protein (g)	Carbohydrate (g)	Fat (g)	Cholesterol (mg)	Sodium (mg)
Dairy Products (*continued*)								
Chocolate milk (commercial)								
Regular	1 cup	250	210	8	26	8	31	149
Low-fat (2% fat)	1 cup	250	180	8	26	5	17	151
Low-fat (1% fat)	1 cup	250	160	8	26	3	7	152
Milk beverages								
Cocoa and chocolate-flavoured beverages								
Prepared (8-oz whole milk plus ¾-oz powder)	1 serving	265	225	9	30	9	33	176
Eggnog (commercial)	1 cup	254	340	10	34	19	149	138
Malted milk, chocolate	¾ oz	21	85		18	1	1	49
Prepared (8 oz whole milk plus ¾-oz powder)	1 serving	265	235	9	29	9	34	168
Shakes, thick								
Chocolate	10-oz container	283	335	9	60	8	30	314
Vanilla	10-oz container	283	315	11	50	9	33	270
Milk desserts, frozen								
Ice cream, vanilla								
Regular (about 11% fat)	1 cup	133	270	5	32	14	59	116
Yogurt								
Made with low-fat milk								
Fruit-flavoured[b]	8-oz container	227	230	10	43	2	10	133
Plain	8-oz container	227	145	12	16	4	14	159
Made with nonfat milk	8-oz container	227	125	13	17	Tr	4	174
Made with whole milk	8-oz container	227	140	8	11	7	29	105
Eggs								
Eggs, large (24 oz per dozen)								
Cooked								
Fried in margarine	1 egg	46	90	6	1	7	211	162
Hard-cooked, shell removed	1 egg	50	75	6	1	5	213	62
Poached	1 egg	50	75	6	1	5	212	140
Scrambled (milk added) in margarine	1 egg	61	100	7	1	7	215	171

[b]Carbohydrate content varies widely because of amount of sugar added and amount of added flavouring. Consult the label if more precise values for carbohydrates and calories are needed.

FOOD ITEM	SERVING SIZE	GRAMS	CALORIES	PROTEIN (g)	CARBOHYDRATE (g)	FAT (g)	CHOLESTEROL (mg)	SODIUM (mg)
Fats and Oils								
Butter (4 sticks per lb)								
Stick	½ cup	113	810	1	Tr	92	247	933[c]
Tablespoon (⅛ stick)	1 tbsp	14	100	Tr	Tr	11	31	116[c]
Pat (1-in square, ⅓ in high; 90 per lb)	1 pat	5	35	Tr	Tr	4	11	41[c]
Margarine								
Regular (about 80% fat)								
Stick	½ cup	113	810	1	1	91	0	1066[d]
Tablespoon (⅛ stick)	1 tbsp	14	100	Tr	Tr	11	0	132
Pat (1-in square, ⅓ in high; 90 per lb)	1 pat	5	35	Tr	Tr	4	0	47[d]
Oils, salad or cooking								
Corn	1 tbsp	14	125	0	0	14	0	0
Olive	1 tbsp	14	125	0	0	14	0	0
Peanut	1 tbsp	14	125	0	0	14	0	0
Safflower	1 tbsp	14	125	0	0	14	0	0
Sunflower	1 tbsp	14	125	0	0	14	0	0
Salad dressings								
Blue cheese	1 tbsp	15	75	1	1	8	3	164
French								
Regular	1 tbsp	16	85	Tr	1	9	0	188
Low-calorie	1 tbsp	16	25	Tr	2	2	0	306
Italian								
Regular	1 tbsp	15	80	Tr	1	9	0	162
Low-calorie	1 tbsp	15	5	Tr	2	Tr	0	136
Mayonnaise								
Regular	1 tbsp	14	100	Tr	Tr	11	8	80
Thousand island								
Regular	1 tbsp	16	60	Tr	2	6	4	112
Low-calorie	1 tbsp	15	25	Tr	2	2	2	150
Fish and Shellfish								
Crab meat, canned	1 cup	135	135	23	1	3	135	1350
Fish sticks, frozen, reheated (stick, 4 by 1 by ½ in)	1 stick	28	70	6	4	3	26	53
Flounder or sole, baked, with lemon juice and butter	3 oz	85	120	16	Tr	6	68	145
Ocean perch, breaded, fried[e]	1 fillet	85	185	16	7	11	66	138
Salmon								
Baked (red)	3 oz	85	140	21	0	5	60	55
Smoked	3 oz	85	150	18	0	8	51	1700
Scallops, breaded, frozen, reheated	6 scallops	90	195	15	10	10	70	298

[c]For salted butter; unsalted butter contains 12 mg sodium per stick, 2 mg per tbsp, or 12 mg per pat.

[d]For salted margarine.

[e]Dipped in egg, milk, and bread crumbs; fried in vegetable shortening.

Food item	Serving size	Grams	Calories	Protein (g)	Carbohydrate (g)	Fat (g)	Cholesterol (mg)	Sodium (mg)
Fish and Shellfish *(continued)*								
Shrimp, French fried (7 medium)[f]	3 oz	85	200	16	11	10	168	384
Trout, broiled, with butter and lemon juice	3 oz	85	175	21	Tr	9	71	122
Tuna, canned, drained solids								
Oil pack, chunk light	3 oz	85	165	24	0	7	55	303
Water pack, solid white	3 oz	85	135	30	0	1	48	468
Tuna salad[g]	1 cup	205	375	33	19	19	80	877
Fruits and Fruit Juices								
Apples								
Raw								
Unpeeled, without cores, 3¼-in diam (about 2 per lb with cores)	1 apple	212	125	Tr	32	1	0	Tr
Peeled, sliced	1 cup	110	65	Tr	16	Tr	0	Tr
Apple juice, bottled or canned	1 cup	248	115	Tr	29	Tr	0	7
Apricots								
Raw, without pits (about 12 per lb with pits)	3 apricots	106	50	1	12	Tr	0	1
Bananas, raw, without peel								
Whole (about 2½ per lb with peel)	1 banana	114	105	1	27	1	0	1
Sliced	1 cup	150	140	2	35	1	0	2
Blueberries, raw	1 cup	145	80	1	20	1	0	9
Cherries, sweet, raw, without pits and stems	10 cherries	68	50	1	11	1	0	Tr
Grapefruit, raw, without peel, membrane, and seeds (3¾-in diam, 1 lb 1 oz, whole, with refuse)	½ grapefruit	120	40	1	10	Tr	0	Tr
Grapes, European type (adherent skin) raw, Thompson seedless	10 grapes	50	35	Tr	9	Tr	0	1

[f]Dipped in egg, milk, and bread crumbs; fried in vegetable shortening.

[g]Made with drained, chunk light tuna, celery, onion, pickle relish, and mayonnaise-type salad dressing.

FOOD ITEM	SERVING SIZE	GRAMS	CALORIES	PROTEIN (g)	CARBOHYDRATE (g)	FAT (g)	CHOLESTEROL (mg)	SODIUM (mg)
Fruits and Fruit Juices *(continued)*								
Melons, raw, without rind and cavity contents								
Cantaloupe, orange-fleshed (5-in diam, 2⅓ lb, whole, with rind and cavity contents)	½ melon	267	95	2	22	1	0	24
Honeydew (6½-in diam, 5¼ lb, whole, with rind and cavity contents)	⅟₁₀ melon	129	45	1	12	Tr	0	13
Nectarines, raw, without pits (about 3 per lb with pits)	1 nectarine	136	65	1	16	1	0	Tr
Oranges, raw, whole, without peel and seeds (2⅝-in diam, about 2½ per lb, with peel and seeds)	1 orange	131	60	1	15	Tr	0	Tr
Orange juice								
Raw, all varieties	1 cup	248	110	2	26	Tr	0	2
Canned, unsweetened	1 cup	249	105	1	25	Tr	0	5
Peaches, raw								
Whole, 2½-in diam, peeled, pitted (about 4 per lb with peels and pits)	1 peach	87	35	1	10	Tr	0	Tr
Sliced	1 cup	170	75	1	19	Tr	0	Tr
Pears, raw, with skin, cored, Bartlett, 2½-in diam (about 2½ per lb with cores and stems)	1 pear	166	100	1	25	1	0	Tr
Pineapple, raw, diced	1 cup	155	75	1	19	1	0	2
Pineapple juice, unsweetened, canned	1 cup	250	140	1	34	Tr	0	3
Plums, without pits, raw, 2⅛-in diam (about 6½ per lb with pits)	1 plum	66	35	1	9	Tr	0	Tr
Raisins, seedless, cup, not pressed down	1 cup	145	435	5	115	1	0	17
Raspberries, raw	1 cup	123	60	1	14	1	0	Tr
Strawberries, raw, capped, whole	1 cup	149	45	1	10	1	0	1

Food item	Serving size	Grams	Calories	Protein (g)	Carbohydrate (g)	Fat (g)	Cholesterol (mg)	Sodium (mg)
Fruits and Fruit Juices *(continued)*								
Watermelon, raw, without rind and seeds, piece (4- by 8-in wedge with rind and seeds; $1/16$ of $32^{2}/_{3}$-lb melon, 10 by 16 in)	1 piece	482	155	3	35	2	0	10
Grain Products								
Bagels, plain or water, enriched, $3^{1}/_{2}$-in diam[h]	1 bagel	68	200	7	38	2	0	245
Breads								
French or vienna bread, enriched[i]								
Slice								
French, 5 by $2^{1}/_{2}$ by 1 in	1 slice	35	100	3	18	1	0	203
Vienna $4^{3}/_{4}$ by 4 by $1/2$ in	1 slice	25	70	2	13	1	0	145
Italian bread, enriched								
Slice, $4^{1}/_{2}$ by $3^{1}/_{4}$ by $3/4$ in	1 slice	30	85	3	17	Tr	0	176
Mixed grain bread, enriched[i]								
Slice (18 per loaf)	1 slice	25	65	2	12	1	0	106
Pita bread, enriched, white, $6^{1}/_{2}$-in diam	1 pita	60	165	6	33	1	0	339
Pumpernickel ($2/3$ rye flour, $1/3$ enriched wheat flour)[j]								
Slice, 5 by 4 by $3/8$ in	1 slice	32	80	3	16	1	0	177
Rye bread, light ($2/3$ enriched wheat flour, $1/3$ rye flour)[j]								
Slice, $4^{3}/_{4}$ by $3^{3}/_{4}$ by $7/16$ in	1 slice	25	65	2	12	1	0	175
Wheat bread, enriched[j]								
Slice (16 per loaf)	1 slice	25	65	2	12	1	0	138
Whole-wheat bread[j]								
Slice (18 per loaf)	1 slice	28	70	3	13	1	0	180
Breakfast cereals								
All-Bran (about $1/3$ cup)	1 oz	28	70	4	21	1	0	320
Cap'n Crunch (about $3/4$ cup)	1 oz	28	120	1	23	3	0	213

[h]Egg bagels have 44 mg cholesterol and 22 IU or 7 RE vitamin A per bagel.
[i]Made with vegetable shortening.
[j]Made with vegetable shortening.

FOOD ITEM	SERVING SIZE	GRAMS	CALORIES	PROTEIN (g)	CARBOHYDRATE (g)	FAT (g)	CHOLESTEROL (mg)	SODIUM (mg)
Grain Products (*continued*)								
Cheerios (about 1¼ cup)	1 oz	28	110	4	20	2	0	307
Corn Flakes (about 1¼ cup)								
Kellogg's	1 oz	28	110	2	24	Tr	0	351
Toasties	1 oz	28	110	2	24	Tr	0	297
40% Bran Flakes								
Kellogg's (about ¾ cup)	1 oz	28	90	4	22	1	0	264
Post (about ⅔ cup)	1 oz	28	90	3	22	Tr	0	260
Froot Loops (about 1 cup)	1 oz	28	110	2	25	1	0	145
Lucky Charms (about 1 cup)	1 oz	28	110	3	23	1	0	201
100% Natural Cereal (about ¼ cup)	1 oz	28	135	3	18	6	Tr	12
Product 19 (about ¾ cup)	1 oz	28	110	3	24	Tr	0	325
Raisin Bran								
Kellogg's (about ¾ cup)	1 oz	28	90	3	21	1	0	207
Post (about ½ cup)	1 oz	28	85	3	21	1	0	185
Special K (about 1⅓ cup)	1 oz	28	110	6	21	Tr	Tr	265
Sugar Frosted Flakes, Kellogg's (about ¾ cup)	1 oz	28	110	1	26	Tr	0	230
Wheaties (about 1 cup)	1 oz	28	100	3	23	Tr	0	354
Cakes prepared from cake mixes with enriched flour[k]								
Angel food, piece, ¹⁄₁₂ of cake	1 piece	53	125	3	29	Tr	0	269
Devil's food with chocolate frosting								
Piece, ¹⁄₁₆ of cake	1 piece	69	235	3	40	8	37	181
Cupcake, 2½-in diam	1 cupcake	35	120	2	20	4	19	92
Cakes prepared from home recipes using enriched flour								
Carrot, with cream cheese frosting[l]								
Piece, ¹⁄₁₆ of cake	1 piece	96	385	4	48	21	74	279
Pound								
Slice, ¹⁄₁₇ of loaf	1 slice	30	120	2	15	5	32	96
Cheesecake								
Piece, ¹⁄₁₂ of cake	1 piece	92	280	5	26	18	170	204

[k]Excepting angel food cake, cakes were made from mixes containing vegetable shortening and frostings were made with margarine.

[l]Made with vegetable oil.

Food item	Serving size	Grams	Calories	Protein (g)	Carbohydrate (g)	Fat (g)	Cholesterol (mg)	Sodium (mg)
Grain Products *(continued)*								
Cookies made with enriched flour								
Brownies with nuts, commercial, with frosting, $1\frac{1}{2}$ by $1\frac{3}{4}$ by $\frac{7}{8}$ in	1 brownie	25	100	1	16	4	14	59
Chocolate chip, commercial, $2\frac{1}{4}$-in diam, $\frac{3}{8}$ in thick	4 cookies	42	180	2	28	9	5	140
Oatmeal with raisins, $2\frac{5}{8}$-in diam, $\frac{1}{4}$ in thick	4 cookies	52	245	3	36	10	2	148
Peanut butter cookie, from home recipe $2\frac{5}{8}$-in diam[m]	4 cookies	48	245	4	28	14	22	142
Corn chips	1-oz package	28	155	2	16	9	0	233
Crackers[n]								
Graham, plain, $2\frac{1}{2}$-in square	2 crackers	14	60	1	11	1	0	86
Melba toast, plain	1 piece	5	20	1	4	Tr	0	44
Saltines[o]	4 crackers	12	50	1	9	1	4	165
Wheat, thin	4 crackers	8	35	1	5	1	0	69
Croissants, made with enriched flour, $4\frac{1}{2}$ by 4 by $1\frac{3}{4}$ in	1 croissant	57	235	5	27	12	13	452
Doughnuts, made with enriched flour								
Cake type, plain, $3\frac{1}{4}$-in diam, 1 in high	1 doughnut	50	210	3	24	12	20	192
Yeast-leavened, glazed, $3\frac{3}{4}$-in diam, $1\frac{1}{4}$ in high	1 doughnut	60	235	4	26	13	21	222
English muffins, plain, enriched	1 muffin	57	140	5	27	1	0	378
French toast, from home recipe	1 slice	65	155	6	17	7	112	257

[m]Made with vegetable shortening.

[n]Crackers made with enriched flour except for rye wafers and whole-wheat wafers.

[o]Made with lard.

FOOD ITEM	SERVING SIZE	GRAMS	CALORIES	PROTEIN (g)	CARBOHYDRATE (g)	FAT (g)	CHOLESTEROL (mg)	SODIUM (mg)
Grain Products *(continued)*								
Macaroni, enriched, cooked (cut lengths, elbows, shells), firm stage (hot)	1 cup	130	190	7	39	1	0	1
Muffins made with enriched flour, 2½-in diam, 1½ in high, from home recipe								
Blueberry^m	1 muffin	45	135	3	20	5	19	198
Bran	1 muffin	45	125	3	19	6	24	189
Corn	1 muffin	45	145	3	21	5	23	169
Noodles (egg noodles), enriched, cooked	1 cup	160	200	7	37	2	50	3
Noodles, chow mein, canned	1 cup	45	220	6	26	11	5	450
Pancakes, 4-in diam								
Buckwheat, from mix (with buckwheat and enriched flours), egg and milk added	1 pancake	27	55	2	6	2	20	125
Plain								
From home recipe using enriched flour	1 pancake	27	60	2	9	2	16	115
From mix (with enriched flour), egg, milk, and oil added	1 pancake	27	60	2	8	2	16	160
Pies, pie crust made with enriched flour, vegetable shortening, 9-in diam								
Apple, piece, ⅙ of pie	1 piece	158	405	3	60	18	0	476
Blueberry, piece, ⅙ of pie	1 piece	158	380	4	55	17	0	423
Cherry, piece, ⅙ of pie	1 piece	158	410	4	61	18	0	480
Lemon meringue, piece, ⅙ of pie	1 piece	140	355	5	53	14	143	395
Pecan, piece, ⅙ of pie	1 piece	138	575	7	71	32	95	305

^m Made with vegetable shortening.

Food item	Serving size	Grams	Calories	Protein (g)	Carbohydrate (g)	Fat (g)	Cholesterol (mg)	Sodium (mg)
Grain Products (*continued*)								
Popcorn, popped								
Air popped, unsalted	1 cup	8	30	1	6	Tr	0	Tr
Popped in vegetable oil, salted	1 cup	11	55	1	6	3	0	86
Sugar syrup coated	1 cup	35	135	2	30	1	0	Tr
Pretzels, made with enriched flour								
Stick, 2¼ in long	10 pretzels	3	10	Tr	2	Tr	0	48
Twisted, dutch, 2¾ by 2⅝ in	1 pretzel	16	65	2	13	1	0	258
Rice								
Brown, cooked, served hot	1 cup	195	230	5	50	1	0	0
White, enriched								
Cooked, served hot	1 cup	205	225	4	50	Tr	0	0
Instant, ready-to-serve, hot	1 cup	165	180	4	40	0	0	0
Rolls, enriched								
Commercial								
Dinner, 2½-in diam, 2 in high	1 roll	28	85	2	14	2	Tr	155
Frankfurter and hamburger (8 per 11½-oz pkg.)	1 roll	40	115	3	20	2	Tr	241
Hard, 3¾-in diam, 2 in high	1 roll	50	155	5	30	2	Tr	313
Hoagie or submarine, 11½ by 3 by 2½ in	1 roll	135	400	11	72	8	Tr	683
Spaghetti, enriched, cooked								
Firm stage, "al dente," served hot	1 cup	130	190	7	39	1	0	1
Tender stage, served hot	1 cup	140	155	5	32	1	0	1
Tortillas, corn	1 tortilla	30	65	2	13	1	0	1
Waffles, made with enriched flour, 7-in diam								
From home recipe	1 waffle	75	245	7	26	13	102	445
From mix, egg and milk added	1 waffle	75	205	7	27	8	59	515
Legumes, Nuts, and Seeds								
Almonds, shelled								
Whole	1 oz	28	165	6	6	15	0	3
Beans, dry								
Black	1 cup	171	225	15	41	1	0	1
Lima	1 cup	190	260	16	49	1	0	4
Pea (navy)	1 cup	190	225	15	40	1	0	13
Pinto	1 cup	180	265	15	49	1	0	3

Food item	Serving size	Grams	Calories	Protein (g)	Carbohydrate (g)	Fat (g)	Cholesterol (mg)	Sodium (mg)
Legumes, Nuts, and Seeds *(continued)*								
Black-eyed peas, dry, cooked (with residual cooking liquid)	1 cup	250	190	13	35	1	0	20
Brazil nuts, shelled	1 oz	28	185	4	4	19	0	1
Cashew nuts, salted								
Dry roasted	1 oz	28	165	4	9	13	0	181[p]
Roasted in oil	1 oz	28	165	5	8	14	0	177[q]
Lentils, dry, cooked	1 cup	200	215	16	38	1	0	26
Mixed nuts, with peanuts, salted								
Dry roasted	1 oz	28	170	5	7	15	0	190[r]
Roasted in oil	1 oz	28	175	5	6	16	0	185[r]
Peanuts, roasted in oil, salted	1 oz	28	165	8	5	14	0	122[s]
Peanut butter	1 tbsp	16	95	5	3	8	0	75
Peas, split, dry, cooked	1 cup	200	230	16	42	1	0	26
Pistachio nuts, dried, shelled	1 oz	28	165	6	7	14	0	2
Refried beans, canned	1 cup	290	295	18	51	3	0	1228
Sesame seeds, dry, hulled	1 tbsp	8	45	2	1	4	0	3
Sunflower seeds, dry, hulled	1 oz	28	160	6	5	14	0	1
Meat and Meat Products								
Beef, cooked[t]								
Cuts braised, simmered, or pot roasted								
Relatively fat, such as chuck blade								
Lean and fat, piece, 2½ by 2½ by ¾ in	3 oz	85	325	22	0	26	87	53
Relatively lean, such as bottom round								
Lean and fat, piece, 4⅛ by 2¼ by ½ in	3 oz	85	220	25	0	13	81	43
Ground beef, broiled, patty, 3 by ⅝ in								
Lean	3 oz	85	230	21	0	16	74	65
Regular	3 oz	85	245	20	0	18	76	70

[p]Cashews without salt contain 21 mg sodium per cup or 4 mg per oz.

[q]Cashews without salt contain 22 mg sodium per cup or 5 mg per oz.

[r]Mixed nuts without salt contain 3 mg sodium per oz.

[s]Peanuts without salt contain 22 mg sodium per cup or 4 mg per oz.

[t]Outer layer of fat was removed to within approximately ½ inch of lean. Deposits of fat within the cut were not removed.

Food item	Serving size	Grams	Calories	Protein (g)	Carbohydrate (g)	Fat (g)	Cholesterol (mg)	Sodium (mg)
Meat and Meat Products *(continued)*								
Roast, oven cooked, no liquid added								
Relatively fat, such as rib								
Lean and fat, 2 pieces, 4⅛ by 2¼ in	3 oz	85	315	19	0	26	72	54
Relatively lean, such as eye of round								
Lean and fat, 2 pieces, 2½ by 2½ by ⅜ in	3 oz	85	205	23	0	12	62	50
Steak								
Sirloin, broiled								
Lean and fat, piece, 2½ by 2½ by ¾ in	3 oz	85	240	23	0	15	77	53
Lamb, cooked								
Chops (3 per lb with bone)								
Arm, braised								
Lean and fat	2.2 oz	63	220	20	0	15	77	46
Loin, broiled								
Lean and fat	2.8 oz	80	235	20	0	16	78	62
Leg, roasted								
Lean and fat, 2 pieces, 4⅛ by 2¼ by ¼ in	3 oz	85	205	22	0	13	78	57
Rib, roasted								
Lean and fat, 3 pieces, 2½ by 2½ by ¼ in	3 oz	85	315	18	0	26	77	60
Pork, cured, cooked								
Bacon								
Regular	3 medium slices	19	110	6	Tr	9	16	303
Canadian-style	2 slices	46	85	11	1	4	27	711
Ham, light cured, roasted								
Lean and fat, 2 pieces, 4⅛ by 2¼ by ¼ in	3 oz	85	205	18	0	14	53	1009
Luncheon meat								
Canned, spiced or unspiced, slice, 3 by 2 by ½ in	2 slices	42	140	5	1	13	26	541
Chopped ham (8 slices per 6-oz pkg)	2 slices	42	95	7	0	7	21	576

FOOD ITEM	SERVING SIZE	GRAMS	CALORIES	PROTEIN (g)	CARBOHYDRATE (g)	FAT (g)	CHOLESTEROL (mg)	SODIUM (mg)
Meat and Meat Products *(continued)*								
Cooked ham (8 slices per 8-oz pkg)								
Regular	2 slices	57	105	10	2	6	32	751
Extra lean	2 slices	57	75	11	1	3	27	815
Pork, fresh, cooked								
Chop, loin (cut 3 per lb with bone)								
Broiled								
Lean and fat	3.1 oz	87	275	24	0	19	84	61
Ham (leg), roasted								
Lean and fat, piece, 2½ by 2½ by ¾ in	3 oz	85	250	21	0	18	79	50
Rib, roasted								
Lean and fat, piece, 2½ by ¾ in	3 oz	85	270	21	0	20	69	37
Shoulder cut, braised								
Lean and fat, 3 pieces, 2½ by 2½ by ¼ in	3 oz	85	295	23	0	22	93	75
Sausages								
Bologna	2 slices	57	180	7	2	16	31	581
Frankfurter	1 frank	45	145	5	1	13	23	504
Pork link	1 link	13	50	3	Tr	4	11	168
Salami								
Cooked type, slice (8 per 8-oz pkg)	2 slices	57	145	8	1	11	37	607
Veal, medium fat, cooked, bone removed								
Cutlet, 4⅛ by 2¼ by ½ in, braised or broiled	3 oz	85	185	23	0	9	109	56
Rib, 2 pieces, 4⅛ by 2¼ by ¼ in, roasted	3 oz	85	230	23	0	14	109	57
Mixed Dishes and Fast Foods								
Mixed dishes								
Beef and vegetable stew, from home recipe	1 cup	245	220	16	15	11	71	292
Beef potpie, from home recipe, baked, piece, ⅓ of 9-in-diam pie	1 piece	210	515	21	39	30	42	596
Chicken à la king, cooked, from home recipe	1 cup	245	470	27	12	34	221	760

FOOD ITEM	SERVING SIZE	GRAMS	CALORIES	PROTEIN (g)	CARBOHYDRATE (g)	FAT (g)	CHOLESTEROL (mg)	SODIUM (mg)
Mixed Dishes and Fast Foods (*continued*)								
Chicken and noodles, cooked, from home recipe	1 cup	240	365	22	26	18	103	600
Chicken chow mein								
Canned	1 cup	250	95	7	18	Tr	8	725
From home recipe	1 cup	250	255	31	10	10	75	718
Chicken potpie, from home recipe, baked, piece, ⅓ of 9-in-diam pie	1 piece	232	545	23	42	31	56	594
Chili con carne with beans, canned	1 cup	255	340	19	31	16	28	1354
Chop suey with beef and pork, from home recipe	1 cup	250	300	26	13	17	68	1053
Macaroni (enriched) and cheese								
Canned	1 cup	240	230	9	26	10	24	730
From home recipe[u]	1 cup	200	430	17	40	22	44	1086
Spaghetti (enriched) in tomato sauce with cheese								
Canned	1 cup	250	190	6	39	2	3	955
From home recipe[u]	1 cup	250	260	9	37	9	8	955
Spaghetti (enriched) with meatballs and tomato sauce								
From home recipe	1 cup	248	330	19	39	12	89	1009
Poultry and Poultry Products								
Chicken								
Fried, flesh, with skin[v]								
Batter dipped								
Breast, ½ breast (5.6 oz with bones)	4.9 oz	140	365	35	13	18	119	385
Drumstick (3.4 oz with bones)	2.5 oz	72	195	16	6	11	62	194
Flour coated								
Breast, ½ breast (4.2 oz with bones)	3.5 oz	98	220	31	2	9	87	74
Drumstick (2.6 oz with bones)	1.7 oz	49	120	13	1	7	44	44
Roasted, flesh only								
Breast, ½ breast (4.2 oz with bones and skin)	3.0 oz	86	140	27	0	3	73	64

[u]Made with margarine.
[v]Fried in vegetable shortening.

Food item	Serving size	Grams	Calories	Protein (g)	Carbohydrate (g)	Fat (g)	Cholesterol (mg)	Sodium (mg)
Poultry and Poultry Products (*continued*)								
Drumstick (2.9 oz with bones and skin)	1.6 oz	44	75	12	0	2	41	42
Turkey, roasted, flesh only								
Dark meat, piece, 2½ by 1⅝ by ¼ in	4 pieces	85	160	24	0	6	72	67
Light meat, piece, 4 by 2 by ¼ in	2 pieces	85	135	25	0	3	59	54
Light and dark meat								
Chopped or diced	1 cup	140	240	41	0	7	106	98
Pieces (1 slice white meat, 4 by 2 by ¼ in and 2 slices dark meat, 2½ by 1⅝ by ¼ in)	3 pieces	85	145	25	0	4	65	60
Soups, Sauces, and Gravies								
Soups								
Canned, condensed								
Prepared with equal volume of milk								
Clam chowder, New England	1 cup	248	165	9	17	7	22	992
Cream of chicken	1 cup	248	190	7	15	11	27	1047
Cream of mushroom	1 cup	248	205	6	15	14	20	1076
Tomato	1 cup	248	160	6	22	6	17	932
Prepared with equal volume of water								
Bean with bacon	1 cup	253	170	8	23	6	3	951
Beef noodle	1 cup	244	85	5	9	3	5	952
Chicken noodle	1 cup	241	75	4	9	2	7	1106
Chicken rice	1 cup	241	60	4	7	2	7	815
Clam chowder, Manhattan	1 cup	244	80	4	12	2	2	1808
Cream of chicken	1 cup	244	115	3	9	7	10	986
Cream of mushroom	1 cup	244	130	2	9	9	2	1032
Minestrone	1 cup	241	80	4	11	3	2	911
Pea, green	1 cup	250	165	9	27	3	0	988
Tomato	1 cup	244	85	2	17	2	0	871
Vegetable beef	1 cup	244	80	6	10	2	5	956

Food Item	Serving Size	Grams	Calories	Protein (g)	Carbohydrate (g)	Fat (g)	Cholesterol (mg)	Sodium (mg)
Soups, Sauces, and Gravies *(continued)*								
Sauces								
From dry mix								
Cheese, prepared with milk	1 cup	279	305	16	23	17	53	1565
Hollandaise, prepared with water	1 cup	259	240	5	14	20	52	1564
Gravies								
Canned								
Beef	1 cup	233	125	9	11	5	7	1305
Chicken	1 cup	238	190	5	13	14	5	1373
Mushroom	1 cup	238	120	3	13	6	0	1357
Sugars and Sweets								
Candy								
Caramels, plain or chocolate	1 oz	28	115	1	22	3	1	64
Chocolate								
Milk, plain	1 oz	28	145	2	16	9	6	23
Milk, with almonds	1 oz	28	150	3	15	10	5	23
Milk, with peanuts	1 oz	28	155	4	13	11	5	19
Milk, with rice cereal	1 oz	28	140	2	18	7	6	46
Fudge, chocolate, plain	1 oz	28	115	1	21	3	1	54
Gum drops	1 oz	28	100	Tr	25	Tr	0	10
Hard candy	1 oz	28	110	0	28	0	0	7
Jelly beans	1 oz	28	105	Tr	26	Tr	0	7
Marshmallows	1 oz	28	90	1	23	0	0	25
Custard, baked	1 cup	265	305	14	29	15	278	209
Honey, strained or extracted	1 cup	339	1030	1	279	0	0	17
	1 tbsp	21	65	Tr	17	0	0	1
Jams and preserves	1 tbsp	20	55	Tr	14	Tr	0	2
	1 packet	14	40	Tr	10	Tr	0	2
Jellies	1 tbsp	18	50	Tr	13	Tr	0	5
	1 packet	14	40	Tr	10	Tr	0	4
Popsicle, 3-fl-oz size	1 popsicle	95	70	0	18	0	0	11
Puddings								
Canned								
Chocolate	5-oz can	142	205	3	30	11	1	285
Tapioca	5-oz can	142	160	3	28	5	Tr	252
Vanilla	5-oz can	142	220	2	33	10	1	305
Dry mix, prepared with whole milk								
Chocolate								
Instant	½ cup	130	155	4	27	4	14	440
Regular (cooked)	½ cup	130	150	4	25	4	15	167
Rice	½ cup	132	155	4	27	4	15	140
Tapioca	½ cup	130	145	4	25	4	15	152

FOOD ITEM	SERVING SIZE	GRAMS	CALORIES	PROTEIN (g)	CARBOHYDRATE (g)	FAT (g)	CHOLESTEROL (mg)	SODIUM (mg)
Sugars and Sweets (*continued*)								
Vanilla								
Instant	½ cup	130	150	4	27	4	15	375
Regular (cooked)	½ cup	130	145	4	25	4	15	178
Sugars								
Brown, pressed down	1 cup	220	820	0	212	0	0	97
White, granulated	1 cup	200	770	0	199	0	0	5
	1 tbsp	12	45	0	12	0	0	Tr
	1 packet	6	25	0	6	0	0	Tr
Syrups								
Chocolate-flavoured syrup or topping								
Thin type	2 tbsp	38	85	1	22	Tr	0	36
Fudge type	2 tbsp	38	125	2	21	5	0	42
Vegetables and Vegetable Products								
Asparagus, green, cooked, drained								
From raw, cuts and tips	1 cup	180	45	5	8	1	0	7
From frozen, cuts and tips	1 cup	180	50	5	9	1	0	7
Beans								
Lima, immature seeds, frozen, cooked, drained, thick-seeded types (Ford hooks)	1 cup	170	170	10	32	1	0	90
Beets, cooked, drained, diced or sliced	1 cup	170	55	2	11	Tr	0	83
Black-eyed peas, immature seeds, cooked and drained, from raw	1 cup	165	180	13	30	1	0	7
Broccoli, raw	1 spear	151	40	4	8	1	0	41
Spears, cut into ½-in pieces	1 cup	155	45	5	9	Tr	0	17
Brussels sprouts, cooked, drained, from raw, 7–8 sprouts, 1¼ to 1½-in diam	1 cup	155	60	4	13	1	0	33
Cabbage, common varieties, raw, coarsely shredded or sliced	1 cup	70	15	1	4	Tr	0	13
Carrots, Raw, without crowns and tips, scraped, whole, 7½ by 1⅛ in, or strips, 2½ to								

Food item	Serving size	Grams	Calories	Protein (g)	Carbohydrate (g)	Fat (g)	Cholesterol (g)	Sodium (mg)	(mg)
Vegetables and Vegetable Products (*continued*)									
Carrots									
3 in long	1 carrot or 18 strips	72	30	1	7	Tr	0	25	
Cooked, sliced, drained, from raw	1 cup	156	70	2	16	Tr	0	103	
Cauliflower									
Raw (florets)	1 cup	100	25	2	5	Tr	0	15	
Cooked, drained From raw (florets)	1 cup	125	30	2	6	Tr	0	8	
Celery, pascal type, raw									
Stalk, large outer, 8 by 1½ in (at root end)	1 stalk	40	5	Tr	1	Tr	0	35	
Corn, sweet, cooked, drained									
From raw, ear 5 by 1¾ in	1 ear	77	85	3	19	1	0	13	
From frozen	1 ear	63	60	2	14	Tr	0	3	
Cucumber, with peel, slices, ⅛ in thick (large, 2⅛-in diam; small, 1¾-in diam)	6 large or 8 small slices	28	5	Tr	1	Tr	0	1	
Eggplant, cooked, steamed	1 cup	96	25	1	6	Tr	0	3	
Lettuce, raw									
Butterhead, as Boston types:									
Head, 5-in diam	1 head	163	20	2	4	Tr	0	8	
Leaves	1 outer or 2 inner leaves	15	Tr	Tr	Tr	Tr	0	1	
Crisphead, as iceberg									
Pieces, chopped or shredded	1 cup	55	5	1	1	Tr	0	5	
Loose leaf (bunching varieties including romaine or cos), chopped or shredded pieces	1 cup	56	10	1	2	Tr	0	5	
Mushrooms									
Raw, sliced or chopped	1 cup	70	20	1	3	Tr	0		
Cooked, drained	1 cup	156	40	3	8	1	0	3	
Onions									
Raw, chopped	1 cup	160	55	2	12	Tr	0	3	
Cooked (whole or sliced), drained	1 cup	210	60	2	13	Tr	0	17	

FOOD ITEM	SERVING SIZE	GRAMS	CALORIES	PROTEIN (g)	CARBOHYDRATE (g)	FAT (g)	CHOLESTEROL (mg)	SODIUM (mg)
Vegetables and Vegetable Products (*continued*)								
Peas, edible pod, cooked, drained	1 cup	160	65	5	11	Tr	0	6
Peas, green								
Canned, drained solids	1 cup	170	115	8	21	1	0	372[w]
Frozen, cooked, drained	1 cup	160	125	8	23	Tr	0	139
Potatoes, cooked								
Baked (about 2 per lb, raw)								
With skin	1 potato	202	220	5	51	Tr	0	16
Flesh only	1 potato	156	145	3	34	Tr	0	8
Boiled (about 3 per 1b, raw)								
Peeled after boiling	1 potato	136	120	3	27	Tr	0	5
Peeled before boiling	1 potato	135	115	2	27	Tr	0	7
French fried, strip, 2 to 3½ in long, frozen								
Oven heated	10 strips	50	110	2	17	4	0	16
Fried in vegetable oil	10 strips	50	160	2	20	8	0	108
Potato products, prepared								
Au gratin								
From dry mix	1 cup	245	230	6	31	10	12	1076
From home recipe	1 cup	245	325	12	28	19	56	1061
Hashed brown, from frozen	1 cup	156	340	5	44	18	0	53
Mashed								
From home recipe								
Milk added	1 cup	210	160	4	37	1	4	636
Milk and margarine added	1 cup	210	225	4	35	9	4	620
Potato salad, made with mayonnaise	1 cup	250	360	7	28	21	170	1323
Scalloped								
From dry mix	1 cup	245	230	5	31	11	27	835
From home recipe	1 cup	245	210	7	26	9	29	821
Potato chips	10 chips	20	105	1	10	7	0	94
Pumpkin, cooked from raw, mashed	1 cup	245	50	2	12	Tr	0	2
Radishes, raw, stem ends, rootlets cut off	4 radishes	18	5	Tr	1	Tr	0	4
Sauerkraut, canned, solids and liquid	1 cup	236	45	2	10	Tr	0	1560

[w]For regular pack; special dietary pack contains 3 mg sodium.

FOOD ITEM	SERVING SIZE	GRAMS	CALORIES	PROTEIN (g)	CARBOHYDRATE (g)	FAT (g)	CHOLESTEROL (mg)	SODIUM (mg)
Vegetables and Vegetable Products (*continued*)								
Spinach								
Raw, chopped	1 cup	55	10	2	2	Tr	0	43
Cooked, drained								
From raw	1 cup	180	40	5	7	Tr	0	126
From frozen (leaf)	1 cup	190	55	6	10	Tr	0	163
Sweet potatoes								
Cooked (raw, 5 by 2 in; about 2½ per lb)								
Baked in skin, peeled	1 potato	114	115	2	28	Tr	0	11
Boiled, without skin	1 potato	151	160	2	37	Tr	0	20
Tomatoes								
Raw, 2⅗-in diam (3 per 12-oz pkg)	1 tomato	123	25	1	5	Tr	0	10
Tomato juice, canned	1 cup	244	40	2	10	Tr	0	881[x]
Tomato products, canned								
Paste	1 cup	262	220	10	49	2	0	170[y]
Sauce	1 cup	245	75	3	18	Tr	0	1482[z]
Vegetable juice cocktail, canned	1 cup	242	45	2	11	Tr	0	883
Miscellaneous Items								
Catsup	1 cup	273	290	5	69	1	0	2845
	1 tbsp	15	15	Tr	4	Tr	0	156
Chili powder	1 tsp	2.6	10	Tr	1	Tr	0	26
Mustard, prepared, yellow	1 tsp or individual packet	5	5	Tr	Tr	Tr	0	63
Olives, canned								
Green	4 medium or 3 extra large	13	15	Tr	Tr	2	0	312
Ripe, Mission, pitted	3 small or 2 large	9	15	Tr	Tr	2	0	68
Pickles, cucumber								
Dill	1 pickle	65	5	Tr	1	Tr	0	928
Sweet	1 pickle	15	20	Tr	5	Tr	0	107
Salt	1 tsp	5.5	0	0	0	0	0	2132

[x]For added salt; if none is added, sodium content is 24 mg.

[y]With no added salt; if salt is added, sodium content is 2070 mg.

[z]With no added salt; if salt is added, sodium content is 998 mg.

Notional information is also available online for items served at many fast food franchises.

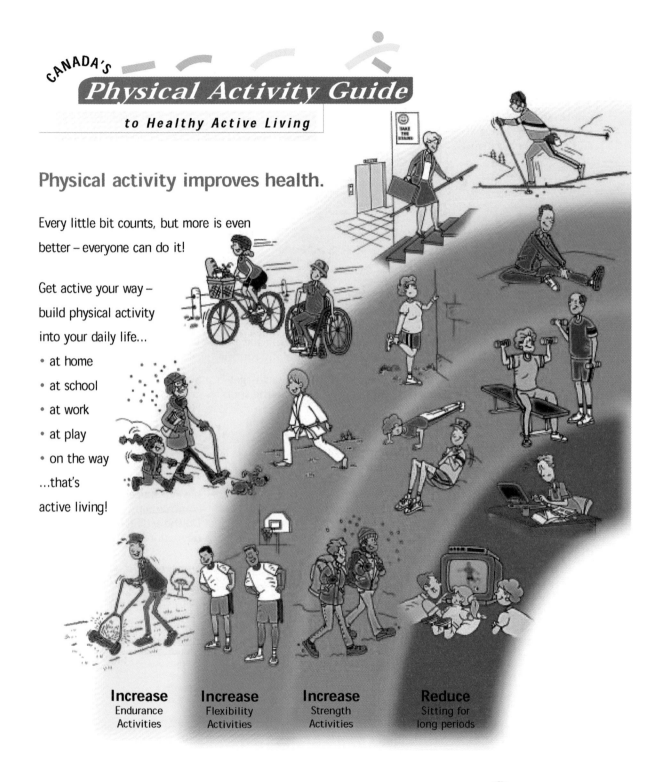

CANADA'S

Physical Activity Guide

to Healthy Active Living

Physical activity improves health.

Every little bit counts, but more is even better – everyone can do it!

Get active your way – build physical activity into your daily life...

• at home
• at school
• at work
• at play
• on the way
...that's active living!

Increase	Increase	Increase	Reduce
Endurance Activities	Flexibility Activities	Strength Activities	Sitting for long periods

 Health Canada Santé Canada

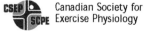 CSEP SCPE Canadian Society for Exercise Physiology

Choose a variety of activities from these three groups:

Endurance

4-7 days a week
Continuous activities for your heart, lungs and circulatory system.

Flexibility

4-7 days a week
Gentle reaching, bending and stretching activities to keep your muscles relaxed and joints mobile.

Strength

2-4 days a week
Activities against resistance to strengthen muscles and bones and improve posture.

Starting slowly is very safe for most people. Not sure? Consult your health professional.

For a copy of the *Guide Handbook* and more information: **1-888-334-9769**, or **www.paguide.com**

Eating well is also important. Follow *Canada's Food Guide to Healthy Eating* to make wise food choices.

Get Active Your Way, Every Day—For Life!

Scientists say accumulate 60 minutes of physical activity every day to stay healthy or improve your health. As you progress to moderate activities you can cut down to 30 minutes, 4 days a week. Add-up your activities in periods of at least 10 minutes each. Start slowly... and build up.

Time needed depends on effort

Very Light Effort	Light Effort *60 minutes*	Moderate Effort *30-60 minutes*	Vigorous Effort *20-30 minutes*	Maximum Effort
• Strolling • Dusting	• Light walking • Volleyball • Easy gardening • Stretching	• Brisk walking • Biking • Raking leaves • Swimming • Dancing • Water aerobics	• Aerobics • Jogging • Hockey • Basketball • Fast swimming • Fast dancing	• Sprinting • Racing

Range needed to stay healthy

You Can Do It – Getting started is easier than you think

Physical activity doesn't have to be very hard. Build physical activities into your daily routine.

- Walk whenever you can– get off the bus early, use the stairs instead of the elevator.
- Reduce inactivity for long periods, like watching TV.
- Get up from the couch and stretch and bend for a few minutes every hour.
- Play actively with your kids.
- Choose to walk, wheel or cycle for short trips.

- Start with a 10 minute walk– gradually increase the time.
- Find out about walking and cycling paths nearby and use them.
- Observe a physical activity class to see if you want to try it
- Try one class to start – you don't have to make a long-term commitment.
- Do the activities you are doing now, more often.

Benefits of regular activity:

- better health
- improved fitness
- better posture and balance
- better self-esteem
- weight control
- stronger muscles and bones
- feeling more energetic
- relaxation and reduced stress
- continued independent living in later life

Health risks of inactivity:

- premature death
- heart disease
- obesity
- high blood pressure
- adult-onset diabetes
- osteoporosis
- stroke
- depression
- colon cancer

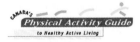

Source: Canada's Physical Activity Guide to Healthy Active Living, Health Canada, (1998). Reproduced with the permission of the Minister of Public Works and Government Services Canada, 2003.

Appendix C

Physical Activity Readiness
Medical Examination for
Pregnancy (2002)

PARmed-X for PREGNANCY PHYSICAL ACTIVITY READINESS MEDICAL EXAMINATION

PARmed-X for PREGNANCY is a guideline for health screening prior to participation in a prenatal fitness class or other exercise.

Healthy women with uncomplicated pregnancies can integrate physical activity into their daily living and can participate without significant risks either to themselves or to their unborn child. Postulated benefits of such programs include improved aerobic and muscular fitness, promotion of appropriate weight gain, and facilitation of labour. Regular exercise may also help to prevent gestational glucose intolerance and pregnancy-induced hypertension.

The safety of prenatal exercise programs depends on an adequate level of maternal-fetal physiological reserve. PARmed-X for PREGNANCY is a convenient checklist and prescription for use by health care providers to evaluate pregnant patients who want to enter a prenatal fitness program and for ongoing medical surveillance of exercising pregnant patients.

Instructions for use of the 4-page PARmed-X for PREGNANCY are the following:

1. The patient should fill out the section on PATIENT INFORMATION and the PRE-EXERCISE HEALTH CHECKLIST (PART 1, 2, 3, and 4 on p. 1) and give the form to the health care provider monitoring her pregnancy.

2. The health care provider should check the information provided by the patient for accuracy and fill out SECTION C on CONTRAINDICATIONS (p. 2) based on current medical information.

3. If no exercise contraindications exist, the HEALTH EVALUATION FORM (p. 3) should be completed, signed by the health care provider, and given by the patient to her prenatal fitness professional.

In addition to prudent medical care, participation in appropriate types, intensities and amounts of exercise is recommended to increase the likelihood of a beneficial pregnancy outcome. PARmed-X for PREGNANCY provides recommendations for individualized exercise prescription (p. 3) and program safety (p. 4).

NOTE: *Sections A and B should be completed by the patient before the appointment with the health care provider.*

A PATIENT INFORMATION

NAME _____
ADDRESS _____
TELEPHONE_____ BIRTHDATE _____ HEALTH INSURANCE No. _____
NAME OF
PRENATAL FITNESS PROFESSIONAL _____   PRENATAL FITNESS PROFESSIONAL'S PHONE NUMBER _____

B PRE-EXERCISE HEALTH CHECKLIST

PART 1: GENERAL HEALTH STATUS

In the past, have you experienced (check YES or NO):

	YES	NO
1. Miscarriage in an earlier pregnancy?	❑	❑
2. Other pregnancy complications?	❑	❑
3. I have completed a PAR-Q within the last 30 days.	❑	❑

If you answered YES to question 1 or 2, please explain:

_____

Number of previous pregnancies? _____

PART 2: STATUS OF CURRENT PREGNANCY

Due Date: _____

During this pregnancy, have you experienced:

	YES	NO
1. Marked fatigue?	❑	❑
2. Bleeding from the vagina ("spotting")?	❑	❑
3. Unexplained faintness or dizziness?	❑	❑
4. Unexplained abdominal pain?	❑	❑
5. Sudden swelling of ankles, hands or face?	❑	❑
6. Persistent headaches or problems with headaches?	❑	❑
7. Swelling, pain or redness in the calf of one leg?	❑	❑
8. Absence of fetal movement after 6th month?	❑	❑
9. Failure to gain weight after 5th month?	❑	❑

If you answered YES to any of the above questions, please explain:

_____

PART 3: ACTIVITY HABITS DURING THE PAST MONTH

1. List only regular fitness/recreational activities:

_____

INTENSITY	FREQUENCY (times/week)			TIME (minutes/day)		
	1-2	2-4	4+	<20	20-40	40+
Heavy	___	___	___	___	___	___
Medium	___	___	___	___	___	___
Light	___	___	___	___	___	___

2. Does your regular occupation (job/home) activity involve:

	YES	NO
Heavy Lifting?	❑	❑
Frequent walking/stair climbing?	❑	❑
Occasional walking (>once/hr)?	❑	❑
Prolonged standing?	❑	❑
Mainly sitting?	❑	❑
Normal daily activity?	❑	❑
3. Do you currently smoke tobacco?*	❑	❑
4. Do you consume alcohol?*	❑	❑

PART 4: PHYSICAL ACTIVITY INTENTIONS

What physical activity do you intend to do?

_____

Is this a change from what you currently do?   ❑ YES   ❑ NO

*NOTE: PREGNANT WOMEN ARE STRONGLY ADVISED NOT TO SMOKE OR CONSUME ALCOHOL DURING PREGNANCY AND DURING LACTATION.

© Canadian Society for Exercise Physiology
Société canadienne de physiologie de l'exercice

Supported by: Health Santé
Canada Canada

423

Physical Activity Readiness
Medical Examination for
Pregnancy (2002)

PARmed-X for PREGNANCY PHYSICAL ACTIVITY READINESS MEDICAL EXAMINATION

C CONTRAINDICATIONS TO EXERCISE: to be completed by your health care provider

Absolute Contraindications

Does the patient have:

	YES	NO
1. Ruptured membranes, premature labour?	❑	❑
2. Persistent second or third trimester bleeding/placenta previa?	❑	❑
3. Pregnancy-induced hypertension or pre-eclampsia?	❑	❑
4. Incompetent cervix?	❑	❑
5. Evidence of intrauterine growth restriction?	❑	❑
6. High-order pregnancy (e.g., triplets)?	❑	❑
7. Uncontrolled Type I diabetes, hypertension or thyroid disease, other serious cardiovascular, respiratory or systemic disorder?	❑	❑

Relative Contraindications

Does the patient have:

	YES	NO
1. History of spontaneous abortion or premature labour in previous pregnancies?	❑	❑
2. Mild/moderate cardiovascular or respiratory disease (e.g., chronic hypertension, asthma)?	❑	❑
3. Anemia or iron deficiency? (Hb < 100 g/L)?	❑	❑
4. Malnutrition or eating disorder (anorexia, bulimia)?	❑	❑
5. Twin pregnancy after 28th week?	❑	❑
6. Other significant medical condition?	❑	❑

Please specify: _____

NOTE: Risk may exceed benefits of regular physical activity. The decision to be physically active or not should be made with qualified medical advice.

PHYSICAL ACTIVITY RECOMMENDATION: ❑ Recommended/Approved ❑ Contraindicated

Prescription for Aerobic Activity

RATE OF PROGRESSION: The best time to progress is during the second trimester since risks and discomforts of pregnancy are lowest at that time. Aerobic exercise should be increased gradually during the second trimester from a minimum of 15 minutes per session, 3 times per week (at the appropriate target heart rate or RPE to a maximum of approximately 30 minutes per session, 4 times per week (at the appropriate target heart rate or RPE).

WARM-UP/COOL-DOWN: Aerobic activity should be preceded by a brief (10-15 min.) warm-up and followed by a short (10-15 min.) cool-down. Low intensity calesthenics, stretching and relaxation exercises should be included in the warm-up/cool-down.

PRESCRIPTION/MONITORING OF INTENSITY: The best way to prescribe and monitor exercise is by combining the heart rate and rating of perceived exertion (RPE) methods.

TARGET HEART RATE ZONES

The heart rate zones shown below are appropriate for most pregnant women. Work during the lower end of the HR range at the start of a new exercise program and in late pregnancy.

Age	Heart Rate Range
< 20	140-155
20-29	135-150
30-39	130-145

RATING OF PERCEIVED EXERTION (RPE)

Check the accuracy of your heart rate target zone by comparing it to the scale below. A range of about 12-14 (somewhat hard) is appropriate for most pregnant women.

6	
7	Very, very light
8	
9	Somewhat light
10	
11	Fairly light
12	
13	Somewhat hard
14	
15	Hard
16	
17	Very hard
18	
19	Very, very hard
20	

F I T T

FREQUENCY	INTENSITY	TIME	TYPE
Begin at 3 times per week and progress to four times per week	Exercise within an appropriate RPE range and/or target heart rate zone	Attempt 15 minutes, even if it means reducing the intensity. Rest intervals may be helpful	Non weight-bearing or low-impact endurance exercise using large muscle groups (e.g., walking, stationary cycling, swimming, aquatic exercises, low impact aerobics)

"TALK TEST" - A final check to avoid overexertion is to use the "talk test". The exercise intensity is excessive if you cannot carry on a verbal conversation while exercising.

The original PARmed-X for PREGNANCY was developed by L.A. Wolfe, Ph.D., Queen's University. The muscular conditioning component was developed by M.F. Mottola, Ph.D., University of Western Ontario. The document has been revised based on advice from an Expert Advisory Committee of the Canadian Society for Exercise Physiology chaired by Dr. N. Gledhill, with additonal input from Drs. Wolfe and Mottola, and Gregory A.L. Davies, M.D.,FRCS(C) Department of Obstetrics and Gynaecology, Queen's University, 2002.

No changes permitted. Translation and reproduction in its entirety is encouraged.

Disponible en français sous le titre «Examination medicale sur l'aptitude à l'activité physique pour les femmes enceintes (X-AAP pour les femmes enceintes)»

Additional copies of the PARmed-X for PREGNANCY, the PARmed-X and/or the PAR-Q can be downloaded from: http://www.csep.ca/forms.asp. For more information contact the:

Canadian Society for Exercise Physiology
185 Somerset St. West, Suite 202, Ottawa, Ontario CANADA K2P 0J2
tel.: 1-877-651-3755 FAX (613) 234-3565 www.csep.ca

Physical Activity Readiness
Medical Examination for
Pregnancy (2002)

PARmed-X for PREGNANCY PHYSICAL ACTIVITY READINESS MEDICAL EXAMINATION

Prescription for Muscular Conditioning

It is important to condition all major muscle groups during both prenatal and postnatal periods.

WARM-UPS & COOL DOWN:
Range of Motion: neck, shoulder girdle, back, arms, hips, knees, ankles, etc.

Static Stretching: all major muscle groups

(DO NOT OVER STRETCH!)

EXAMPLES OF MUSCULAR STRENGTHENING EXERCISES

CATEGORY	PURPOSE	EXAMPLE
Upper back	Promotion of good posture	Shoulder shrugs, shoulder blade pinch
Lower back	Promotion of good posture	Modified standing opposite leg & arm lifts
Abdomen	Promotion of good posture, prevent low-back pain, prevent diastasis recti, strengthen muscles of labour	Abdominal tightening, abdominal curl-ups, head raises lying on side or standing position
Pelvic floor ("Kegels")	Promotion of good bladder control, prevention of urinary incontinence	"Wave", "elevator"
Upper body	Improve muscular support for breasts	Shoulder rotations, modified push-ups against a wall
Buttocks, lower limbs	Facilitation of weight-bearing, prevention of varicose veins	Buttocks squeeze, standing leg lifts, heel raises

PRECAUTIONS FOR MUSCULAR CONDITIONING DURING PREGNANCY

VARIABLE	EFFECTS OF PREGNANCY	EXERCISE MODIFICATIONS
Body Position	• in the supine position (lying on the back), the enlarged uterus may either decrease the flow of blood returning from the lower half of the body as it presses on a major vein (inferior vena cava) or it may decrease flow to a major artery (abdominal aorta)	• past 4 months of gestation, exercises normally done in the supine position should be altered • such exercises should be done side lying or standing
Joint Laxity	• ligaments become relaxed due to increasing hormone levels • joints may be prone to injury	• avoid rapid changes in direction and bouncing during exercises • stretching should be performed with controlled movements
Abdominal Muscles	• presence of a rippling (bulging) of connective tissue along the midline of the pregnant abdomen (diastasis recti) may be seen during abdominal exercise	• abdominal exercises are not recommended if diastasis recti develops
Posture	• increasing weight of enlarged breasts and uterus may cause a forward shift in the centre of gravity and may increase the arch in the lower back • this may also cause shoulders to slump forward	• emphasis on correct posture and neutral pelvic alignment. Neutral pelvic alignment is found by bending the knees, feet shoulder width apart, and aligning the pelvis between accentuated lordosis and the posterior pelvic tilt position.
Precautions for Resistance Exercise	• emphasis must be placed on continuous breathing throughout exercise • exhale on exertion, inhale on relaxation using high repetitions and low weights • Valsalva Manoevre (holding breath while working against a resistance) causes a change in blood pressure and therefore should be avoided • avoid exercise in supine position past 4 months gestation	

✂ -

PARmed-X for Pregnancy - Health Evaluation Form
(to be completed by patient and given to the prenatal fitness professional after obtaining medical clearance to exercise)

I, _____ PLEASE PRINT (patient's name), have discussed my plans to participate in physical activity during my current pregnancy with my health care provider and I have obtained his/her approval to begin participation.

Signed: _____   Date: _____
           (patient's signature)

                                      HEALTH CARE PROVIDER'S COMMENTS:

Name of health care provider: _____   _____

Address: _____   _____

_____   _____

Telephone: _____   _____
                                            (health care provider's signature)

Physical Activity Readiness
Medical Examination for
Pregnancy (2002)

Advice for Active Living During Pregnancy

Pregnancy is a time when women can make beneficial changes in their health habits to protect and promote the healthy development of their unborn babies. These changes include adopting improved eating habits, abstinence from smoking and alcohol intake, and participating in regular moderate physical activity. Since all of these changes can be carried over into the postnatal period and beyond, pregnancy is a very good time to adopt healthy lifestyle habits that are permanent by integrating physical activity with enjoyable healthy eating and a positive self and body image.

Active Living:

➤ see your doctor before increasing your activity level during pregnancy

➤ exercise regularly but don't overexert

➤ exercise with a pregnant friend or join a prenatal exercise program

➤ follow FITT principles modified for pregnant women

➤ know safety considerations for exercise in pregnancy

Healthy Eating:

➤ the need for calories is higher (about 300 more per day) than before pregnancy

➤ follow Canada's Food Guide to Healthy Eating and choose healthy foods from the following groups: whole grain or enriched bread or cereal, fruits and vegetables, milk and milk products, meat, fish, poultry and alternatives

➤ drink 6-8 glasses of fluid, including water, each day

➤ salt intake should not be restricted

➤ limit caffeine intake i.e., coffee, tea, chocolate, and cola drinks

➤ dieting to lose weight is not recommended during pregnancy

Positive Self and Body Image:

➤ remember that it is normal to gain weight during pregnancy

➤ accept that your body shape will change during pregnancy

➤ enjoy your pregnancy as a unique and meaningful experience

For more detailed information and advice about pre- and postnatal exercise, you may wish to obtain a copy of a booklet entitled *Active Living During Pregnancy: Physical Activity Guidelines for Mother and Baby* © 1999.   Available from the Canadian Society for Exercise Physiology, 185 Somerset St. West, Suite 202, Ottawa, Ontario Canada K2P 0J2   Tel. 1-877-651-3755 Fax: (613) 234-3565 Email: info@csep.ca (online: www.csep.ca). Cost: $11.95

For more detailed information about the safety of exercise in pregnancy you may wish to obtain a copy of the Clinical Practice Guidelines of the Society of Obstetricians and Gynaecologists of Canada and Canadian Society for Exercise Physiology entitled *Exercise in Pregnancy and Postpartum* © 2003. Available from the Society of Obstetricians and Gynaecologists of Canada online at www.sogc.org

For more detailed information about pregnancy and childbirth you may wish to obtain a copy of *Healthy Beginnings: Your Handbook for Pregnancy and Birth* © 1998. Available from the Society of Obstetricians and Gynaecologists of Canada at 1-877-519-7999 (also available online at www.sogc.org) Cost $12.95.

For more detailed information on healthy eating during pregnancy, you may wish to obtain a copy of *Nutrition for a Healthy Pregnancy: National Guidelines for the Childbearing Years* © 1999.   Available from Health Canada, Minister of Public Works and Government Services, Ottawa, Ontario Canada (also available online at www.hc-sc.gc.ca).

SAFETY CONSIDERATIONS

◆ Avoid exercise in warm/humid environments, especially during the 1st trimester

◆ Avoid isometric exercise or straining while holding your breath

◆ Maintain adequate nutrition and hydration — drink liquids before and after exercise

◆ Avoid exercise while lying on your back past the 4th month of pregnancy

◆ Avoid activities which involve physical contact or danger of falling

◆ Know your limits — pregnancy is not a good time to train for athletic competition

◆ Know the reasons to stop exercise and consult a qualified health care provider immediately if they occur

REASONS TO STOP EXERCISE AND CONSULT YOUR HEALTH CARE PROVIDER

◆ Excessive shortness of breath

◆ Chest pain

◆ Painful uterine contractions (more than 6-8 per hour)

◆ Vaginal bleeding

◆ Any "gush" of fluid from vagina (suggesting premature rupture of the membranes)

◆ Dizziness or faintness

Index

Photo Credits